Primer on the
Autonomic
Nervous System

Primer on the
Autonomic
Nervous System

Edited by

David Robertson
Clinical Research Center
Vanderbilt University
Nashville, Tennessee

Phillip A. Low
The Mayo Clinic
Department of Neurology
Rochester, Minnesota

Ronald J. Polinsky
Sandoz Research Institute
East Hanover, New Jersey

Academic Press

San Diego   New York   Boston   London   Sydney   Tokyo   Toronto

Cover photograph (paperback edition only): Thoracic positron emission tomography scan in a normal volunteer after intravenous injection of 6-[^{18}F]-fluorodopamine. Note intense reconstructed radioactivity derived from positron emission in the left ventricular myocardium. The upper right section of the picture corresponds to the left front of the patient. Photograph courtesy of David S. Goldstein of NIH.

Copyright © 1996 by ACADEMIC PRESS

Academic Press
A Division of Harcourt Brace & Company
525 B Street, Suite 1900, San Diego, California 92101-4495

United Kingdom Edition published by
Academic Press Limited
24-28 Oval Road, London NW1 7DX

Library of Congress Cataloging-in-Publication Data

Primer on the autonomic nervous system / [edited] by David Robertson,
  Phillip A. Low, Ronald J. Polinsky.
        p.   cm.
  Includes index.
  ISBN 0-12-589760-X (hb: alk. paper). -- ISBN 0-12-589761-8 (pb :
alk. paper)
  1. Autonomic nervous system--Physiology. 2. Autonomic nervous
system--Pathophysiology. I. Robertson, David, date. II. Low,
Phillip A. III. Polinsky, Ronald J.
  [DNLM: 1. Autonomic Nervous System Diseases--physiopathology.
2. Autonomic Nervous System--physiology. WL 600 P953 1996]
QP368.P75 1996
612.8'9--dc20
DNLM/DLC
for Library of Congress   95-25734
                                                 CIP

PRINTED IN THE UNITED STATES OF AMERICA
        98 99 00 01 QW 9 8 7 6 5 4 3

Contents

PART III

Pharmacology

PART IV

Clinical Evaluation of Autonomic Function

PART V

Environmental and Physical Stresses

PART VI

Cardiovascular and Cerebrovascular Disorders

PART **VII**

Paroxymal Autonomic Syncopes

PART **VIII**

Catecholamine Disorders

PART **IX**

Central Autonomic Disorders

PART **X**

Peripheral Autonomic Disorders

PART XI

Orthostatic Intolerance Syndrome

PART XII

Other Clinical Conditions

PART XIII

Management of Autonomic Disorders

Contributors

Numbers in parentheses indicate the pages on which the authors' contributions begin.

Felicia B. Axelrod (242), Departments of Neurology and Pediatrics, Carl Seamon Family Center for Dysautonomia Treatment and Research, Pediatrics, New York University School of Medicine, New York, New York 10016

Eduardo E. Benarroch (226), Department of Neurology, Mayo Clinic, Rochester, Minnesota 55905

Italo Biaggioni (332), Department of Medicine and Pharmacology, Vanderbilt University, Nashville, Tennessee 37232

Vernon S. Bishop (125), Department of Physiology, The University of Texas Health Science Center, San Antonio, Texas 78284

Frans Boomsma (205), Department of Internal Medicine I, University Hospital Dijkzigt, Rotterdam, The Netherlands

Alba Larre Borges (271), Department of Neurology, School of Medicine, Montevideo 11300, Uruguay

Xandra Breakefield (210), Neuroscience Program, Harvard Medical School, Molecular Neurogenetics Unit, Massachusetts General Hospital, Charlestown, Massachusetts 02129

Beverley A. Britt (138), Department of Anaesthesia and Pharmacology, Toronto General Division, The Toronto Hospital, Toronto, Ontario, Canada M6G 2C4

Daniel Bulla (271), Department of Neurology, School of Medicine, Montevideo 11300, Uruguay

Geoffrey Burnstock (99), Department of Anatomy and Developmental Biology, University College London, London WC1E 6BT, United Kingdom

David A. Calhoun (143), Department of Medicine, Vascular Biology and Hypertension Program, The University of Alabama at Birmingham, Birmingham, Alabama 35294

Michael Camilleri (33), Department of Medicine, Gastroenterology Research Unit, Mayo Clinic, Rochester, Minnesota 55905

P. David Charles (134), Division of Movement Disorders, Department of Neurology, Vanderbilt University, Nashville, Tennessee 37212

Sudhansu Chokroverty (304), Department of Neurology, VA Medical Center, Lyons, New Jersey 07939; Departments of Neurology and Neurophysiology, St. Vincent's Hospital and Medical Center of New York; Robert Wood Johnson Medical School, Piscataway, New Jersey; and New York Medical College, Valhalla, New York

H. Cecil Coghlan (283), Division of Cardiovascular Diseases, Department of Medicine, Uihlein Autonomic Research Laboratory, The University of Alabama, Birmingham, Alabama 35294

Victor A. Convertino (183), Armstrong Laboratory, Physiology Research Branch, Brooks Air Force Base, Texas 78235

Allen W. Cowley, Jr. (42, 49), Department of Physiology, Medical College of Wisconsin, Milwaukee, Wisconsin 53226

Thomas L. Davis (134, 219), Division of Movement Disorders, Department of Neurology, Vanderbilt University, Nashville, Tennessee 37212

Dwain L. Eckberg (59), Department of Medicine and Physiology, Hunter Holmes McGuire Department of Veterans Affairs Medical Center, Medical College of Virginia, Richmond, Virginia 23249

Murray Esler (164), Baker Medical Research Institute, Melbourne, Australia

Robert Fealey (293), Department of Neurology, Mayo Medical Center, Rochester, Minnesota 55905

Fetnat M. Fouad-Tarazi (286), Department of Cardiology, The Cleveland Clinic Foundation, Cleveland, Ohio 44195

Kleber G. Franchini (42, 49), Hypertension Unit, Heart Institute, University of São Paulo, 05403-000 São Paulo, Brazil

Roy Freeman (326), Harvard Medical School, Deaconess Hospital, Boston, Massachusetts 02215

Ray W. Gifford, Jr. (187), Dept. of Nephrology and Hypertension, Cleveland Clinic Foundation, Cleveland, Ohio 44195; and Department of Internal Medicine, Ohio State University College of Medicine, Columbus, Ohio 43210

Eugene V. Golanov (56), Department of Neurobiology and Neuroscience, Cornell University Medical College, New York, New York 10021

David S. Goldstein (91), Clinical Neurochemistry Section, National Institute of Neurological Disorders and Stroke, National Institutes of Health, Bethesda, Maryland 20892

Blair P. Grubb (179), Division of Cardiology, Department of Medicine, Medical College of Ohio, Toledo, Ohio 43699

Robert W. Hamill (12), Department of Neurology, Fletcher Allen Health Care, The University of Vermont College of Medicine, Burlington, Vermont 05401

Yadollah Harati (249, 255), Department of Neurology, Baylor College of Medicine, Houston, Texas 77030

Robert Hoeldtke (39, 208), Division of Endocrinology/Metabolism and Nutrition, Department of Medicine, West Virginia University Medical School, Morgantown, West Virginia 26506

Keith Hyland (201), Institute of Metabolic Disease, Baylor University Medical Center, and Department of Neurology, University of Texas Southwestern Medical Center, Dallas, Texas 75226

Timothy J. Ingall (130), Department of Neurology, Mayo Clinic Scottsdale, Scottsdale, Arizona 85259

Joseph L. Izzo, Jr. (116), Department of Medicine, Millard Fillmore Hospitals, State University of New York at Buffalo, Buffalo, New York 14209

Garry Jennings (164), Baker Medical Research Institute, Alfred and Baker Medical Unit, Alfred Hospital, Melbourne, Australia

Michael J. Joyner (69), Department of Anesthesiology and Physiology and Biophysics, Mayo Clinic, Rochester, Minnesota 55905

Horacio Kaufmann (173), Department of Neurology, Autonomic Nervous System Laboratory, Mt. Sinai School of Medicine, New York, New York 10029

David Kaye (164), Division of Cardiology, Brigham and Women's Hospital, Boston, Massachusetts 02115

Ramesh K. Khurana (266), Department of Neurology, University of Maryland School of Medicine, Baltimore, Maryland 21218; and Division of Neurology, The Johns Hopkins University School of Medicine, Baltimore, Maryland 21218

Irwin J. Kopin (87), Clinical Neuroscience Branch, National Institute of Neurological Disorders and Stroke, National Institutes of Health, Bethesda, Maryland 20892

Daniel J. Kosinski (179), Division of Cardiology, Department of Medicine, Medical College of Ohio, Toledo, Ohio 43699

Otto Kuchel (212), Department of Medicine, Clinical Research Institute of Montreal, University of Montreal and McGill, Montreal, Quebec, Canada H2W 1R7

Gavin Lambert (164), Baker Medical Research Institute, Melbourne, Victoria, Australia

Lewis A. Lipsitz (79), Department of Medicine, Harvard Medical School, Hebrew Rehabilitation Center for Aged, Boston, Massachusetts 02131

Phillip A. Low (279), Mayo Medical School, Mayo Clinic, Rochester, Minnesota 55905

Arie J. Man in't Veld (205), Department of Internal Medicine I, Hypertension Unit, University Hospital Dijkzigt, Rotterdam, The Netherlands

William M. Manger (187), Department of Clinical Medicine, New York University Medical Center, New York, New York 10016; and Columbia Medical Center and National Hypertension Association, New York, New York 10016

Allyn L. Mark (65), Department of Internal Medicine, College of Medicine, The University of Iowa, Iowa City, Iowa 52242

Christopher J. Mathias (230), Cardiovascular Medicine Unit, Department of Medicine, St. Mary's Hospital Medical School/Imperial College of Science, Technology and Medicine; and Autonomic Unit, University Department of Clinical Neurology, National Hospital and Institute of Neurology, University of London, London WC1N 3BG, United Kingdom

James G. McLeod (269, 273), Division of Neurology, Department of Medicine, The University of Sydney, Sydney, N.S.W., Australia

Mario Medici (271), Department of Neurology, School of Medicine, Montevideo 11300, Uruguay

Douglas F. Milam (300), Department of Urology, D-4314 MCN, Vanderbilt University, Nashville, Tennessee 37232

Jere H. Mitchell (26), Department of Internal Medicine, Harry S. Moss Heart Center, University of Texas Southwestern Medical Center, Dallas, Texas 75235

Rogelio Mosqueda-Garcia (3), Department of Medicine and Pharmacology, Vanderbilt University, Nashville, Tennessee 37232

James E. Muller (157), Cardiovascular Division, Deaconess Hospital, Harvard Medical School, Boston, Massachusetts 02215

Katherine T. Murray (149), Division of Clinical Pharmacology, Department of Medicine and Pharmacology, Vanderbilt University, Nashville, Tennessee 37232

James L. Netterville (192), Department of Otolaryngology, Vanderbilt University Medical Center, Nashville, Tennessee 37232

Suzanne Oparil (143), Vascular Biology and Hypertension Program, Division of Cardiovascular Disease, University of Alabama at Birmingham, Birmingham, Alabama 35294

Bruce C. Paton (128), Department of Surgery, University of Colorado, Denver, Colorado 80237

Michael Pfeifer (260), Division of Endocrinology and Metabolism, Southern Illinois University, School of Medicine, Springfield, Illinois 62702

Ronald J. Polinsky (222), Drug Safety Department, Clinical Pharmacology, Sandoz Research Institute, East Hanover, New Jersey 07936

Raquel Ponce De Leon (271), Department of Neurology, School of Medicine, Montevideo 11300, Uruguay

S. Regunathan (107), Department of Neurology and Neuroscience, Cornell University Medical College, New York, New York 10021

Donald J. Reis (56, 107), Department of Neurology and Neuroscience, Cornell University Medical College, New York, New York 10021

L. Jackson Roberts II (313), Department of Medicine and Pharmacology, Vanderbilt University, Nashville, Tennessee 37232

David Robertson (111, 324), Departments of Medicine, Pharmacology, and Neurology, Vanderbilt University, Nashville, Tennessee 37232

Rose Marie Robertson (197), Department of Medicine, Division of Cardiology, Vanderbilt University, Nashville, Tennessee 37232

Dan M. Roden (149), Department of Medicine and Pharmacology, Division of Clinical Pharmacology, Vanderbilt University, Nashville, Tennessee 37232

Irwin J. Schatz (239), Department of Medicine, University of Hawaii John A. Burns School of Medicine, Honolulu, Hawaii 96813

Ronald Schondorf (279), Department of Neurology, McGill University, Jewish General Hospital, Montreal, Quebec, Canada H3T 1E2

Aziz Taher Shaibani (249, 255), Department of Neurology, Baylor College of Medicine, Houston, Texas 77030

Robert Sinard (192), Department of Otolaryngology, University of Texas, Dallas, Texas 75235

James E. Skinner (153), Totts Gap Medical Research Institute, Bangor, Pennsylvania 18013

Virend K. Somers (65), Department of Internal Medicine, Cardiovascular Division, The University of Iowa College of Medicine, Iowa City, Iowa 52242

John D. Stewart (31), Department of Neurology and Neurosurgery, McGill University, Montreal Neurological Institute and Hospital, Montreal, Quebec, Canada H3A 2B4

David H. P. Streeten (309), Section of Endocrinology, Department of Medicine, State University of New York Health Science Center, Syracuse, New York 13210

William T. Talman (104), Department of Neurology, The University of Iowa and Department of Veterans Affairs Medical Center, Iowa City, Iowa 52242

Peter Y. D. Taylor (157), Cardiovascular Division, Deaconess Hospital, Harvard Medical School, Boston, Massachusetts 02215

H. Stanley Thompson (74), Department of Ophthalmology, Neuro-ophthalmology Service, The University of Iowa, Iowa City, Iowa 52242

Anton H. van den Meiracker (205), Department of Internal Medicine I, University Hospital Dijkzigt, Rotterdam, The Netherlands

Richard L. Verrier (157), Institute for the Prevention of Cardiovascular Disease, Deaconess Hospital, Harvard Medical School, Boston, Massachusetts 02215

Wouter Wieling (319), Department of Internal Medicine, Academic Medical Center, 1105 AZ Amsterdam, The Netherlands

Peter R. Wilson (311), Department of Anesthesiology, Mayo Clinic, Rochester, Minnesota 55905

Preface

The goal of this book is to present the canon of autonomic neuroscience to students, scientists, and physicians in a concise and accessible manner. The idea for this *Primer* was conceived as an educational project of the American Autonomic Society. Topics for inclusion were selected with input from many leading clinicians and scientists. In spite of the small size of the text, more contributors were engaged in its preparation than in any previous treatise on the autonomic nervous system.

The editors and I thank the many individuals who contributed to the development of the *Primer,* all of whom agreed to do so without compensation in order to keep the cost of the book as low as possible. We are especially grateful for the unprecedented speed with which the contributors and reviewers responded in order that the finished product would be as up-to-date as humanly possible. We also want to acknowledge the pivotal roles of Mrs. Dorothea Boemer at Vanderbilt University and Dr. Jasna Markovac at Academic Press for their unflagging help in bringing this endeavor to a successful conclusion.

We want future editions of this *Primer* to be as helpful to our readership as possible. For this reason, we would be grateful for comments and suggestions of ways it can be improved. These can be sent to me at david.robertson@mcmail.vanderbilt.edu.

David Robertson

PART I

Anatomy

1 Central Autonomic Regulation

Rogelio Mosqueda-Garcia
Vanderbilt University
Nashville, Tennessee

Adaptation to environmental change is regulated by the **autonomic nervous system.** Accordingly, sensory, visceral, motor, and neuroendocrine functions can be modulated by this system. The autonomic nervous system can be subdivided into three major components: the sympathetic, the parasympathetic, and the enteric nervous system. Entities regulating these branches can be found both inside and outside the **central nervous system (CNS).** This section presents an overview of the main components, functions, and interrelations of CNS autonomic regulation.

Central autonomic regulation is achieved through interrelated neuronal cell groups located in the **brainstem** (medulla oblongata, pons, and midbrain), **diencephalon,** and **telencephalon** (see Fig. 1). Prominent areas that constitute major autonomic relay or integrative centers include the **ventrolateral medulla,** the **nucleus tractus solitarii** (NTS), the **parabrachial nucleus,** the **periaqueductal gray** matter in the midbrain, the **hypothalamus,** the **amygdala,** and the **insular** and **prefrontal cortex.** These structures can affect autonomic function either by reflex changes of the end-organ response or by neurohumoral mechanisms that may involve multiple sites and release of different substances. **Reflex autonomic mechanisms** involve the activation of neuronal circuits that result in rapid modulation of sympathetic and/or parasympathetic tone. In contrast, **neurohumoral mechanisms** often involve a variety of neuronal structures that process and then affect neuroendocrine and autonomic behavioral and motor responses.

Several features underlie central autonomic regulation: (1) major relay cell groups in the brain process that regulate afferent and efferent information, (2) confluence (or convergence) of autonomic information (cardiovascular, respiratory, gastrointestinal, etc.) occurs onto discrete brain nuclei, (3) autonomic function is modulated by changes in preganglionic sympathetic or parasympathetic tone and/or by changes in neuroendocrine effectors, (4) neuronal interconnections among different components of central autonomic regulation are reciprocally innervated, (5) parallel pathways carry autonomic information to other structures, and (6) multiple chemical substances mediate transduction of neuronal information.

Nucleus Tractus Solitarii

One of the most important sites of autonomic regulation is the **nucleus tractus solitarii** (NTS) (Figs. 1 and 2). This structure, located in the dorsal surface of the medulla oblongata, receives visceroceptive information from cardiovascular, respiratory, and gastrointestinal sites. The NTS is an ovoid-

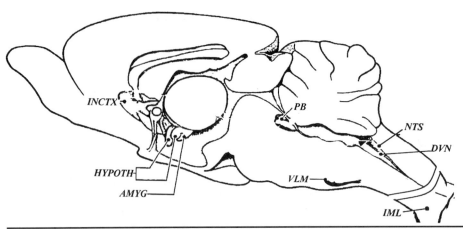

Figure 1. Prominent central autonomic regulatory centers. Schematic representation of major autonomic centers in the rat brain. AMYG, amygdala; DVN, dorsal motor nucleus of the vagus; IML, intermediolateral cell column of the spinal cord; INCTX, insular cortex; NTS, nucleus tractus solitarii; PB, parabrachial nucleus; VLM, ventrolateral medulla.

shaped nucleus located in the dorsal aspect of the medulla oblongata. Rostral to the obex, the NTS is bilateral, while at the level of the area postrema, the bilateral components of the NTS merge to form the **commissural subnucleus** of the NTS. Other subnuclei have been identified in the NTS. These subnuclei have been classified according to their position relative to the solitary tract (a central fiber bundle comprising the axons of the **VIIth, IXth,** and **Xth** cranial nerves). Accordingly, NTS subnuclei can be described as medial or lateral to the solitary tract. The medial subnuclei lie dorsal and dorsolateral to the motor nucleus of the vagus and comprise the **medial,** the **intermediate,** and the **parvicellular** subnuclei. The lateral subnuclei include the **interstitial,** the **ventral,** the **ventrolateral,** and the **dorsolateral subnuclei.** Functionally, these subnuclei can be classified according to the distribution of afferent inputs or type of end-organ response affected. For instance, cardiovascular afferents predominantly terminate in the **dorsal NTS** while many gastrointestinal afferents, including gustatory fibers, segregate in the **parvicellular subnucleus.** While pulmonary fibers synapse in the **ventral** and **ventrolateral subnuclei,** afferents from respiratory structures such as the trachea or bronchi project to the interstitial NTS. In contrast, the **commissural NTS,** and to a lesser extent the **medial NTS,** receive afferents from most of the major visceral components. For instance, spinal inputs conveying somatic and visceral afferents project mainly to this NTS subdivision and may represent a sensory connection whereby visceral and somatic information is relayed to higher brain centers.

The NTS projects to brainstem and forebrain nuclei that in turn regulate preganglionic sympathetic and parasympathetic activity and/or neuroendocrine functions. Many of these structures (such as the noradrenergic A5 cell group, caudal raphe nuclei, rostral ventrolateral medulla, central gray matter, and paraventricular and lateral hypothalamic areas) send, in turn, afferents to the

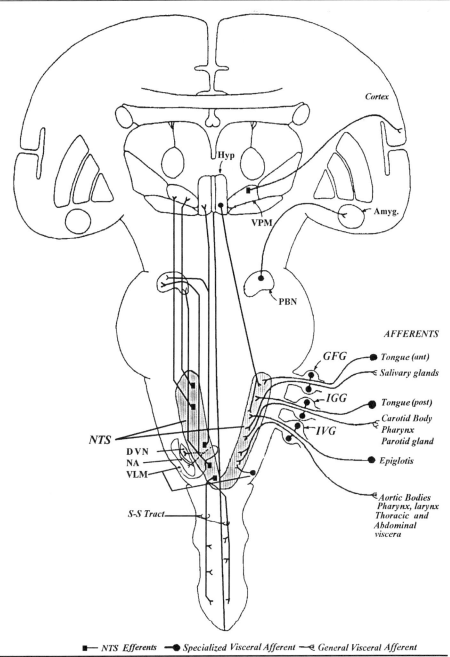

Figure 2. Neuronal connections of the nucleus of the solitary tract in the human brain. Diagrammatic representation of most prominent afferent and efferents of the NTS. Amyg, amygdala; DVN, dorsal motor nucleus of the vagus; GFG, geniculate offacial ganglia; Hyp, hypothalamus; IGG, inferior of glosopharyngeal ganglia; IVG, inferior of the vagus ganglia; NA, nucleus ambiguus; NTS, nucleus tractus solitarii; PBN, parabrachial nucleus; S-S tract, solitariospinal tract; VLM, ventrolateral medulla; VPM, ventral posteromedial nucleus of thalamus. (■) NTS efferents, (●) specialized visceral afferent, (ε) general visceral afferent.

NTS; these reciprocal connections may serve as feedback regulatory mechanisms. In addition, several of these projections have functional or visceral selectivity. For instance, baroreceptor and chemoreceptor information relays from the NTS to the **central nucleus of the amygdala** and to the **paraventricular hypothalamic nucleus.** Cardiac parasympathetic activity can be altered by the NTS projections to the **motor nucleus of the vagus** and to the **nucleus ambiguus.** Sympathetic vascular activity can be altered by NTS projections terminating in the **rostral** or **caudal** part of the **ventrolateral medulla.** Information affecting fluid and osmotic balance projects from the NTS to the **median preoptic nucleus** (affecting the release of **vasopressin**), the paraventricular hypothalamic nucleus, the lateral hypothalamic area, and the zona incerta.

The NTS is the first relay area for several reflexes that control respiration and circulation. This nucleus can initiate multiple medullary reflexes that directly affect blood pressure, heart rate, respiration, and other autonomic functions or it can provide viscerosensory inputs to higher autonomic nuclei. One of the best studied examples is the **baroreceptor reflex.** Sudden increases or decreases in arterial blood pressure activate or inhibit, respectively, stretch receptors or baroreceptors. These receptors, which have been identified in the aortic arch, carotid sinus, lungs, and heart, relay information to the NTS through the **glossopharyngeal** and **vagus nerves.** It has been proposed that an excitatory amino acid, such as glutamate, is the primary neurotransmitter of the first synapse of the baroreceptor reflex. Substances like adenosine, angiotensin II, endogenous opioid peptides, and **gamma aminobutyric acid (GABA)** serve as baroreceptor reflex modulators within the NTS. Through appropriate neuronal connections, the NTS evokes reciprocal changes in sympathetic (**vascular tone**) and parasympathetic activity (**heart rate rhythm**) that aim to preserve arterial blood pressure within narrow ranges. The crucial role of the NTS is illustrated by ablation of the NTS, which produces **fulminating hypertension** or excessive **blood pressure variability** with some degree of chronic hypertension depending on the animal species.

The **ventrolateral medulla** plays a critical role in the control of vasomotor tone. At a simple level, it has been subdivided into the rostral (**RVLM**) and the caudal ventrolateral medulla (**CVLM**). The RVLM receives baroreceptor information from projections originating in the NTS and probably releasing glutamate as neurotransmitter. In addition, afferent fibers from the area postrema and the CVLM have been described. Reciprocal connections between the RVLM and other nuclei (the central gray matter, lateral hypothalamic area, paraventricular hypothalamic nucleus, and the parabrachial nucleus) may constitute an autonomic regulatory network. One of the main outputs from RVLM neurons goes to the thoracolumbar **intermediolateral cell column** of the spinal cord which is the origin of preganglionic fibers modulating sympathetic tone. **Glutamate** has been proposed as the neurotransmitter of this projection. Aminergic (particularly adrenergic neurons in the **C1 area**) and noncatecholaminergic neurons in the RVLM participate in vasomotor function. Some of these neurons exhibit **intrinsic pacemaker properties.** Increase in RVLM–neuronal activity results in release of **catecholamines** and **vasopressin** and increases in blood pressure and heart rate. Reduction of neuronal activity in the RVLM, on the other hand, results in pronounced **hypotension**.

The CVLM is a circumscribed region in the medullary reticular formation that extends caudally from the obex close to the ventral surface of the medulla. At different rostrocaudal levels, the cardiovascular neurons in this area overlap or are located either ventrolateral or medial to the **A1 noradrenergic cell group**. The CVLM contains neurons that reduce arterial blood pressure by a **reduction in sympathetic tone**. These neurons are concentrated in a region of the reticular formation that lies between the nucleus ambiguus and the lateral reticular nucleus. Afferent projections to the CVLM from the NTS are thought to be involved in the processing of baroreflex information. Unlike the RVLM, neurons from the CVLM do not project directly to the spinal cord. The CVLM inhibits sympathetic activity through a short inhibitory projection to the RVLM that probably uses GABA as neurotransmitter.

The Parabrachial Nucleus

Located also in the brainstem, the **parabrachial nucleus (PBN)** rests in the dorsal aspect of the medulla oblongata. Several subdivisions of this nucleus have been described including the medial, lateral, and ventral aspects. The major afferents to this nucleus arise from specific NTS regions and also exhibit some visceral distribution. While the ventral aspect of the PBN receives respiratory information relayed from the ventral and ventrolateral NTS, gastrointestinal pathways from the parvicellular NTS synapse in the medial parabrachial nucleus. General visceroceptive information from the commissural NTS projects to the lateral parabrachial area. The PBN has been implicated in regulation of food intake and cortical and gustatory functions.

Major efferent connections from the lateral PBN include the **cerebral cortex** (indirectly through thalamic pathways and directly to the frontal, infralimbic, and **insular areas** of the cerebral cortex), ventromedial hypothalamic nucleus, lateral hypothalamic area, paraventricular hypothalamic nucleus, substantia innominata, the median preoptic nucleus, the central nucleus of the amygdala, and the bed nucleus of the stria terminalis. The medial PBN projects to the ventroposterior thalamic nucleus, zona incerta, central nucleus of the amygdala, bed nucleus of the stria terminalis, and infralimbic cortex. In contrast, the ventral PBN projects to nuclei in the brainstem that control respiration.

Locus Coeruleus

Although the exact function of the locus coeruleus is not known, it has been proposed that this center integrates information from both the external and internal environment. Accordingly, the neuronal activity in the locus coeruleus relates to the state of consciousness. Chemical stimulation of locus coeruleus neurons results in decreases in blood pressure and heart rate. Two main projections have been identified: one arising from the nucleus prepositus hypoglossi and the other from the ventrolateral medulla. Through multisynaptic pathways, the locus coeruleus also receives afferent information from areas such as the splanchnic, pelvic, and vagal nerves.

Hypothalamus

The hypothalamus integrates autonomic and neuroendocrine function and serves as an important homeostatic center. It is a bilateral paired structure that occupies the side walls and floor of the third ventricle. In the coronal plane, it has been divided into lateral, medial, and periventricular regions. These regions contain at least 15 nuclei. The **lateral zone** is believed to modulate behavior and integrate autonomic responses during **feeding and reproduction.** The **medial zone** seems to integrate autonomic and motor responses during **homeostasis.** The **periventricular zone** seems to participate in autonomic and neuroendocrine control as well as in the generation of **biological rhythms.** Two extensively studied hypothalamic areas include the **supraoptic (SO)** and **paraventricular hypothalamic nuclei (PVH).** The magnocellular portions of these nuclei contain both **vasopressin** and **oxytocin.** Afferents projecting to these nuclei carry information concerning water balance, reflex cardiovascular function, and perhaps activity from chemoreceptor and muscle afferents. Major inputs to the PVH and SO nuclei include the subfornical organ, the median preoptic nucleus, the pedunculopontine nucleus, the laterodorsal tegmental nucleus, the rostral and caudal ventrolateral medulla, and the NTS.

Distinct PVH areas affect endocrine and autonomic responses. While some PVH neurons contain peptides that regulate pituitary function (i.e., cortico-tropin-releasing hormone), some release vasopressin to the circulation and others give rise to autonomic pathways projecting to the brainstem and spinal cord. These include projections to the central gray matter, locus coeruleus, parabrachial nucleus, NTS, dorsal vagal nucleus, nucleus ambiguus, and inter-mediolateral cell column of the spinal cord. It has been suggested that the PVH regulates the amplitude of general sympathetic outflow in addition to specific autonomic and visceral functions.

Amygdala

The amygdala participates in different behavioral, neuroendocrine, and au-tonomic functions. The central nucleus of the amygdala contributes to auto-nomic control. Relevant afferents to this nucleus include those from the cerebral cortex (orbital, frontal, and insular), the NTS, and the parabrachial nucleus. In turn, the central nucleus of the amygdala projects to the lateral hypothalamic area, central gray matter, RVLM, parabrachial nucleus, NTS, and vagal mo-tor nuclei.

Cerebral Cortex

The **insular** and **medial prefrontal cortex** areas are known to participate in autonomic regulation. The **insular cortex** receives afferents from the thalamus, the lateral hypothalamic area, and the parabrachial nucleus. Efferent projec-tions from the insular cortex are to the parabrachial nucleus, lateral hypothala-mic area, thalamus, central nucleus of the amygdala, and NTS. Neuronal activation in the insular cortex increases blood pressure and heart rate, evokes piloerection and pupillary dilatation and affects respiration, gastric motility, and salivation. Since this area has been implicated in gustatory function, the insular cortex may be considered as a visceral sensorimotor area.

The **medial prefrontal cortex** has been implicated in cardiovascular and gastrointestinal motor function. Particularly relevant are the prelimbic and infralimbic areas, which constitute the medial bank of the prefrontal cortex. The infralimbic area receives afferents from the hippocampus, amygdala, and other cortex areas. Infralimbic efferents project to the thalamus, hypothalamus, parabrachial nucleus, and NTS. The prelimbic cortex has reciprocal connections with the limbic system and spare projections to the parabrachial nucleus and hypothalamus. Electrical stimulation of the prelimbic and infralimbic areas results in **hypotensive** and **bradycardic** effects. Ablation of the medial prefrontal cortex blunts renovascular hypertension, conditioned heart rate responses, and baroreflex activation. Also, changes in gastric motility have been recorded.

The **somatic sensory cortex** processes autonomic information from sympathetic fibers. These fibers enter the thoracic spinal cord with somatic sensory afferents in the dorsal horn and then project as a part of the thoracic somatic sensory pathway. The integration of autonomic and sensory signals may be relevant in the cardiovascular and gastrointestinal responses to pain and stress (i.e., emotional syncope or hypertension evoked by stress). For instance, it has been proposed that **spinothalamic projections** (carrying information from cardiac afferents) to the sensory cortex participate in **referred cardiac pain** in humans. In some species, these projections are known to carry information from cardiac chemical receptors and from somatic sensory peripheral fields.

Circumventricular Organs

High-molecular-weight substances in the systemic circulation normally do not gain access to the central nervous system. Their penetration is prevented by an elaborate system of **tight junctions** in the endothelial layer. This system, which is present throughout the central nervous system, is known as the **blood–brain barrier.** In some areas along the third and fourth ventricles of the brain, however, the capillaries are fenestrated (therefore, an incomplete blood–brain barrier is present) and contain specialized ependymal cells (tanycytes) which have prolongations extending to the ventricular surface or to the surrounding neural tissue. These regions are called circumventricular organs and are thought to be important for sensing the chemical environment in plasma and the cerebrospinal fluid and for transmitting this information to the CNS. Circumventricular organs include the **organum vasculosum of the lamina terminalis (OVLT), subfornical organ (SFO), median eminence, posterior pituitary, intermediate lobe of the pituitary, subcomissural organ, pineal gland,** and the **area postrema (AP)** (Fig. 3). Among these, the OVLT, the AP, and the SFO are thought to participate in the integration of neuroendocrine and autonomic functions.

Area postrema. The AP is the most caudal of the circumventricular organs. It lies at the end of the fourth ventricle. While in humans it is a bilateral structure, in other species (i.e., rodents) it is a midline organ positioned dorsal to the site where the fourth ventricle communicates with the central canal. The AP is a highly vascularized area which, in addition, receives neuronal afferents from the **carotid sinus nerve, vagus nerve,** and **hypothalamic nuclei.** Among others, the AP projects to the NTS, lateral parabrachial nucleus, nucleus ambiguus, and the RVLM. The AP has been implicated in **cardiovascular regulation,** in **fluid homeostasis,** and in a chemoreceptive sensing area triggering **vomiting.**

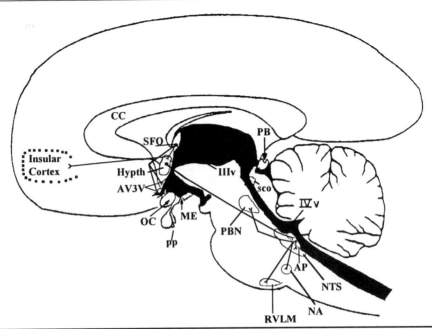

Figure 3.   Anatomical location and most prominent neural connections of the circumventricular organs of the rat. The circumventricular organs are highlighted in gray in the figure and in bold in the text. AP, area postrema; AV3V region, area including the median preoptic nucleus, the preoptic periventricular nucleus, and the anteroventral periventricular nucleus; CC, corpus callosum; Hypth, hypothalamus; ME, median eminence; NA, nucleus ambiguus; NTS, nucleus tractus solitarii; PB, pineal body; PBN, parabrachial nucleus; pp, posterior pituitary; OC, optic chiasm; RVLM, rostral ventrolateral medulla; SCO, subcommisural organ; SFO, subfornical organ; IIIv, third ventricle; IVv, fourth ventricle.

It is not clear whether AP lesions affect resting blood pressure or whether this circumventricular organ mediates the cardiovascular effects of some peptides (angiotensin II or vasopressin). Ablation of the AP abolishes or greatly attenuates drug-induced vomiting and in humans surgical destruction of this area abolishes idiopathic vomiting.

The subfornical organ. Anatomically positioned at the roof of the third ventricle, the SFO has been increasingly studied for its potential role in autonomic and neuroendocrine function. Relevant projections from the SFO include those to the paraventricular and supraoptic nuclei, to the anteroventral third ventricular (AV3V) region, to the lateral hypothalamic area, and to the infralimbic cerebral cortex. The SFO participates in the regulation of salt and water balance affecting drinking behavior. In addition, neuronal function within the SFO seems to mediate the cardiovascular responses of peptides like angiotensin II, endothelin, and vasopressin.

The organum vasculosum of the lamina terminalis. This structure is situated in the ventral portion of the rostral wall of the third cerebral ventricle in between the optic chiasm and the ventral median preoptic nucleus. In the rat, the OVLT, the median preoptic nucleus, the preoptic periventricular nucleus, and the anteroventral periventricular nucleus form the **AV3V region.** Proposed

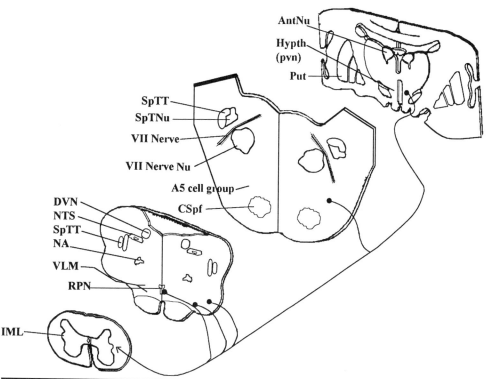

Figure 4.   Major sources of sympathetic outflow. Main centers of sympathetic outflow have been located in the hypothalamus and in the brainstem. These include the paraventricular nucleus of the hypothalamus (pvn), the noradrenergic A5 cell group, the caudal raphe nuclei (RPN), and the ventrolateral medulla (VLM). These projections terminate in sympathetic preganglionic nuclei (i.e., intermedilateral cell column, IML) of the spinal cord, from where sympathetic outflow is regulated. AntNu, anterior nucleus of the thalamus; Put, putamen; SpTT, spinal trigeminal tract; SpTNu, spinal trigeminal nucleus; VII Nerve Nu, facial nerve nucleus; CSpf, corticospinal fibers; DVN, dorsal motor nucleus of the vagus; NTS, nucleus tractus solitarii; NA, nucleus ambiguus; IML, intermediolateral column.

afferent connections to the OVLT include some from the SFO, anterior hypothalamus, posterior hypothalamus, arcuate nucleus, and locus coeruleus. The OVLT appears to send projections to the supraoptic nucleus, paraventricular nucleus, dentate gyrus, stria medullaris, basal ganglia, and septum. The OVLT is thought to be involved in osmotic and sodium balance. Lesions of the AV3V region (including the OVLT) result in cessation of water ingestion, impairment of vasopressin secretion, and changes in the development of hypertension in some animal models. In addition, it may subserve a modulatory role in sexual function.

   The final common pathways: Centers regulating sympathetic and parasympathetic outflow. Homeostatic responses mediated by the autonomic nervous system are achieved by altering the balance among sympathetic, parasympathetic, and different hormonal systems (i.e., vasopressin, renin). Main centers affecting efferent sympathetic flow are located in the hypothalamus and brainstem (Fig. 4). These include the paraventricular hypothalamic nucleus, the A5 noradrenergic cell group (located in the most rostral portion of the ventrolateral medulla), caudal raphe region, RVLM, and ventromedial medulla. Projections from these areas terminate in the **intermediolateral (IML) cell column** of the spinal thoracolumbarcord. The IML gives rise to sympathetic preganglionic neurons and represents the final CNS output of the **autonomic network.**

Centers regulating parasympathetic tone include the **nucleus ambiguus** and the **dorsal motor nucleus of the vagus.** Fibers originating in these centers innervate parasympathetic ganglia whose axons terminate in near proximity or within the walls of viscera located in the cervical, thoracic, and abdominal regions.

References

1. Spyer KM. The central nervous organization of reflex circulatory control. In: Loewy AD, Spyer KM, eds. Central regulation of autonomic functions. New York: Oxford University Press, 1990: 168–88.
2. Loewy AD. Central autonomic pathways. In: Loewy AD, Spyer KM, eds. Central regulation of autonomic functions. New York: Oxford University Press, 1990: 88–103.
3. Various. Functional morphology and chemical neuroanatomy of the NTS. In: Barraco IR, ed. Nucleus of the solitary tract. Boca Raton FL: CRC Press, 1993:1–92.
4. Mosqueda-Garcia R. β-Endorphin in central cardiovascular control. Cardiovasc Rev Rep 1987;8:39–45.
5. Mosqueda-Garcia R, Tseng C-J, Appalsamy M, Robertson D. Modulatory effects of adenosine on baroreflex activation in the nucleus of the solitary tract. Eur J Pharmacol 1989;174:119–22.
6. Mosqueda-Garcia R, Inagami T, Appalsamy M, Robertson RM. Endothelin as a neuropeptide: cardiovascular effects in the brainstem. Circ Res 1993;72:20–35.

2   Peripheral Autonomic Nervous System

Robert W. Hamill
Department of Neurology
The University of Vermont College of Medicine
Fletcher Allen Health Care
Burlington, Vermont

The **autonomic nervous system** (ANS) is structurally and functionally positioned to interface between the internal and external milieu, coordinating bodily functions to ensure normal **homeostasis** (cardiovascular control, thermal regulation, gastrointestinal motility, urinary and bowel excretory functions, reproduction, and normal metabolic and endocrine physiology), and adaptive responses to stress (flight or fight response). Thus, the ANS has the daunting task of ensuring the survival as well as the procreation of the species. These complex roles require complex responses, and depend upon the integration of behavioral and physiological responses that are coordinated centrally and peripherally. Langley, a Cambridge University physiologist, coined the term "autonomic nervous system" and identified three separate components (**sympathetic, parasympathetic, and enteric**) around the turn of the century. This chapter focuses on the first two aspects of the peripheral ANS: the sympathetic nervous system (SNS), including the adrenal medulla, and the parasympathetic nervous system (PNS). The following précis will address the neuroanatomy of the SNS, adrenal medulla, and PNS, and then present a more detailed, albeit brief, review of the functional neuroanatomy, physiology, and pharmacology of the peripheral autonomic nervous system. This information will serve as a framework from which to view the more detailed descriptions in the chapters that follow.

Sympathetic Nervous System

The SNS (see Fig. 1) is organized at a spinal and peripheral level such that cell bodies within the **thoracolumbar** sections of the spinal cord provide **preganglionic** efferent innervation to postsynaptic sympathetic neurons that reside in ganglia dispersed in three arrangements: **paravertebral** ganglia, **prevertebral** ganglia, and **previsceral** or terminal ganglia. Paravertebral ganglia are paired structures which are located bilaterally along the vertebral column and extend from the rostrally situated **superior cervical ganglia** (SCG), located at the bifurcation of the internal carotid arteries, to ganglia located in the sacral region. All told, there are 3 cervical ganglia (the SCG, middle cervical ganglion, and inferior cervical ganglion, which is usually termed the cervicothoracic or **stellate ganglion** because it is a fused structure combining the inferior cervical and first thoracic paravertebral ganglia), 11 thoracic ganglia, 4 lumbar ganglia, and 4 or 5 sacral ganglia. More caudally, the 2 paravertebral ganglia join to become the **ganglion impar.** Prevertebral ganglia are midline structures located anterior to the aorta and vertebral column, and are represented by the celiac ganglia, aortico-renal ganglia and the superior and inferior mesenteric ganglia. Previsceral ganglia are small collections of sympathetic ganglia located close to target structures; they are also referred to as short noradrenergic neurons since their axons cover limited distances. Generally, the preganglionic fibers are relatively short and the postganglionic fibers are quite long in the SNS. The axons of these postsynaptic neurons are generally unmyelinated and of small diameter (<5 μm). The target organs of sympathetic neurons include smooth muscle and cardiac muscle, glandular structures, and parenchymal organs (e.g., liver, kidney, bladder, reproductive organs, muscles) (see Fig. 1) as well as other cutaneous structures.

The spinal cells of origin for the presynaptic input to sympathetic peripheral ganglia are located from the first thoracic to the second lumbar level of the cord, although minor variations exist. The principal neurons generally have been viewed as located in the lateral horn of the spinal gray matter (**intermediolateral cell column, IMC**), but four major groups of autonomic neurons exist: intermediolateralis pars principalis (ILP), intermediolateralis pars funicularis (ILF), nucleus intercalatus spinalis (IC), and the central autonomic nucleus (CAN) or dorsal commissural nucleus (DCN) [anatomical nomenclature is nucleus intercalatus pars paraependymalis (ICPE)]. For paravertebral ganglia,

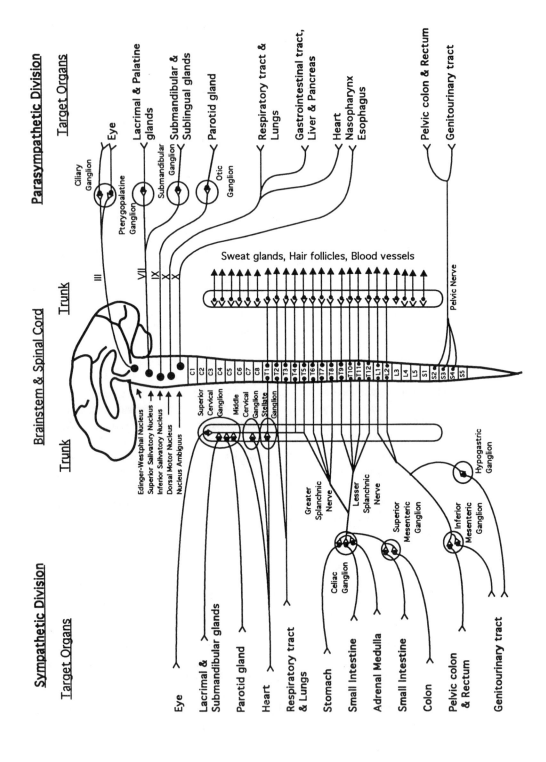

>85–90% of the presynaptic fibers originate from cell bodies in ILP or ILF. Prevertebral ganglia and terminal ganglia receive a larger proportion of preganglionic terminals from the CAN/DCN. The nucleus intercalatus also contributes preganglionic fibers, but the exact extent of these is not fully understood and is probably limited. These spinal autonomic nuclei receive substantial supraspinal input from multiple transmitter systems located at multiple levels of the neuraxis; diencephalon (hypothalamus) and brainstem (raphe, locus coeruleus, reticular formation, and ventral lateral medulla) provide the largest input and the pattern of innervation viewed in horizontal sections reveals a ladder-like arrangement of the distribution of nerve terminals (4). Without detailing the source or course of specific systems, it is important to point out that the following different neurotransmitter systems impinge on preganglionic neurons within this ladder-like structure: **monoamines**—epinephrine, norepinephrine, serotonin; **neuropeptides**—substance P, thyrotropin–release hormone (TRH), metenkephalin, vasopressin, oxytocin, and neuropeptide Y; **amino acids**—glutamate, GABA, and glycine. Undoubtedly, others exist and will be found. It is apparent that dysfunction of these supraspinal systems, or alterations of these neurotransmitters by disease or pharmacological agents, will alter the spinal control of peripheral ganglia and result in clinical dysfunction.

The outflow from the spinal cord to peripheral ganglia is segmentally organized with some overlap. Retrograde tracing studies indicate that there is a rostral–caudal gradient: SCG receives innervation from spinal segments T1 to T3; stellate ganglia, T1–T6; adrenal gland, T5–T11; celiac and superior mesenteric ganglia, T5–T12; inferior mesenteric and hypogastric ganglion, L1–L2. These presynaptic fibers, which are small in diameter (2–5 μm) and thinly myelinated, exit the ventral roots and via the **white rami communicantes** join the paravertebral chain either directly innervating their respective ganglion at the same level or traveling along the chain to innervate a target ganglion many levels away (Fig. 2). The distribution of postsynaptic fibers also follows a regional pattern with the head, face, and neck receiving innervation from the **cervical ganglia** (spinal segments T1–T4), the upper limb and thorax from the **stellate and upper thoracic ganglia** (spinal segments T1–T8), the lower trunk and abdomen from lower thoracic ganglia (spinal segments T4–T12), and the pelvic region and lower limbs from lumbar and sacral ganglia (spinal segments T10–L2). More recently, with the introduction of transneuronal tracing techniques, using such molecules as the pseudorabies virus, it has been possible to inject ganglia in the periphery and examine the transneuronal passage of tracer. Thus, supraspinal neurons projecting to the specific sets of preganglionic neurons which innervate the peripheral ganglia injected may be examined. Interestingly, a surprisingly common set of central pathways

---

Figure 1.   Schematic diagram of the sympathetic and parasympathetic divisions of the peripheral autonomic nervous system. The paravertebral chain of the sympathetic division is illustrated on both sides of the spinal outflow in order to demonstrate the full range of target structures innervated. Although the innervation pattern is diagrammatically illustrated to be direct connects between preganglionic outflow and postganglionic neurons, there is overlap of innervation such that more than one spinal segment provides innervation to neurons within the ganglia.

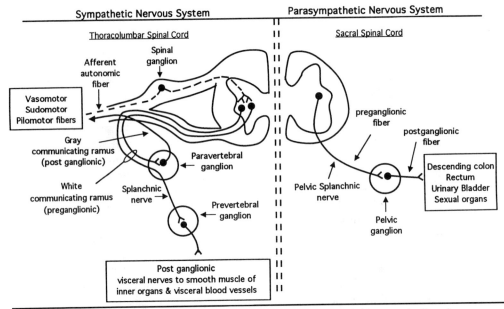

Figure 2.   Schematic illustration of the segmental spinal arrangement of the sympathetic and parasympathetic nervous system. Although segmental interactions exist, they are polysynaptic operating via interneurons; the primary input to spinal preganglionic neurons is supraspinal originating from brainstem structures (not shown).

influencing the thoracolumbar sympathetic outflow was labeled. For instance, following injections in either the SCG, stellate or celiac ganglia, or the adrenal gland, the following five brain areas are labeled: **ventromedial and rostral ventrolateral medulla, caudal raphe nuclei, A5 noradrenergic cell group,** and the **paraventricular nucleus** of the hypothalamus (5,6). Apparently, these central loci must share regulatory functions which are coordinated through similar pathways of thoracolumbar outflow. These same studies indicate that other brain areas are only labeled from specific ganglia; thus, site-specific central control exists as well. Of additional interest is that numerous small **interneurons** in Rexed laminae VII and X of the spinal cord were labeled, providing structural support for the observation that spinal intersegmental and intrasegmental autonomic interactions (including autonomic reflexes) exist.

It is apparent that the structural organization of the sympathetic nervous system permits the integration and dissemination of responses depending on the need. Multiple supraspinal descending pathways provide a dense innervation of all four major autonomic cell groups in the spinal cord, but clearly specific topographic responses exist as well. In turn, each preganglionic neuron innervates anywhere from 4 to 20 postganglionic sites (estimates), and each spinal outflow level may reach multiple peripheral ganglia which in turn supply multiple targets, permitting additional dispersion of sympathetic responses when indicated. At each thoracic level there are an estimated **5000 preganglionic neurons** (these counts have generally been limited to the cells located in the ILP). Since preganglionic output to prevertebral ganglia originates from more medially placed cell bodies, it is conceivable that a greater number of neurons at certain segmental levels contribute to the output. Thus, a given spinal segment has a powerful base to influence greater than **100,000 postganglionic neurons.** Although original thinking suggested that responses were "all or none and widespread," anatomical studies have continued to reveal subtleties of structural arrangements that indicate that the system not only is poised for generalized activation of the peripheral sympathetic nervous system, but also is able to exert control of relatively specific sites and functions.

The **postganglionic fibers** in the SNS travel quite lengthy paths to arrive at target organs. For instance, fibers from the SCG traverse the extracranial and intracranial vasculature to reach such targets as the lacrimal glands, parotid glands, pineal gland, and pupils. Fibers from the stellate ganglia course through the branchial plexus to reach vascular and cutaneous targets in the upper limb and hand. Within the abdomen axons originating from the paravertebral ganglia supply the viscera as well as the mesenteric vasculature. Lumbar and sacral paravertebral ganglia course distally along peripheral nerves and blood vessels to reach the distal vasculature and cutaneous structures in the feet. In humans, the innervation to the leg requires a sympathetic axon to be **50 cm long,** and with an estimated overall diameter of 1.2 m, the axonal volume is approximately **565,000 μm^3.** This axonal cytoskeleton and its metabolic requirements are supported by a perikaryon of about 30 μm with a somal volume of 14,000 μm^3. With this structural architecture to maintain, it may not be too surprising that these neurons are **vulnerable to various metabolic and structural insults.** Although most preganglionic fibers have a relatively short course to their ganglion targets, the upper thoracic preganglionic fibers travel relatively long distances to reach the stellate and SCG, and preganglionic fibers to the adrenal medulla and prevertebral ganglia course through the paravertebral chain reaching these visceral targets as the splanchnic nerves. Along the course fiber systems may be interrupted, resulting in local autonomic dysfunction, such as **Horner's syndrome,** which results from lesion of either preganglionic fibers to the SCG or the postganglionic axons which leave the SCG to innervate the upper lid, pupil, facial vasculature, and sudomotor structures of the face (see Fig. 1).

The **autonomic neuroeffector junction** is generally not a well defined synaptic structure with pre- and postjunctional specializations that are observed in the central nervous system or skeletal muscle motor end plates. The unmyelinated highly branched postganglionic fibers become beaded with **varicosities** as they approach their targets. The varicosities are not static; they move along as structures with a diameter of 0.5 to 2 μm, and a length of approximately 1.0 μm. The number of varicosities varies from 10,000 to over 2 million per mm^3 depending on the target being innervated. The varicosities are packed with mitochondria and vesicles containing various transmitters, and are at varying distances from their target organs. For instance, for smooth muscle targets, this distance varies from 20 nm in the vas deferens to 1–2 μm in large arteries. In a sense the release of transmitter is accomplished in *en passage* as the impulse travels along an autonomic axon. The lack of a restrictive synaptic arrangement permits the released NT to diffuse various distances along a target organ and activate multiple receptors, again expanding the overall effect of sympathetic activation. Between **100** and **1000 vesicles** exist in each varicosity in noradrenergic fibers. Traditional teaching suggests that vesicle characteristics indicate the transmitter system: **small granular vesicles** are noradrenergic, **small agranular vesicles** are cholinergic, **large granular vesicles** are peptidergic. However, exceptions to these correlations exist.

The principal neuronal phenotype in peripheral sympathetic ganglia is the noradrenergic neuron, which is generally multipolar in character with synapses mainly located on dendrites, although axosomatic synaptic junctions do exist. Depending on which ganglia are examined, studies indicate that from 80 to 95% of ganglion cells will stain positively for **tyrosine hydroxylase,** the rate-limiting enzyme in catecholamine biosynthesis, or have positive catecholamine fluorescence. The remaining cells have a mixture of transmitters, or are postganglionic cholinergic cells (the sudomotor component of sympathetic function). Within sympathetic ganglia there is a small group of neurons which fluoresce intensely and are termed SIF (small intensely fluorescent) cells. The transmitters identified in SIF cells include dopamine, epinephrine, and serotonin. As will be described later, the original concept that preganglionic neurons in the SNS are cholinergic and postganglionic neurons are noradrenergic has given way to new information that a whole array of transmitter molecules (catecholaminergic, monoaminergic, peptidergic, "noncholinergic, nonadrenergic," and gaseous) appear to be involved in neurotransmission either as agents themselves or as neuromodulators (*vide infra*).

Sympathoadrenal Axis and the Adrenal Gland

A most apparent and critical link between the autonomic and endocrine systems is manifested by interactions between the adrenal cortex and adrenal medulla. The adrenal cortex, which is largely regulated by the hypothalamic–pituitary–adrenocortical axis, and the adrenal medulla, which is primarily under neural control, have shared responsibilities in responding to stress and metabolic aberrations. The coordinated response of elevated plasma cortisol and catecholamines during stress indicates that central limbic and hypothalamic centers exert combined influences to ensure the needed neurohumoral adaptations. The interdependence of these two components of the adrenal gland exist from development: migrating **sympathoblasts** require the presence of the cortical tissue to change their developmental fate from neurons to that of **chromaffin cells.** These cells, named because they exhibit brown color when treated with "chrome salts," do not develop neural processes but instead serve an endocrine function by releasing their neurohumors (epinephrine and norepinephrine) into the blood stream. During adulthoood the presence of the cortex is critical for maintaining the levels of epinephrine since the induction of the enzyme **phenylethanolamine-*n*-methyltransferase** is dependent on local levels of cortisol. Although traditional teaching emphasizes the preganglionic cholinergic splanchnic innervation, there is also evidence that postganglionic sympathetic fibers, vagal afferents, and other sensory afferents supply the adrenal gland.

Retrograde tracing studies indicate that dye placed within the adrenal medulla will distribute itself in a somewhat bell-shaped curve within spinal **preganglionic sympathetic neurons** from approximately T_2 to L_1 with the predominant innervation originating T_7–T_{10}. Neuronal cell bodies are primarily within the nucleus intermediolateralis pars principalis (ILP) with the pars funicularis and pars intercalatus providing a relatively small portion of the innervation. The exiting nerve roots pass through the sympathetic chain, join to form the **greater splanchnic nerve**, and distribute themselves beneath the capsule and within the medulla. A small number of nerve cells are labeled in ganglia within the sympathetic chain, suggesting that postganglionic sympathetic fibers innervate the gland. Whether these terminals are labeled as they pass along blood vessels within the gland or whether they innervate medullary or cortical cells is not fully resolved. Also, at least in the guinea pig, tracing studies indicate that the parasympathetic system may contribute a small efferent innervation to the gland since neurons in the **dorsal motor nucleus of the vagus** are labeled after injections in the medulla. Cell bodies within the **dorsal root ganglia** and **vagal sensory ganglia (nodose)** are also labeled after tracer studies of the adrenal medulla, indicating an afferent innervation as well. Lastly, although not a prominent innervation pattern, there appears to be an **intrinsic innervation** that arises from ganglion cells sparsely populating the subcapsular, cortical, and medullary regions of the gland. The innervation pattern of the adrenal medulla is thus more complex than the traditionally listed thoracolumbar preganglionic cholinergic outflow, although the major adaptive responses depend on the preganglionic cholinergic innervation since surgical section of these nerves, or pharmacological blockade with cholinergic antagonists, precludes the induction of tyrosine hydroxylase and appropriate release of catecholamines following various stress paradigms.

Morphological studies of the adrenal medulla have revealed the presence of two basic types of granules in chromaffin cells. A diffuse spherical granule contains the predominant monoamine secreted by medullary cells, **epinephrine**, whereas eccentrically located dense core granules contain **norepinephrine**. As indicated above for ganglion neurons, chromaffin cells of the adrenal medulla also co-contain other molecules. For instance, the **opioid** molecules are well represented: **enkephalin** is co-contained in vesicles with the **monoamines**. The signaling cascade responsible for enhancing the synthesis and release of these neurohormonal agents is complicated and includes preganglionic innervation, steroid hormones (**glucocorticoids**), and **growth factors** (NGF).

Parasympathetic Nervous System

The craniosacral outflow is the source of central neuronal pathways providing the efferent innervation of peripheral ganglia of the parasympathetic nervous system (PNS) (see Fig. 1). The cranial nerves involved include **cranial nerves III, VII, IX, and X,** and the sacral outflow is largely restricted to **sacral cord levels 2,3, and 4.** As indicated for the SNS, the preganglionic innervation is largely cholinergic with these terminals releasing **acetylcholine** (ACh) at the ganglion synapses. In contrast to the SNS, the major transmitter postsynaptically is also ACh. These cholinergic neurons also co-contain other transmitter substances: preganglionic neurons contain **enkephalins,** and postsynaptic cholinergic neurons frequently contain **vasoactive intestinal peptide** and **NPY**. The parasympathetic fibers in cranial nerve III originate in the **Edinger–Westphal nuclei** of the midbrain and travel in the periphery of the nerve (where they are subject to dysfunction secondary to nerve compression), exiting along with the nerve to the inferior oblique to supply the **ciliary ganglion.** Second-order postganglionic fibers exit in the ciliary nerves and supply the pupiloconstrictor fibers of the iris and the ciliary muscle where their combined action permits the near response, including accommodation. The salivatory nuclei, located near the pontomedullary junction, provide the preganglionic parasympathetic innervation for cranial nerves VII and IX. The superior salivatory nucleus sends preganglionic fibers, which leave the **facial nerve** at the level of the geniculate ganglion (non-parasympathetic sensory ganglion) to form the greater superficial petrosal nerve to the pterygopalatine (sphenopalatine) ganglia, which provides postganglionic secretomotor and vasodilator fibers to the lacrimal glands via the maxillary nerve. Other preganglionic fibers in the facial nerve continue and subsequently leave via the chorda tympani to join the lingual nerve, eventually synapsing in the submandibular ganglion. Postsynaptic cholinergic fibers supply the sublingual and submandibular glands. Postganglionic fibers from the pterygopalatine and submandibular ganglia also supply glands and vasculature in the mucosa of the sinuses, palate, and nasopharynx. The inferior salivatory nucleus sends preganglionic fibers via the **glossopharyngeal nerve** (cranial nerve IX) to the otic ganglion which in turn relays postganglionic fibers to the parotid gland via the auriculotemporal nerve. The preganglionic fibers in cranial nerve IX branch from the nerve at the jugular foramen, and contribute to the tympanic plexus and form the lesser superficial petrosal nerve. This nerve exits the intracranial compartment via the foramen ovale along with the third division of the trigeminal nerve to reach the otic ganglion.

The most caudal cranial nerve participating in the preganglionic parasympathetic system is the **vagus nerve** (cranial nerve X). The **dorsal motor nucleus of the vagus** is located in the medulla and sends preganglionic fibers to innervate essentially all organ systems within the chest and abdomen, including the gastrointestinal tract as far as the left colonic flexure (splenic flexure). Also, the **nucleus ambiguus** supplies preganglionic fibers to the vagus; these fibers are believed to be involved mostly with regulating visceral smooth muscle whereas the dorsal motor vagus neurons may be secretomotor in nature. The glossopharyngeal and vagus nerves also contain a substantial number of afferent fibers (in the vagus afferent exceed the efferent fiber system by a great amount) so that a sensory component related to autonomic control exists within cranial nerves IX and X. These afferents provide a critical component of the **baroreceptor reflex** arc relaying information regarding the systemic blood pressure to central cardiovascular areas in the **nucleus tractus solitarii** and other medullary centers involved in blood pressure and heart rate control.

The **parasympathetic cell bodies** in the spinal cord are located in the **intermediolateral cell column** of second, third, and fourth sacral segments (see Fig. 2). These neurons send preganglionic nerve fibers via the pelvic nerve to ganglia located close to or within the pelvic viscera. Postganglionic fibers are relatively short, in contradistinction to their length in the SNS, and supply cholinergic terminals to structures involved in excretory (bladder and bowel) and reproductive (fallopian tubes and uterus, prostate, seminal vesicles, vas deferens, and erectile tissue) functions. Of interest, the pelvic ganglia involved in some of these functions appear to be mixed ganglia (especially in rodents) where sympathetic and parasympathetic neurons are components of the same pelvic ganglion. They appear to receive their traditional preganglionic input, but may have local interconnections which are not fully revealed by current studies. As indicated below, there is clear evidence that the **cholinergic postganglionic neurons** in the pelvic ganglion in the rodent co-contain **vasoactive intestinal peptide** and **nitric oxide** as two other transmitter molecules. These neurons are believed to be integrally involved in sexual functions in the male, permitting the development and maintenance of potency. The exact regulatory factors controlling the synthesis and release of these transmitter molecules, and the specific receptor systems involved, remain to be fully explored.

The Concept of Plurichemical Transmission and Chemical Coding

The notion of the presence of multiple transmitters and a chemical coding system of autonomic neurons is now quite firmly established. Originally it was posited that principal neurons were only **noradrenergic** (contained norepinephrine), but over the last decade it has become clear that within a single neuron multiple transmitter systems may exist, and that within a given ganglion the variety and pattern of neurotransmitters may be quite extensive (see Table 1).

Table 1. **Neurotransmitter Phenotypes in Autonomic Neurons**

Autonomic neurons	Transmitter characteristics (not all inclusive)[a]
Sympathetic neurons	
Paravertebral ganglia	NE, CCK, somatostatin
Prevertebral ganglia	SP, Enk, Ach
Terminal ganglia (previsceral ganglia)	VIP, 5-HT, NPY, DYN1-8, DYN-1-17
Parasympathetic neurons	Ach, VIP, SP, CAs–SIF, NPY, NO
Major parasympathetic ganglia	
Ciliary	
Sphenopalatine	
Otic	
Submandibular/sublingual	
Pelvic ganglia	
Terminal parasympathetic ganglia (previsceral ganglia)	
Enteric neurons Myenteric plexus	
(Auerbach's)	GABA, Ach, VIP, 5-HT, Sp, Enk, SRIF,
Submucosal plexus (Meisner's)	motilin-like peptide, bombesin-like
Enteric ganglia	peptide
Chromaffin cells of adrenal medulla	E, NE, Enk, NPY, APUD
Paraganglia-chromaffin	5-HT, DA, E
Small intensely fluorescent (SIF) cells, ganglia	5-HT, DA, E

[a] NE, norepinephrine; CCK, cholecystokinin; SP, substance P; Enk, enkephalin; Ach, acetylcholine; VIP, vasoactive intestinal polypeptide; 5-HT, 5-hydroxyltryptamine; CAs–SIF, catecholamines–small intensity fluorescent; GABA, gamma aminobutyric acid; SRIF, somatostatin; NPY, neuropeptide Y; NO, nitric oxide; APUD, amine precursor uptake and decarboxylation; DA, dopamine; E, epinephrine; DYN, dynorphin A (DYN 1-8, or DYN 1-17) (neurons with dynorphin A also contain dynorphin B and α-neo-endorphin).

Also, the composition of neurotransmitters (NT) may change depending on the location of the ganglia: paravertebral ganglia tend to have fewer transmitters whereas prevertebral and terminal ganglia may have various NT, although as noted for the guinea pig SGC (Fig. 3), some paravertebral ganglia have a broad array of transmitters. The exact colocation and functions of these multiple transmitters are not fully understood, but some general principles exist. **Neuropeptide Y** is probably the most prominent peptide in sympathetic ganglia and is highly colocalized with **norepinephrine** (NE). The sudomotor component of ganglia is dependent upon a population of cells which are cholinergic in character [contain acetylcholine (ACh) as the NT], and the most frequent peptide colocalized with ACh is **vasoactive intestinal peptide** (VIP). The distribution of these cholinergic cells varies: in paravertebral ganglia they may represent 10–15% of the neuronal population whereas they represent <1% of the neurons in prevertebral ganglia. NE, NPY, ACh, and VIP are believed to be released together, but some degree of activity–chemical coding exists. That is, at lower levels of activation NE is preferentially released, whereas higher levels of stimulation result in NPY being released. Both agents have vasoconstrictor properties and are integral in cardiovascular control, especially in the maintenance of blood pressure. Of course, the eventual action and effect of a transmitter rests with the receptor system that is activated (vide infra).

Chemical coding also reveals that ganglion neurons with specific transmitter molecules innervate specific targets or receive specific afferent inputs. Apparently, anterograde and retrograde **transsynaptic information** appears to determine the **transmitter phenotype** of the neuron. Thus, studies of neuronal circuitry indicate that pathway–specific combinations determine the presence and combinations of specific peptides within autonomic neurons. This is particularly so in the prevertebral ganglia, but studies in the guinea pig SCG demonstrate that the transmitter molecules will vary depending on the target organ supplied (see Fig. 3). Although all principal cells portrayed are noradrenergic in character (as indicated by NA), the neuropeptides co-contained in neurons vary depending on whether the targets are secretory (salivary and lacrimal glands), vascular (small vs large arteries, arterioles vs arterio-venous anastomoses), pupil, or skin. Detailed pictures of these chemically coded circuits are beginning to emerge from studies of paravertebral (SCG), prevertebral (superior mesenteric), and previsceral (pelvic) ganglia. This phenomenon pertains to both the SNS and PNS.

Preganglionic sympathetic neurons in the spinal cord have traditionally been viewed as cholinergic neurons. More recently, it has been recognized that neuronal cell bodies in the cat ILP may contain a variety of transmitters including **enkephalin, neurotensin, somatostatin,** and **substance P.** In rodents, VIP- and calcitonin gene-related peptide (CGRP)-containing neurons have also been localized to the ILP by immunocytochemistry. Also, preganglionic fibers in the sacral parasympathetic outflow of co-contain enkephalin. It is apparent that preganglionic and postganglionic neurotransmission are plurichemical.

Functional Neuroanatomy and Biochemical Pharmacology

The peripheral ANS is well structured to provide the physiological responses critical for homeostasis and acute adaptations to stressful, perhaps life-threaten-

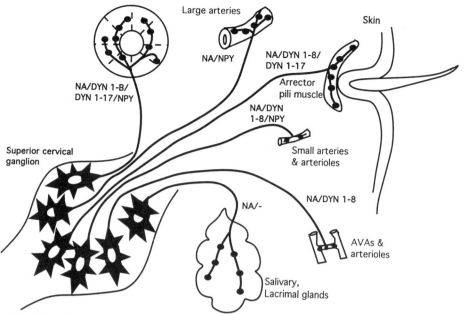

Figure 3. Chemical coding and target organization. Chemical coding of sympathetic neurons projecting from the superior cervical ganglion to various targets in the head of guinea pigs. Each population of neurons has a specific combination of neuropeptides. Note that all neurons containing a form of dynorphin A also contain dynorphin B and α-neoendorphin. No neuropeptides have been found in neurons projecting to secretory tissue in the salivary or lacrimal glands. Neurons with similar peptide combinations also occur in other paravertebral ganglia of guinea pigs, except that the salivary secretomotor neurons are absent. Conversely, the paravertebral ganglia have many nonnoradrenergic vasodilatory neurons containing prodynorphin derived peptides, arterio venous anastomoses; NA, noradrenaline; NPY, neuropeptide Y. (See Elfvin, Lindh and Hokfelt, 1993; Gibbins, 1995). Adapted with permission from Elfvin L-G, Lindh B, Hokfelt TL. Ann Rev Neurosci 1993;16:471–507.

ing, circumstances. As outlined in Fig. 1 and indicated in Table 2, multiple organ systems respond to neurotransmitter release from autonomic endings, and circulating catecholamine release from the adrenal medulla. Traditional teaching indicates that the effects of activation of the SNS and PNS are generally antagonistic; this is still largely the case. However, viewed more specifically, the relationships between these two major components of the ANS is far from simple. For instance, not all organs receive an equal number of both sets of fibers, and in some situations, both SNS and PNS responses are in the same direction. It is important to remember that receptor systems, including the signal transduction components, on the target organs are the critical molecular proteins that determine the actual effects of ligand–receptor interactions on the cell membrane. Thus, when the SNS is stimulated with its capability to produce a widespread response, a host of receptor systems are activated to effect the necessary and desired change. An example of these responses include the following aspects of SNS activation: dilatation of the pupil, slight increase in glandular secretions, bronchodilatation, increased heart rate and force of contraction, decreased gastrointestinal tract motility, decreased function of the

Table 2.   Autonomic Nervous System Functions

Organ	SNS	PNS
Eye		
Pupil	Dilatation	Constriction
Ciliary muscle	Relax (far vision)	Constrict (near vision)
Lacrimal gland	Slight secretion	Secretion
Parotid gland	Slight secretion	Secretion
Submandibular gland	Slight secretion	Secretion
Heart	Increased rate	Slowed rate
	Positive inotropism	Negative inotropism
Lungs	Bronchodilation	Bronchodilation
Gastrointestinal tract	Decreased motility	Increased motility
Kidney	Decreased output	None
Bladder	Relax detrusor, contract sphincter	Contract detrusor, relax sphincter
Penis	Ejaculation	Erection
Sweat glands	Secretion	Palmar sweating
Piloerector muscles	Contraction	None
Blood vessels		
Arterioles	Constriction	None
Muscle		
Arterioles	Constriction or dilatation	None
Metabolism	Glycogenolysis	None

reproductive organs, and mobilization of energy substrates to meet demands. The **receptor systems** mediating these responses include α_1, α_2, β_1, β_2, and β_3. α-Receptor activation occurs following interaction with NE: α_1 mediates smooth muscle contraction in the vasculature and iris, and has a limited positive inotropic effect on the heart. Smooth muscle of the gut is relaxed and salivary gland secretion is activated. α_2 receptors serve as autoreceptors on sympathetic nerve terminals and inhibit the release of NE as part of a negative feedback loop. These receptors also mediate metabolic and endocrine changes such as inhibition of lipolysis in adipose tissue and reduction of insulin release from the pancreas. β_1 receptors provide positive inotropic and chronotropic effects on the heart and stimulate renin release from the kidney. β_2 receptors relax smooth muscle of the bronchi and pelvic organs as well as the vascular structures of the gut and skeletal muscle. β_2 receptors located in liver and skeletal muscle elicit activation of glycogenolysis and gluconeogenesis. This receptor system is particularly activated by epinephrine rather than norepinephrine.

The **parasympathetic nervous system** is poised for more focal responses, but some effects may be quite broad, particularly with the wide-ranging innervation of the vagus nerve. Activation of parasympathetic pathways leads to pupillary constriction, substantial secretion from lacrimal and salivary glands, slowed cardiac rate and negative inotropism, bronchoconstriction, enhanced gastrointestinal motility, and contraction of the detrusor muscle of the bladder. In contrast to the SNS, the PNS does not appear to influence metabolic or endocrine processes in any major way. However, recent evidence indicates that preganglionic vagal fibers originating in the dorsal motor nucleus innervate postganglionic parasympathetic ganglia in the pancreas, and appear to influence exocrine and endocrine function. Thus, as new data emerge, the integrated roles of the SNS and PNS will continue to expand.

An understanding of the **receptor systems** mediating the response of the PNS is not fully developed. Preganglionic cholinergic receptors, which exist in the SNS as well as PNS, are **nicotinic** in character whereas postganglionic cholinergic receptors are **muscarinic**. Recently, molecular cloning studies have indicated multiple subtypes of both sets of receptors. The subtypes of muscarinic receptors, which are termed M_1, M_2, M_3, M_4, and M_5, are more fully understood (at least for the first three subtypes): M_1 receptors are excitatory to neurons in ganglia and lead to noradrenaline release in sympathetic neurons; M_2 receptors mediate the bradycardia and decreased contractility of the heart following vagal activation; M_3 stimulation leads to contraction of smooth muscle and enhanced secretion from glandular tissues. The recent discovery that multiple subtypes of nicotinic receptors also exist will lead to new understanding of how these cholinergic receptor systems function with both the presynaptic and postsynaptic components of the peripheral ANS.

The recent discoveries that a number of neurotrophic factors (**neurotrophins**) and their receptors are part and parcel of the development and integrity of the SNS and PNS expand the horizons regarding how anatomical pathways are established and maintained, and how they adapt to intrinsic and extrinsic demands. Because of its relatively simple anatomical architecture, the peripheral ANS continues to serve as a model system to understand neuronal development, structural and functional linkages among neurons and their targets, and the integrative role(s) these "little brains" (6,000–30,000 neurons) serve. It becomes clear that as data continue to emerge regarding the structure–function relationships and molecular pharmacology of the peripheral ANS, new approaches to understanding its myriad functions and treatment of maladies related to disease and dysfunction will undoubtedly emerge. The following chapters will expand on these issues.

References

1. Elfvin L-G, Lindh B, Hokfelt TL. The chemical neuroanatomy of sympathetic ganglia. Ann Rev Neurosci 1993;16:471–507.
2. Dinner DS, ed. The autonomic nervous system (review articles). J Clin Neurophysiol 1993;10:1–82.
3. Gibbins I. Chemical neuroanatomy of sympathetic ganglia. In: McLachlan EM, ed. Autonomic ganglia. Luxembourg: Harwood Academic Publishers, 1995:73–121.
4. Lowey AD. Anatomy of the autonomic nervous system: an overview. In: Loewy AD, Spyer KM, eds. Central regulation of autonomic functions. New York: Oxford University Press, 1990:3–16.
5. Romagnano MA, Hamill RW. Spinal sympathetic pathway: an enkephalin ladder. Science 1984;225:737–9.
6. Strack AM, Sawyer WG, Hughes JH, et al. A general pattern of CNS innervation of the sympathetic outflow demonstrated by transneuronal pseudorabies viral infections. Brain Res 1989;491:156–62.
7. Strack AM, Sawyer WG, Platt KB, et al. CNS cell groups regulating the sympathetic outflow to adrenal gland as revealed by transneuronal cell body labelling with pseudorabies virus. Brain Res 1989;491:274–96.

3

Skeletal Muscle Afferents and Cardiovascular Control

Jere H. Mitchell
Harry S. Moss Heart Center
University of Texas Southwestern Medical Center
Dallas, Texas

During **exercise** important changes occur in the heart, resistance vessels, and capacitance vessels to provide appropriate blood flow to the contracting skeletal muscle. Changes in activity of the autonomic nervous system underlie these cardiovascular responses. With exercise there is an overall increase in the activity of the sympathetic nervous system and a decrease in the activity of the parasympathetic nervous system. Skeletal muscle contraction causes activation of afferent fibers that play a role in regulating the autonomic nervous system, and this neural mechanism has been termed the **exercise pressor reflex.**

Skeletal muscle afferent fibers have been classified by the diameter or the conduction velocity of the fibers. There are four types of muscle afferent fibers. The larger myelinated fibers with faster conduction velocities (Group I and II) are concerned with regulation of skeletal muscle function. When these fibers are electrically or chemically activated there is little or no change in heart rate and blood pressure. However, the finely myelinated fibers (Group III) and the unmyelinated fibers (Group IV) do cause cardiovascular responses when activated, and they are the muscle afferents involved in the exercise pressor reflex.

The anatomy of the Group III and Group IV receptor endings has been studied with great detail by serial electron microscopic sections. The receptor endings of these fibers have been termed "free" or "naked" nerve terminals. However, the fine afferent fibers terminate in very specialized structures without a perineural sheath surrounding the specific receptive area. A better terminology for these receptive areas is **unencapsulated nerve endings.** In general, receptive endings of the Group III muscle afferents are closely associated with collagen structures in the skeletal muscle, and those of Group IV afferents are closely associated with blood and lymphatic vessels.

The discharge characteristics of the Group III and Group IV muscle afferents have also been carefully studied. In general, the receptor endings of these fibers have been termed **ergoreceptors** and **nociceptors. Ergoreceptors** are defined as those activated by muscle contraction; **nociceptors** are those activated by noxious stimuli and are responsible for the sensation of muscle pain (e.g., claudication).

A large majority of the Group III fibers are activated by deformation charges that occur in a contracting skeletal muscle and are termed **mechanoreceptors.** These afferent fibers discharge immediately when the muscle contracts or is stretched. These receptors are rapidly adaptive and the discharge frequency quickly declines. Most of the Group IV fibers appear to be activated by chemical changes that occur in the contracting muscle and are called **metaboreceptors.** These afferents do not fire immediately when the muscle contracts and are not stimulated by muscle stretch. However, as a muscle contraction continues the discharge of these fibers increases. This suggests that they are being activated by some increasing chemical change that is occurring in the contracting muscle.

The question of what stimulus activates the unencapsulated nerve endings of the Group IV is being actively investigated. These receptors appear to monitor the effectiveness of blood flow to meet the increased metabolic needs in a contracting skeletal muscle. Several metabolic consequences of a discrepancy between muscle blood flow and metabolic needs have been shown to increase the activity of Group IV muscle afferents. Among these are an increase in H^+, K^+, **bradykinin, prostaglandins,** and **adenosine.** However, is is unlikely that any one of these is "the factor"; a more likely scenario is that many chemical factors are involved.

The Group III and IV afferents from skeletal muscle make their first synapse in the **dorsal horn** of the spinal cord. Two peptides, **substance P** and **somatostatin,** may be involved in transmission at this first synapse. In addition, **glutamate** may play an important role in the transmission of signals from group III and IV muscle afferents in the spinal cord.

The important areas for the full expression of the exercise pressor reflex are located in the **ventrolateral medulla,** which includes the **lateral reticular nucleus.** Electrical and chemical stimulation of this region of the medulla causes cardiovascular responses similar to those seen during exercise. Also, bilateral electrolytic lesioning of this area markedly attenuates the **exercise pressor reflex,** and this same area has been shown by radioactive glucose studies to become more metabolically active during the expression of this reflex. In addition, recordings from cell bodies in the ventrolateral medulla show the same discharge characteristics as those seen from either a Group III or a Group IV muscle afferent during induced static contraction; this activity is also correlated with efferent sympathetic discharge. Thus it seems clear that areas in the ventrolateral medulla are important in the exercise pressor reflex, which plays a role in controlling the cardiovascular system during exercise.

During muscle contraction there may be activation of both **mechanoreceptors** and **metaboreceptors.** This activation causes an increase in blood pressure, heart rate, cardiac output, and left ventricular contractility. In addition, there tends to be redistribution of cardiac output to the contracting skeletal muscle. The hemodynamic responses and autonomic neural activity changes that occur during muscle contraction cannot be separated into those caused by activation of mechanoreceptors and those caused by metaboreceptors. However, muscle stretch can be used to isolate the effects of muscle mechanoreceptors and postexercise circulatory arrest can be used to isolate the effects of muscle metaboreceptors. In addition, fatiguing contractions, in which muscle tension (and thereby, activation of mechanoreceptors) decreases, can be used to isolate the effects of muscle metaboreceptors.

In general, stimulation of the metaboreceptors in skeletal muscle causes an activation of the sympathetic nervous system and little or no effect on the parasympathetic nervous system. The heart rate increase that occurs during exercise returns to resting values during postexercise ischemia when muscle metaboreceptors are still activated. However, it has been shown that activation of muscle mechanoreceptors causes both an increase in sympathetic efferent activity and a decrease in parasympathetic efferent activity to the heart.

In man, sympathetic efferent nerve activity has been recorded to skeletal muscle and to skin; studies have shown that muscle **metaboreceptor activity** causes a marked increase in sympathetic activity to skeletal muscle but has little to no effect on sympathetic activity to skin. Muscle sympathetic nerve activity starts to increase about 1 min after the start of a static contraction and remains elevated during postexercise ischemia. In contrast, muscle mechanoreceptor activity causes an increase in sympathetic efferent nerve activity to skin but has little or no effect on muscle sympathetic activity. Skin sympathetic activity increases immediately with the onset of muscle contraction and returns to resting levels during postexercise ischemia. Sympathetic efferent nerve activity to other areas during exercise has not been studied in man.

In animals, sympathetic efferent nerve activity has been measured to the kidney, heart, and adrenal gland during muscle contraction. Studies demonstrate that both mechanoreceptor activity and metaboreceptor activity increase sympathetic efferent activity to the **kidney.** Also, activation of only the muscle mechanoreceptors by stretch increases sympathetic nerve activity. However, a reduction in renal blood flow is produced only by a muscle contraction that activates both mechanoreceptors and metaboreceptors. Muscle mechanoreceptors appear to have a greater effect on **cardiac sympathetic nerve activity** than do the metaboreceptors. Finally, sympathetic efferent nerve activity to the **adrenal glands,** which normally causes the release of epinephrine, is primarily controlled by the muscle **mechanoreceptors** with little effect by metaboreceptors.

References

1. Mitchell JH, Schmidt RF. Cardiovascular reflex control by afferent fibers from skeletal muscle receptors. In: Handbook of physiology. The cardiovascular system Vol. III. Bethesda, MD: American Physiological Society, 1983: 623–58.
2. Mitchell JH, Kaufman MP, Iwamoto GA. The exercise reflex: its cardiovascular effects, afferent mechanisms, and central pathways. Ann Rev Physiol 1983;45:229–42.
3. Mitchell JK, Joseph B. Wolffe Memorial Lecture. Neural control of the circulation during exercise. Med Sci Sports Exer 1990;22:141–54.
4. Kaufman MP, Forster HV. Reflexes controlling circulatory, ventilatory and airway responses to exercise. In: Rowell L, Shepherd J, eds. Handbook on exercise: integration of motor, circulatory, respiratory, and metabolic control during exercise. American Physiology Society 187–197.
5. Hansen J, Victor RG, Mitchell JH. Control of regional sympathetic nerve activity during exercise: integration of studies in humans and animals. In: Jordon D, ed. Central control of the autonomic nervous system. London: Harwood Academic Publishers, in press.

PART II

Physiology

4

Sexual Function

John D. Stewart
Department of Neurology and Neurosurgery
McGill University
Montreal Neurological Institute and Hospital
Montreal, Quebec, Canada

The physiological events of the sexual act are mediated by the combined and integrated activities of the **somatic** and **autonomic** nervous systems. In spite of the obvious anatomic differences between males and females, many of the physiological sexual responses are similar: **erectile tissue engorgement** and detumescence, **glandular secretion,** and **contraction of smooth and striated muscles.**

The erectile tissue of the penis and clitoris consists of the **corpora cavernosa.** These comprise many blood filled spaces called lacunae. The walls of the lacunae are the trabeculae which consist of, like blood vessels, smooth muscle and fibro-elastic tissue. Within each cavernosum lies a **cavernosal artery** which gives off numerous **helicine arteries** that open directly into the lacunar spaces. Small veins lie among the lacunae and drain into the deep dorsal vein of the penis (or clitoris).

In the central nervous system, hypothalamic and limbic areas and pathways are important in **sexual arousal.** The **medial preoptic-anterior hypothalamic area** is of particular importance. Descending pathways travel in the **medial forebrain bundle** in the tegmentum of the midbrain, in the ventrolateral pons and medulla, and then in the lateral column of the spinal cord. They terminate in the lower thoracic, lumbar, and sacral areas of the spinal cord.

Three sets of peripheral nerves are involved: (a) thoracolumbar **sympathetic** nerves, (b) sacral **parasympathetic** nerves, and (c) pudendal **somatic** nerves. The sympathetic and parasympathetic nerves join to form the **pelvic plexus.** From this arise adrenergic, cholinergic and nonadrenergic, noncholinergic nerves. These innervate erectile tissue, nonerectile smooth muscle, glandular tissue, and blood vessels. The pudendal somatic nerves supply the bulbocavernosus and ischiocavernosus muscles, and are the sensory nerves of the genitalia.

The following sequence of events during penile erection and clitoral engorgement is now known to occur. Relaxation of the smooth muscle of the cavernosal and helicine arteries and of the cavernosal trabeculae occurs from both a reduction of tonic smooth muscle contraction and active relaxation. **Noradrenergic nerves** release norepinephrine that acts on α_1 receptors to cause arterial and trabecular smooth muscle contraction, thereby maintaining flaccidity; a reduction in this activity contributes to erection. Other substances such as **adenosine triphosphate** (ATP) and neuropeptides are cotransmitters in these neurons. **Cholinergic nerves** do not directly dilate or constrict smooth muscle but modulate other neuroeffector systems and/ or the vascular endothelium. Acetylcholine (ACh) release may act prejunctionally to inhibit the (vasoconstrictor) activity of noradrenergic nerves, and to excite the (vasodilator) nonadrenergic, noncholinergic nerves. ACh also reacts with muscarinic receptors on endothelial cells to release **nitric oxide** (NO) which relaxes vascular and trabecular smooth muscle cells. NO release may also be stimulated by other mechanisms, including local physical effects on the endothelium such as increased blood flow. The vascular endothelium likely produces **vasoconstrictor** peptides, for example the very potent constrictor **endothelin;** this may play a role in the maintenance of penile flaccidity. The **nonadrenergic, noncholinergic nerves** probably contain principally vasoactive intestinal polypeptide (VIP), a powerful relaxer of vascular and trabecular smooth muscle.

The result of these physiological events is that there is increased arterial blood flow into expanding lacunae. This is accompanied by reduced venous drainage. Venous occlusion occurs passively as the engorged corpora cavernosa press against the surrounding tunica albuginea, occluding the subtunical veins. Detumescence occurs from a reversal of these processes.

Emission of semen occurs by smooth muscle contraction in the epididymis, vas deferens, seminal vesicles, and the prostate gland. This deposits spermatozoa and seminal fluid into the proximal urethra. Contraction of the bladder neck sphincters prevents backflow of semen into the bladder (retrograde ejaculation). These events are principally mediated by the sympathetic nerves. Ejaculation consists of the semen being rapidly transmitted down the urethra and released in spurts. This is accomplished by rhythmic contractions of the bulbocavernosus, ischiocavernosus, and periurethral striated muscles supplied by the pudendal nerve.

The physiology of many of the events in the female sexual response cycle is similar to that in the male.

References

1. Creed KE, Carati CJ, Keogh EJ. The physiology of penile erection. Oxf Rev Reprod Biol 1991;13:73–95.
2. Tong Y-C, Broderick G, Hypolite J, Levin RM. Correlations of purinergic, cholinergic and adrenergic functions in rabbit corporal cavernosal tissue. Pharmacology 1992;45: 241–9.
3. Trigo-Rocha F, Hsu GL, Donatucci CF, Lue TF. The role of cyclic adenosine monophosphate, cyclic guanosine monophosphate, endothelium and nonadrenergic, noncholinergic neurotransmission in canine penile erection. J Urol 1993;149:872–7.
4. Lerner SE, Melman A, Christ GJ. A review of erectile dysfunction: new insights and more questions. J Urol 1993;149:1246–55.

5

Gastrointestinal Function

Michael Camilleri
Gastroenterology Research Unit
Mayo Clinic
Rochester, Minnesota

Proper function of the gastrointestinal tract is essential for the orderly digestion, absorption, and transport of food and residue. Digestion requires secretion
of endogenous fluids from the salivary glands, stomach, pancreas, and small
bowel to facilitate intraluminal breakdown of foods; fluids, electrolytes, and
smaller building blocks of the macronutrients are then absorbed, leaving nondigestible residue to be excreted.

The motor activity of the gut is one of the integrated functions that is essential
for the normal assimilation of food. Gut motility facilitates the transport of
nutrients, brings together digestive enzymes and their substrates, temporarily
stores content, particularly in the distal small bowel and right colon, for optimal
absorption, and finally, excretes nondigestible residue by defecation in a well-
coordinated function under voluntary control. The extrinsic **autonomic nervous
system** is critically important for almost all **secretory and motor functions** in
the digestive tract (Fig. 1).

Salivary Secretion

Presentation of food to the mouth and olfactory stimulation trigger afferent
nerves that stimulate secretory centers in the medulla. These reflexly stimulate
efferent fibers along parasympathetic and sympathetic pathways: parasympathetic fibers course along the **facial** nerve to **sublingual and submaxillary glands,**
and the **glossopharyngeal** nerve to the **parotid gland.** Synapse with postganglionic fibers occurs in or near the glands. Sympathetic fibers reach the salivary
glands through the cervical sympathetic trunk, but the brainstem centers are
unclear. Parasympathetic efferents stimulate secretion; sympathetic fibers serve
to cause contraction of myoepithelial cells in the duct.

The human salivary glands secrete 0.5–1.0 liters of saliva per day, at a
maximal rate of 4 ml/min. Saliva facilitates speech, lubricates food for swallowing, and contains the α-amylase **ptyalin** which begins the digestion of starch.
Bicarbonate in saliva neutralizes noxious acidic ingesta.

Gastric secretion is stimulated by the act of eating (**cephalic phase**) and the
arrival of food in the stomach (**gastric phase**). Arrival of the food in the intestine
also controls gastric secretion (**intestinal phase**). The secreted fluid contains
hydrochloric acid, pepsinogen, intrinsic factor, bicarbonate, and mucus. Gastric
secretion of acid and pepsinogen follows stimulation of oral and gastric vagal
afferents. **Efferent vagal pathways** synapse with submucous plexus neurons

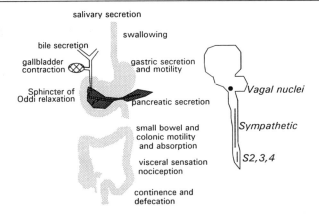

Figure 1.   Gastrointestinal physiology: functions under extrinsic autonomic control.

which innervate secretory cells via several important bioactive molecules including **gastrin, histamine,** and **somatostatin.** In the stomach, there is some digestion of carbohydrate and protein, but very little absorption except for some fat-soluble substances. The mucus–bicarbonate layer protects the stomach lining from auto digestion by acid.

Pancreaticobiliary Secretion

Pancreatic juice consists of alkaline (chiefly bicarbonate) fluid and enzymes; 200–800 ml is produced each day. The enzymes **trypsin, lipase,** and **amylase** are essential for digestion of most of the protein, fat, and carbohydrate in the meal. The pancreas consists of exocrine and endocrine portions: bicarbonate and fluid are secreted by ductular cells, chiefly under the influence of **secretin;** enzymes are produced by acinar cells in response to vagal stimulation of intrapancreatic cholinergic neurons. Recent data suggest that **cholecystokinin** (CCK) activates enzyme secretion by stimulating vagal afferents.

Bile is continuously secreted by the liver as two fractions: the bile salt-independent fraction, controlled by secretin and CCK, is similar to pancreatic juice; the bile salt-dependent fraction contains bile salts. Bile flow is controlled by storage in the gall bladder and by the sphincter of Oddi. Postprandially, the gall bladder contracts under vagal and CCK stimulation, and the basal sphincter tone within the ampulla of Vater falls to allow bile to enter the duodenum. There is evidence for interdigestive cycling of pancreaticobiliary secretion that is synchronous with the main phases of the gut's cyclical migrating motor complex (vide infra).

Intestinal Secretion and Absorption

The small bowel produces about 5 liters of fluid per day during the equilibration of osmotic loads, induced by ingested nutrients, and during intraluminal digestion. Yet most of the 7 liters entering the digestive tract each day is reabsorbed (about 80% in small bowel, 20% in colon) during the organized flow of chyme through the small bowel and colon, thereby ensuring a stool weight below 200 g/day in health. Water and electrolyte fluid fluxes are generally independent of extrinsic neural control; on the other hand, the submucosal plexus is increasingly recognized as a key factor influencing mucosal blood flow and enterocyte function.

Absorption of macro- and micronutrients is generally determined by concentration gradients or active carrier-mediated, energy-requiring transport processes. These are indirectly influenced by the autonomic nervous system through its effects on the secretion of salivary, gastric, and pancreaticobiliary juices and by the motor processes of mixing and delivery of substrate to sites of preferential absorption, e.g., vitamin B_{12} to the ileum.

Control of Gut Motility

The function of the gastrointestinal smooth muscle is intimately controlled by release of peptides and transmitters by the intrinsic (or enteric) nervous system; modulation of the latter input arises in the extrinsic autonomic nerves, the **craniospinal** (vagus, and $S_{2,3,4}$ nerves) parasympathetic excitatory input, and the thoracolumbar sympathetic outflow, which is predominantly inhibitory to the gut, but excitatory to the sphincters (Fig. 2). Gastrointestinal smooth muscle forms an electrical syncytium whereby the impulse that induces contraction of the first muscle cell results in efficient transmission to a sheet of sequentially linked cells in the transverse and longitudinal axes of the intestine.

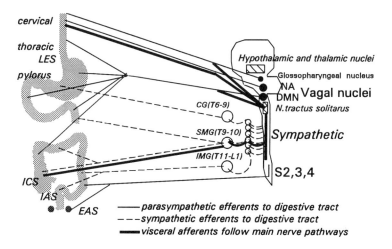

Figure 2. Neural pathways with sympathetic and parasympathetic nervous systems to the gastrointestinal tract. LES, lower esophageal sphincter; ICS, ileocecal sphincter; IAS, internal anal sphincter; EAS, external anal sphincter; NA, nucleus ambiguus; DMN, dorsal motor nucleus of vagus; S, sacral roots.

In several species, including man, the enteric nervous system is formed of a series of ganglionated plexuses, such as the **submucosal (Meissner's)**, **myenteric (Auerbach)**, **deep muscular** (Cajal), **mucosal,** and **submucosal** plexuses. Together these enteric nerves number **almost 100 million neurons;** this number is roughly equivalent to the number of neurons in the spinal cord.

At the level of the diaphragm, the **vagus** nerve consists predominantly of **afferent fibers.** Thus, the classical concept that preganglionic vagal fibers synapse with a few motor neurons is not tenable, in view of the overwhelmingly larger number of effector cells that would need to be innervated by the smaller number of preganglionic nerves. The current concept (Fig. 3) is that each **vagal command fiber** supplies an integrated circuit that is hard-wired in the intestinal wall and results in a specific motor or secretory response. These hard-wired circuits in the enteric nervous system are also important in many of the automated responses of the gut, such as the peristaltic reflex, which proceed even in a totally extrinsically denervated intestine. The enteric nerves also control pacemaker activity such as those located on the greater curve of the gastric corpus and the duodenal bulb. As in the heart, malfunction of the pacemaker with the highest frequency results in "takeover" of pacemaker function by the region with the next highest intrinsic contractile frequency. Derangement of the extrinsic neural control of the gastrointestinal smooth muscle forms the basis for disorders of motility, such as **diabetic gastroparesis** or anal **incontinence** following obstetric trauma, which are encountered in clinical practice. Other diseases result from disorders of enteric neural function including **achalasia** or **Hirschsprung's disease.**

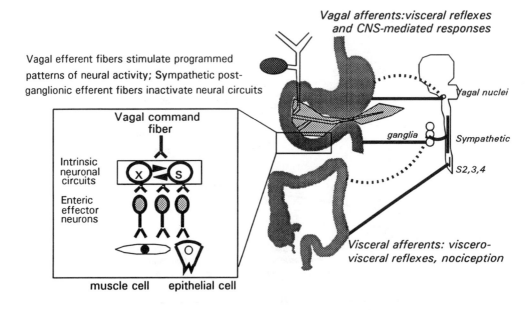

Figure 3.   Integration between extrinsic and intrinsic (or enteric) neural control. Hardwired programs controlling such functions of peristalsis are modulated by efferents in the vagus and sympathetic nerves, which also contain afferent fibers mediating visceral sensation, nociception, and reflex responses.

Normal Gastrointestinal Motor Function

Swallowing involves chewing of food, transfer from the oral cavity to the hypopharynx, ejection of the bolus into the esophagus and esophageal peristalsis. The lower esophageal sphincter relaxes at the onset of the swallowing reflex and remains open for a period of about 8 sec until the bolus passes through the entire esophagus. Then the sphincter contracts to prevent gastroesophageal reflux. Reflux is also prevented by the positive intra-abdominal pressure that occludes the short intra-abdominal portion of the esophagus. Extrinsic neural control reaches the esophagus through efferent pathways in the **glossopharyngeal** (upper esophagus) and **vagus** nerves.

The motor functions of the **stomach** and **small bowel** differ greatly between the fasting and postprandial periods. During fasting, cyclical motor events sweep through the stomach and small bowel and are associated with similarly cyclical secretion from the biliary tract and pancreas. The cyclical motor activity is called the **interdigestive migrating motor complex;** this consists of a phase I of **quiescence,** phase II of **intermittent pressure activity,** and phase III or the **activity front,** when contractions of the maximal frequency typical of each region (3 per minute in stomach, 12 per minute in the small bowel) sweep through the gut like a housekeeper, transporting nondigestible residue, products of digestion, and epithelial debris toward the colon for subsequent excretion. The pacemaking functions, cyclical motor activity, and peristalsis are essentially controlled by intrinsic neural pathways, but they can be modulated by extrinsic nerves.

Postprandially, this cyclical activity is abolished, and the different regions of the gut subserve specific functions. Tonic contractions in the gastric fundus result in the emptying of liquids; antral contractions sieve and triturate solid food and propel particles that are less than 2 mm in size from the stomach. Irregular, frequent contractions in the postprandial period serve to mix food with digestive juices in the duodenum and jejunum and to propel it aborally. The duration of small bowel transit is on average about 3 hr, and the ileum is a site of temporary storage of chyme, allowing salvage of nutrients, fluids, and electrolytes that were not absorbed upstream. Residues are finally discharged from the ileum to the colon in bolus transfers that probably result from prolonged propagated contractions or reestablished interdigestive cyclical motor activity. The vagus nerve is critically important in efferent control of the fed phase; sympathetic and vagal afferents convey signals from the gut to the brain and spinal cord to evoke reflex responses and coordination of secretory and motor functions.

In the dog, the **colon** also demonstrates cyclical activity, but this is not observed in humans, and is less understood than in the small bowel. The proximal colon (ascending and transverse regions) stores solid residue. The ascending colon has variable patterns of emptying: relatively linear, or constant; intermittent; or sudden mass movements. The descending colon is mainly a conduit, and the rectosigmoid functions as a terminal reservoir leading to the call to defecate and empty under voluntary control.

Defecation results from a well-coordinated series of motor responses (Fig. 4). The rectoanal angle is maintained relatively acute by the puborectalis muscle

Resting

Straining

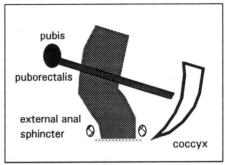

Relaxation of puborectalis
Straightening of rectoanal angle
Relaxation of external anal sphincter

Rectoanal Angle

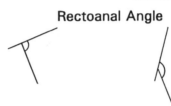

Figure 4.   Dynamics of normal defecation: note the straightening of the rectoanal angle by relaxation of the puborectalis to facilitate evacuation.

sling or pelvic floor, and this is important to maintain continence. For defecation to occur, this sling relaxes, thereby opening the rectoanal angle to allow a straighter rectal conduit; the anal sphincters are inhibited by parasympathetic (pudendal nerve, $S_{2,3,4}$) input, and intracolonic pressure increases predominantly by a rise in intra-abdominal pressure associated with straining. In contrast, continence is maintained by contraction of the puborectalis (parasympathetic pudendal nerve), contraction of the internal sphincter (sympathetic lumbar colonic nerves), and contraction of the external sphincter (parasympathetic pudendal nerve).

References

1. Davenport HW. Physiology of the digestive tract, fifth edition, Chicago: Year Book Med. Pub., 1982.
2. Camilleri M. Autonomic regulation of gastrointestinal motility. In: Low PA, ed. Clinical autonomic disorders: evaluation and management. Boston: Little, Brown and Company, 1992: 125–32.
3. Camilleri M. Gastrointestinal motor mechanisms and motility: hormonal and neural regulation. In: Singer MV, Ziegler R, Rohr G., eds. The gastrointestinal tract and endocrine system. Dordrecht: Kluwer Academic, 1995;237–53.
4. Cooke HJ. Role of "little brain" in the gut in water and electrolyte homeostasis. FASEB J 1989;3:127–38.

6 Regulation of Metabolism

Robert Hoeldtke
Department of Medicine
Division of Endocrinology
West Virginia University Medical School
Morgantown, West Virginia

Epinephrine, the adrenal medullary hormone, and **norepinephrine,** the sympathetic neurotransmitter, have multiple effects on intermediary metabolism, most of which act synergistically to mobilize stored fuels. In addition to direct effects on target organs (primarily liver, adipose, and muscle), catecholamines act on the pancreatic islets where they regulate the secretion of insulin and glucagon. The most important effect on the islet is to suppress insulin secretion by α-adrenergic mechanisms. Thus, the direct catabolic effects of catecholamines are amplified by their suppression of the predominant anabolic hormone, insulin.

Catecholamines and Glucose Metabolism

Catecholamines activate β-adrenergic receptors in the liver and stimulate hepatic glucose production by multiple mechanisms. **Glycogenolysis** and **gluconeogenesis** are enhanced, whereas glycogen synthesis is inhibited. In addition to stimulating the entry of glucose into the bloodstream, catecholamines decrease plasma glucose clearance by both direct (β) and indirect (α) adrenergic mechanisms as illustrated in Fig. 1. These multiple catecholamine effects are synergistic insofar as they all serve to raise plasma glucose concentrations. These mechanisms become physiologically important in the setting of **hypoglycemia,** the classical stimulus to epinephrine secretion by the adrenal medulla. Thus, the autonomic activation associated with hypoglycemia serves the ultimate purpose of mobilizing endogenous substrates for glucose production and increasing glucose concentrations in the bloodstream so that central nervous system demand for its obligatory fuel can be met.

The autonomic mechanisms for correcting hypoglycemia are well established; nevertheless, glucose counterregulation remains intact in adrenalectomized patients as well as in those subjected to combined (α plus β) adrenergic blockade. This is because the **glucagon** response to hypoglycemia, although probably mediated by the autonomic nervous system, is relatively unaffected by most adrenergic blocking drugs. Since glucagon's effects on carbohydrate metabolism are nearly identical to those of the catecholamines, glucose counterregulation is preserved even when adrenergic mechanisms are inoperative.

The redundancy of the mechanisms for acute glucose counterregulation becomes clinically important in patients with insulin-dependent diabetes, most of whom lose their ability to secrete glucagon in response to hypoglycemia

Primer on the Autonomic Nervous System

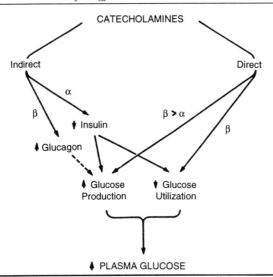

CATECHOLAMINES

Indirect

Direct

α

β

Insulin

β > α

β

Glucagon

Glucose
Production

Glucose
Utilization

PLASMA GLUCOSE

Figure 1.   Mechanisms for catecholamine induced increments in plasma glucose concentrations.

during the first decade of their illness; they therefore become dependent on adrenergic mechanisms for acute glucose counterregulation. These also fail eventually in some patients because of autonomic neuropathy and other factors. Inadequate acute glucose counterregulation places many patients with long-standing type I diabetes at risk for developing severe hypoglycemia.

Catecholamines and Fat Metabolism

Catecholamines act directly on adipose tissue to stimulate fat breakdown. This is a β_1-adrenergic effect involving adenyl cyclase-mediated activation of hormone-sensitive triacylglycerol lipase, the enzyme that cleaves triglyceride in adipose tissue into fatty acids and glycerol. Insulin inhibits catecholamine-induced lipolysis; thus, catecholamine-mediated suppression of insulin secretion is synergistic with the direct catecholamine effects on adipose tissue.

It is unknown whether circulating or locally released catecholamines are more important physiologically in regulating lipolysis. In patients with diabetic ketoacidosis circulating catecholamines become high enough to stimulate both lipolysis and ketogenesis.

Catecholamines and Thermogenesis

Obligatory thermogenesis (**basal metabolic rate**) is regulated by thyroid hormones whereas facultative thermogenesis (total heat production minus basal) is regulated by the adrenergic nervous system predominantly through β_3 adrenoreceptors. Cold exposure and exercise stimulate the adrenergic nervous system and thereby enhance facultative thermogenesis. The increase in heat production associated with eating (dietary-induced thermogenesis) cannot be fully attributed to the energy cost of eating. In addition to the energy expenditure associated with the digestion, absorption, and metabolism of nutrients, food ingestion activates the sympathetic nervous system, stimulates thermogenesis, and may serve to protect against obesity in patients who overeat chronically. The sympathetic nervous system may also mediate the increased thermogenesis associated with trauma, shock, infections, tetanus, and withdrawal from addicting drugs (alcohol and opiates).

Insulin and Autonomic Function

There are complex interactions between insulin and the autonomic nervous system. In patients with autonomic neuropathy insulin acts as a vasodilator and may aggravate orthostatic hypotension. On the other hand, in patients with intact autonomic function insulin stimulates the sympathetic nervous system and causes **sodium retention** and **high blood pressure**. There is increasing evidence, particularly in children and young adults, that **hyperinsulinemia** mediates the **hypervolemia, sympathetic stimulation,** and **hypertension** associated with obesity.

Miscellaneous Effects

Sympathoadrenal stimulation increases **renal tubular sodium reabsorption,** an effect which opposes the **natriuresis** produced by **dopamine.** Epinephrine has a biphasic effect on serum **potassium.** A transient increase in potassium efflux from liver is followed by a β-adrenergic stimulation of potassium uptake into muscle and liver and ultimately **hypokalemia.**

Catecholamines tend to increase serum **calcium** and lower **magnesium,** but these effects are small and not always evident. Catecholamines lower serum **phosphate;** this effect probably explains the **hypophosphatemia** which occurs postoperatively or following a myocardial infarction.

References

1. Landsberg L, Young JB. Catecholamines and the adrenal medulla. In: Wilson JD, Foster DW, eds. Williams textbook of endocrinology, 8th ed. Philadelphia: W.B. Saunders, 1992: 621–707.
2. Cryer E. Diseases of the sympathochromaffin system. In: Felig P, Baxter AE, Broadus LA, Frohman, eds. Endocrinology and metabolism, 2nd ed. NewYork: McGraw–Hill, 1987: 651–91.
3. Gerich JE, Mokan M, Veneman T, Korytkowski M, Mitrakou A. Hypoglycemia unawareness. Endocr Rev 1991;12:356–71.
4. Hoeldtke RD, Boden G. Epinephrine secretion, hypoglycemia unawareness, and diabetic autonomic neuropathy. Ann Int Med 1994;120:512–7.
5. Rocchini AP, Key J, Bondie D, Chico R, Moorehead C, Katch V, Martin M. The effects of weight loss on the sensitivity of blood pressure to sodium in obese adolescents. N Engl J Med 1989;321:580–5.

7 Autonomic Control of Cardiac Function

Kleber G. Franchini
Heart Institute
University of São Paulo
São Paulo, Brazil

Allen W. Cowley, Jr.
Department of Physiology
Medical College of Wisconsin
Milwaukee, Wisconsin

The autonomic neural regulation of cardiovascular function is of great importance for survival. The centrally orchestrated sympathetic and parasympathetic neural pathways enable the cardiovascular system to optimize its delivery of blood flow and satisfy the requirements of different physiological and behavioral stimuli such as eating, sleeping, and the many conditions of exercise and stress to which the body is subjected. It has long been recognized that each of the components of the cardiovascular system can operate and respond independently of neural and hormonal control systems. The classic example for this was the demonstration by Starling early in the 20th century that an **isolated heart** is capable of increasing its **contractile state** and **stroke volume** simply by increasing the volume preload into the right ventricle. Thus, when a greater amount of blood returns to the heart under conditions such as exercise, the heart is intrinsically capable of increasing its work load and responding with an elevation of cardiac output. It is recognized, however, that this intrinsic length-tension mechanism of the cardiac muscle is only capable of increasing cardiac output from resting levels of about 5 liters/min in humans to a maximum permissive pumping level of about 13 liters/min. This is far less than the maximum permissive pumping level of normal individuals who can achieve levels of nearly 20 liters/min during sustained exercise. These optimum levels of cardiac pumping ability can be achieved only in the presence of the increased force of contraction and an increased heart rate brought about through the coordinated activities of the sympathetic and parasympathetic nervous system, as described below.

Although blood flow to many regions of the systemic circulation may be regulated by local mechanisms (**autoregulation**) independent of the nervous system, optimization of blood flow to the various regions of the body during conditions such as exercise, underwater submersion, high altitudes, temperature stress such as fever, frost bite, and hypothermia, hypotensive hemorrhage, systemic hypertension, congestive heart failure, and emotional behavior such as excitement and aversion cannot be achieved without complex sensors, central coordination, and effectors of the autonomic nervous system.

Anatomy of Autonomic Nerves Innervating the Mammalian Heart

The cell bodies of the preganglionic cardiac sympathetic neurons are located in three major ganglia, the **superior** and **middle cervical** ganglia, and the **stellate** ganglion (Fig. 1). The postganglionic sympathetic fibers course to the heart in a **mixed neural plexus** with the preganglionic parasympathetic fibers. Efferent sympathetic axons innervate the S-A and A-V node, the conduction system, and the myocardial fibers. The myocardial fibers receive their innervation from nerves that run parallel with the larger coronary arteries from which they are distributed to the myocardial structures and the coronary main vessels and branches. Although the sympathetic innervation of the S-A and A-V node is abundant, the density of terminals is not significantly different from that in the surrounding cardiac tissue. The sympathetic terminal fibers are characterized by fine varicosities containing the neurotransmitter vesicles but there is no specialization particular to the neuroeffector junction.

The cell bodies of **vagal preganglionic** neurons innervating cardiac ganglia are located mainly in the area of the nucleus ambiguus within the ventrolateral medulla, and to a lesser extent in the dorsal motor nucleus of the vagus.

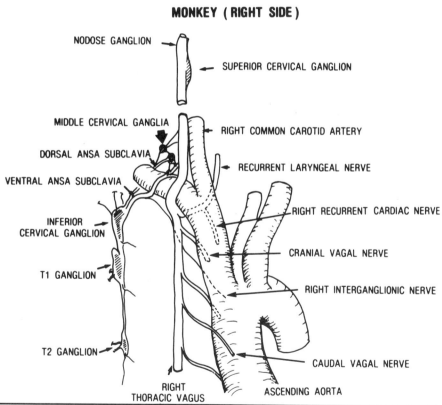

MONKEY (RIGHT SIDE)

Figure 1. Schematic drawing of the rhesus monkey right cardiopulmonary nerves seen from the ventral aspect. Note that there are a number of small ganglia which have been designated collectively as middle cervical ganglia. The major sympathetic ganglia are indicated by shading. (Reprinted, with permission, from *Nervous Control of Cardiovascular Function*, edited by W.C. Randall, Oxford University Press.)

In the thorax, the efferent vagal fibers join the **cardiac neural plexus** and reach the intracardiac ganglia, which are the origin of the short postganglionic neurons. Abundant nerve terminals from the postganglionic vagal fibers innervate the region of the S-A and A-V node, but a small to moderate number of cholinergic nerves, compared to many adrenergic nerves, are distributed within the atrial and ventricular myocardium. The majority of efferent vagal fibers en route to innervate the ventricles cross the A-V groove within 0.25–0.5 mm of the epicardial surface, at which point innervation to this region occurs.

The Autonomic Nervous System and Cardiac Function

The resting activity of the **sympathetic** postganglionic neurons is determined by the interaction between **intrinsic rhythms** generated in the central nervous system and the **cyclic baroreceptor input.** Under different conditions, however, the activity may be influenced by inputs from other peripheral reflexes and from central areas involved in the coordination of the cardiovascular responses to complex behaviors. Tonic and reflex activity of the sympathetic efferents results in release of **norepinephrine** and other neurotransmitters like **neuropeptide Y (NPY)** and ATP. Norepinephrine is responsible for most, if not all, of the postsynaptic effects of the cardiac sympathetic activation, which include the positive inotropic and chronotropic effects and coronary vasoconstriction. During stimulation of the cardiac sympathetic nerves, the heart rate and cardiac contraction begin to increase after a latent period of 1–3 sec, approaching a steady-state level in about 30 sec. After cessation of stimulation, the return toward the control level takes place much more gradually than at the onset of stimulation. The slow return of the heart rate and cardiac contraction to the normal levels after cessation of the sympathetic stimulation is related to the relatively slow rate of metabolism of norepinephrine by the cardiac tissue.

Radioligand binding techniques have shown that both β_1- and β_2-adrenergic receptors coexist in the heart. Physiological studies indicate that β_1 receptors are predominantly linked to the inotropic response, whereas both β_1 and β_2 receptors are linked to the chronotropic response. In the heart, the α receptors are almost exclusively α_1 subtype, and their stimulation usually causes a modest inotropic effect by increasing transarcolemmal calcium influx. In coronary vessels the α_1-receptor stimulation causes vasoconstriction, but usually its effects are overshadowed by the simultaneous increase in the oxygen consumption that stimulates local mechanisms to increase blood flow. As illustrated in Fig. 2, β-adrenergic receptors are members of a large multigene family of the **G-protein-coupled receptors,** which have a secondary structure consisting of seven transmembrane spanning domains and transduce signal through a G protein (G_s). The positive inotropic effect of the sympathetic nervous system (see Fig. 3) is partly mediated by an increase in the **voltage-gated Ca^{2+} current** (I_{Ca}). This increase is generally attributed to a β-adrenergic receptor-stimulated cyclic AMP-dependent **phosphorylation of the calcium channel.** The positive effects of β stimulation on heart rate are related to a stimulation of the slow calcium

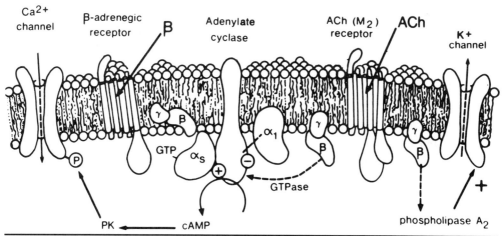

Figure 2. A simplified scheme of sarcolemma-related receptors and channels. The two receptors shown are the β-adrenergic receptor and the cholinergic muscarinic (M_2-receptor), the latter for acetylcholine (ACh). At left, the β-adrenergic receptor is coupled to adenylate cyclase via the activated G-protein subunit α_S-GTP. Consequent formation of cAMP activates the calcium channel to increase calcium entry. Activity of adenylate cyclase can be decreased by the inhibitory subunits of the ACh-associated G-protein (α_i; β-γ). Also note activation of acetylcholine-operated potassium channel via β-γ G and phospholipase A_2. (Reprinted, with permission, from *The Heart* by Lionel H. Opie, Raven Press.)

channel by the increased intracellular cyclic AMP on the S-A and A-V node, bundle of His, and Purkinje fibers.

NPY is a 36 amino acid peptide which is costored and coreleased with norepinephrine during sympathetic stimulation. NPY may act postjunctionally to affect the mechanical and electrophysiological properties of cardiac tissues. However, its principal cardiac action appears to be the prejunctional modula-

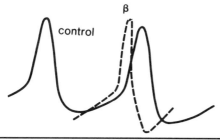

Figure 3. Mechanism whereby β-adrenergic stimulation (β) leads to a sinus tachycardia. First, the inward calcium current I_{Ca} is stimulated. Then, by steps still not fully understood, β-receptor occupancy leads to hyperpolarization. When the diastolic membrane potential is low enough, the current I_f is fired. This current responds to β-adrenergic but not to vagal stimulation. Firing of the current rapidly leads to a loss of membrane polarity to reach the normal activation threshold that allows I_{Ca} to become even more active and to enhance the depolarization process. The total extent of depolarization is greater as a result of the combined activity of these two currents. The earlier depolarization leads to earlier activation of I_K with a greater rate of repolarization. (Reprinted, with permission, from *The Heart* by Lionel H. Opie, Raven Press.)

tion of the release of various neurotransmitters from autonomic nerve endings. It is well known that NPY attenuates the vagal effects on heart rate, A-V conduction, and atrial contractility, presumably by inhibiting the release of acetylcholine from vagal nerve endings. NPY also modulates sympathetic neurotransmission but its physiological role is not well established.

The sympathetic nervous system is the primary mediator of the left ventricular inotropic response to **stress.** Sympathetic activation simultaneously increases heart rate and cardiac contractility through β-adrenergic receptors. One of the most severe physiological stresses that the cardiovascular system encounters is **maximum exercise,** during which heart rate in normal humans may increase to 200 beats per minute. Approximately half of this heart rate response is due to β-adrenergic stimulation since prior β-adrenergic blockade limits the increase in heart rate to about half the maximum response. The other half is due to withdrawal of parasympathetic tone, direct effects of increased blood temperature, and stretch stimulus of the S-A node by the increase in the volume preload. The inotropic response of the heart is virtually eliminated by β-adrenergic receptor blockade, indicating that nearly all of this response is due to β-adrenergic receptor stimulation. Autonomic mechanisms appear important in mediating the rapid onset of the initial hemodynamic responses to dynamic exercise because these changes are delayed in animals after cardiac denervation. The large left ventricular inotropic response to exercise overrides the usual opposing cardiovascular reflexes.

Under normal conditions, cardiac **parasympathetic** neurons fire in synchrony with the cardiac cycle, due to an excitatory input arising from peripheral baroreceptors. They can also be excited powerfully by inputs arising from peripheral chemoreceptors, cardiac receptors, and trigeminal receptors activated during the **diving reflex.** Activation of the vagus nerve releases acetylcholine and vasoactive intestinal peptide (VIP) in the heart. Although VIP may exert some presynaptic effect on the autonomic transmission, the parasympathetic influence on cardiac function occurs predominantly through the binding of acetylcholine to **muscarinic receptors.** As illustrated in Fig. 2, muscarinic receptors are also members of the G-protein-coupled receptors and the M_2 muscarinic receptor subtype is found in the heart. Acetylcholine binding to the muscarinic receptors stimulates the G_i protein to combine with GTP which in turn **inhibits adenylate cyclase** activity. These events result in the decrease of the intracellular cyclic AMP, which is apparently responsible for the negative inotropic effect of acetylcholine, through the **inhibition of the calcium current** (I_{Ca}).

Also, **muscarinic receptors** are directly coupled to specific sarcolemmal **potassium channels** ($I_{K, Ach}$) apparently by G_i or G_0. Activation of acetylcholine activated potassium channels (K_{Ach}) induces a membrane hyperpolarization that occurs within 100 msec of the initiation of vagal stimulation. The flow of potassium current and the accompanying hyperpolarization results in a longer time required to reach the activation threshold for spontaneous firing of the nodal action potential at the S-A and A-V nodes (see Fig. 4).

The net effect of **cholinergic activation** is a decrease in the heart rate due to a decrease in the conductivity of the pathways of the intracardiac conduction system and a decrease in the excitability of the pacemaker cells. The chrono-

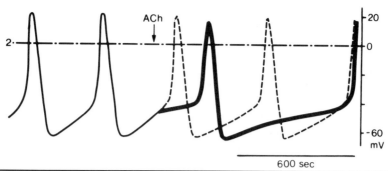

Figure 4. Mechanism for sinus bradycardia in response to increased vagal tone. At the terminal neurons of the vagal system, acetylcholine (ACh) is released, which acts on the muscarinic receptor to stimulate the intracellular protein G, which in turn opens the activation gate of I_{KACh}. The result is flow of potassium current and hyperpolarization, and a longer time is needed to reach the activation threshold for spontaneous firing of the nodal action potential. The result is a sinus bradycardia. (Reprinted, with permission, from *The Heart*, by Lionel H. Opie, Raven Press.)

tropic response of the heart depends on the timing of the vagal stimuli relative to the phase of the cardiac cycle. This **phase dependency** to repetitive vagal stimulation confers a peculiar characteristic to each stimulation such that the stimuli tend **to entrain** the SA nodal pacemaker cells and coordinate the automatic activity of diverse cell clusters within the S-A node. The changes in heart rate produced by a vagal stimulus appear after a brief latent period, reach a steady-state response within a few beats, and decay rapidly back to the control level once stimulation is discontinued. This rapid decay is attributed to the large quantities of acetylcholinesterase present in close proximity to the automatic cells in the S-A node. Electrophysiological studies have revealed that the initial prolongation of the cardiac cycle length evoked by **brief vagal stimulus** is a result of **prolongation of the S-A conduction time** rather than a true reduction in firing rate of the automatic cells in the S-A node. Vagal stimulation also decreases the contractile force of myocardial cells of left and right ventricles and atria. This was clearly demonstrated in experiments in which the effects of vagal stimulation on isovolumic contractions were examined in an externally paced heart maintained with a constant coronary perfusion pressure. In this preparation, vagal stimulation reduced the peak of left ventricular pressure by as much as 30%, an effect potentiated if the sympathetic tone was kept elevated.

One of the most dramatic contributions of the parasympathetic efferents to the adaptation of the cardiovascular system during stress is observed during the **diving reflex.** In this situation, reflexes originating mainly in the **trigeminal afferents** and in the peripheral chemoreceptors elicit simultaneously a potent sympathetic and parasympathetic activation. The **sympathetic activation** is responsible for an increase in the vascular resistance in all organs, except the heart and the brain. Simultaneously, the **cardiac–vagal activation** elicits an intense bradycardia and a decrease in the cardiac contraction, which allows a relative decrease in the energy demand by the heart in a situation of precarious oxygen availability.

Interactions between Sympathetic and Parasympathetic Nerves to the Heart

The tonic inhibitory effects of the vagus nerves on the heart oppose the facilitatory influence of the sympathetic nerves. Changes in heart rate and A-V nodal conduction result not simply from an increase or decrease in either sympathetic or vagal tone, but from opposing variations in the tone of both branches of the autonomic nervous system. Although antagonism between the two divisions of the autonomic nervous system is a well known phenomenon, other more complex interactions may occur. For example, simultaneous activation of sympathetic nerve fibers may exaggerate or blunt cardiovascular responses to parasympathetic activity, depending on the circumstances. The functional interaction between the cardiac sympathetic and parasympathetic control has been demonstrated to occur through presynaptic interneuronal and postsynaptic intracellular mechanisms. Interneuronal interactions occur between the terminal postganglionic vagal and sympathetic fibers, which often lie in close apposition to each other in the heart. Acetylcholine liberated at vagal endings is able to reduce the quantity of norepinephrine released at the sympathetic terminals at any given level of sympathetic neural activity. In addition, NPY released by sympathetic activation may exert inhibitory influence on vagal cholinergic transmission. At the postsynaptic level, the interactions occur via effects on the sarcolemmal membrane receptor sites. Activation of β-adrenergic and muscarinic receptors influence ionic currents, adenylate cyclase activity, and changes in the concentrations of cyclic AMP, cyclic GMP, and other cellular processes, generally in opposite directions, and probably in more complex ways than are currently understood.

References

1. Randall WC. Nervous control of cardiovascular function. New York: Oxford University Press, 1984.
2. Vatner SF. Sympathetic mechanisms regulating myocardial contractility in conscious animals. In: Fozzard HA, *et al.,* eds. The heart and cardiovascular system: scientific foundations, 2nd edition. New York: Raven Press, 1992.
3. Schwinn DA, Caron M, Lefkowitz R. The beta-adrenergic receptors as a model for molecular structure-function relationship in G-protein coupled receptors. In: Fozzard HA, *et al.,* eds. The heart and cardiovascular system: scientific foundations, 2nd edition. New York: Raven Press, 1992.
4. Vatner SF, Franklin D, Higgens CB, Patrick T, Braunwald E. Left ventricular response to severe exertion in untethered dogs. J Clin Invest 1972;51:3052–60.
5. Levy MN, Martin PJ. Neural control of the heart. In: Berne RM, Sperelakis N, Geiger SR, eds. Handbook of physiology, section 2, the cardiovascular system, Vol. 1, Bethesda: American Physiological Society, 1979.

8 Neurogenic Control of Blood Vessels

Allen W. Cowley, Jr.
Department of Physiology
Medical College of Wisconsin
Milwaukee, Wisconsin

Kleber G. Franchini
Heart Institute
University of São Paulo
São Paulo, Brazil

The small arteries (**arterioles**) with thick muscular walls and diameters of 250 μm or less are responsible for the major resistance to blood flow in the circulatory system. Normally these vessels are maintained in a state of functional constriction (**vascular tone**) determined by the interaction between **intrinsic** (myogenic tone) and **extrinsic** (neurotransmitters, hormones, and autacoids) factors. **Myogenic tone** is a property of arteriolar smooth muscle that is independent of any neural or humoral influences and is the reference point around which various neural, humoral, and local metabolic influences are expressed. The importance of the contribution of the sympathetic nervous system to normal vascular tone is apparent by the drop of nearly 50 mm Hg in mean arterial pressure following pharmacological blockade of the α-adrenergic receptors or surgical sympathectomy in normal subjects or animals.

Vasodilatation and **vasoconstriction** are fundamental physiological adjustments to increased and decreased metabolic demands of the tissue. The intrinsic and extrinsic factors cooperate in a complex manner to fulfill the requirements for increased or decreased blood flow to different organs during various physiological situations. However, in the cardiovascular adjustments which occur in many conditions of physiological stress (exercise, diving, hemorrhage, thermal stress, etc), the vascular sympathetic efferents dominate and coordinate the degree of vasoconstriction in many regions of the systemic circulation. These neural responses enable the rapid redistribution of blood flow to areas functionally important to specific activities. This redistribution of blood flow, coordinated by a combination of centrally driven sympathetic activity and its modulation by cardiovascular receptors (mainly the arterial baroreceptors), allows, for example, a person to stand up after awakening without exhibiting hypotension and syncope. In exercise, it enables optimization of skeletal muscle blood flow by diverting cardiac output away from the splanchnic and renal circulation.

Finally, it should be recognized that the **regulation of venous capacity** by the nervous system is an important determinant of systemic blood volume distribution and is of critical importance in the regulation of venous return to the heart and thereby in the regulation of cardiac output. Most of the blood in the body is contained in the veins (approximately 70%) and venules which are relatively flaccid and of larger diameter compared to arteries and arterioles at normal distending pressures. Smooth muscle lines the wall of much of the venous system and its volume can be altered by sympathetic venoconstriction.

Vascular Neuroeffector Innervation of Arteries and Arterioles

The precapillary resistance vessels (arterioles) which are in a constant state of partial constriction (basal tone) are well-innervated by autonomic nerves. The venous capacitance vessels, on the other hand, show much less intrinsic tone, and are largely dependent on extrinsic sympathetic vasoconstrictor influences. There is evidence that contractile proteins are also present in the capillary bed which is supplied with autonomic nerve endings, indicating that capillaries also might play a role in the distribution of blood flow within tissues.

The general organization of the peripheral **autonomic neuroeffector system** has been studied in great detail (see Figs. 1 and 2). The postganglionic autonomic nerves innervating blood vessels ramify into small bundles which form a primary plexus located in the loose adventitia of the blood vessels. These bundles give rise to fibers which form the terminal effector plexus located on the surface of the medial layer. These bundles exhibit a beaded effect (**varicosities**) where the fibers are partly or entirely devoid of their Schwann cell sheaths. It is at this point that the fibers approach the surface of the smooth muscle cell and establish neuromuscular contact. Compared to central synaptic clefs which are not wider than 20 nm, the peripheral neuroeffector units are generally no closer than 100 nm distance to the membrane of the smooth muscle cells. The concentration of norepinephrine in the nerve cell body is on the order of

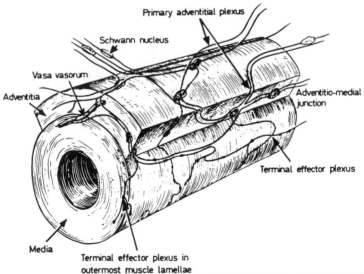

Figure 1. Arrangement of vascular neuroeffector apparatus. Postganglionic autonomic nerves ramify into small bundles forming a primary plexus, which is located in loose adventitia. Bundles consist of axons with smooth appearance characteristic of preterminal portion of nerve fiber. Bundles give rise to beaded (varicosed) fibers forming terminal effector plexus, located on surface of medical layer. A few terminals may sometimes extend, but only for a short distance, into outermost layer of the media. Thus, only smooth muscle cells located in adventitia–media junction receive direct autonomic innervation. (Reprinted, with permission, from Verity MA. Morphologic studies of the vascular neuroeffector apparatus. In: JA Bevan, RF Furchgott, RA Maxwell, and AA Somlyo, eds. Physiology and pharmacology of vascular neuroeffector systems. Basel: Karger, 1971: 2–12.)

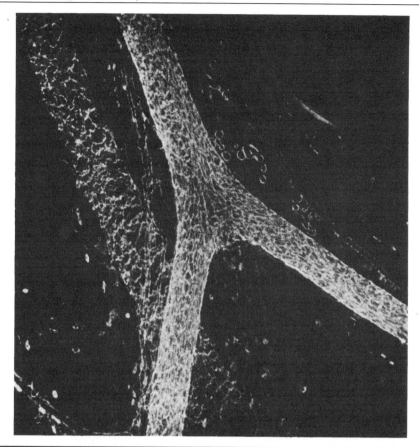

Figure 2. Fluorescence photomicrograph of whole mount of rat mesentery showing perivascular sympathetic nerves demonstrated by Falck–Hillarp formaldehyde technique. Very dense plexus of green-fluorescent, noradrenergic fibers supplies a small artery, whereas corresponding vein has less well-developed innervation. Nerve terminals are seen to accompany small vessels of arteriolar caliber. × 155. (Reprinted, with permission, from Falck B. Observations on the possibilities of the cellular localization of monoamines by a fluorescence method. Acta Physiol Scan Suppl 1962; 197:1–25.

10–100 μg/g wet wt; amine synthesis and storage occur in this part of the neuron, where turnover has been calculated as 1–5 hrs. A varicosity forming contact with vascular smooth muscle cells contains from 500 to 1500 synaptic vesicles, and the norepinephrine concentration in each synaptic vessel has been estimated to be about 2.4 M.

Release of Transmitter and Effector Action

Norepinephrine is released from varicosities of sympathetic nerves which are located in a two-dimensional array 1–10 μm apart. The smooth muscle cell membrane is located at varying distances from the release site (100–200 nm), and subsequent smooth muscle cells appear to be spaced 2–4 μm apart. The variations in distance between autonomic nerve terminals and smooth muscle cells vary depending on vessel size and location (see Table 1). In the smallest arterioles and venules, only one or two muscle cells may be present, but in large arteries, the media thickness may be as great as 500 μm or more. The concentration of norepinephrine in the extracellular space has been difficult to estimate during nerve activation, but in extracellular spaces where the axon varicosity is at close contact to the vascular smooth muscle, it appears to be on the order of 10^{-6} to 10^{-5} g/ml. Only a small fraction of the cells in the vascular smooth musculature is directly innervated by autonomic nerves, so it appears that individual smooth muscle cells probably are electrically and also mechanically coupled. **Gap juntions** have been identified between the opposing membranes between adjacent smooth muscles which offer pathways for low electrical resistance and electrical **coupling** between adjacent muscle cells.

Released norepinephrine binds to lipoprotein sites called **receptors** on the vascular smooth muscle membrane where the vasoconstrictor response is initiated. Norepinephrine is removed from the junctional cleft by **active reuptake** by the neuronal cell membrane (active carrier coupled to Na^+, K^+, ATPase), and by leakage into the capillaries. Nearly 80% of the norepinephrine released is incorporated back into the nerve terminal for **storage**. The amount which is spilled into the capillaries, if widespread, can serve as a rough **index of total sympathetic nervous activity.**

In the vasculature, norepinephrine mostly binds to α **receptors** causing an increase in permeability to Ca^{2+} in the cell membrane and sarcoplasmic reticulum. Calcium entry initiates contraction of vascular smooth muscle. Arterioles in some regions also have β-**adrenergic** receptors which, when activated by agonists such as isoproterenol, cause vasodilatation. The vascular β receptors are designated as β_2. When norepinephrine is infused intravenously into tissues that contain both α and β receptors (e.g., skeletal muscle), the effect on α receptors predominates and the arterioles constrict. Only when α receptors are blocked with an antagonist such as phenoxybenzamine or phentolamine do β-adrenergic effects predominate, and arteriolar dilatation is observed. It is interesting that when norepinephrine is released from nerve endings, there is

Table 1.   **Distance Between Autonomic Nerve Terminals and Smooth Muscular Media Layer in Arterial Vessels**

Blood vessel	External diameter (μm)	Neuromuscular interval (nm)
Precapillary arteriole	~20	20
Renal cortex arteriole	25–35	200–400
Pancreatic arteriole	20–50	<400
Coronary arteriole	~50	300–700
Auricular artery	~1500	~500
Mesenteric artery	100–200	~500
Pulmonary artery	>5000	~2000

Note that mean neuromuscular interval roughly parallels vessel diameter. Reprinted with permission from Verity MA. Morphologic studies of the vascular neuroeffector apparatus. In JA Bevan, RF Furchgott, RA Maxwell, AP Somlyo, eds. "Physiology and pharmacology of vascular neuroeffector systems." Basel: Karger, 1971: 2–12.

little or no β-adrenergic effect even when α receptors are blocked. Thus, neurally released norepinephrine acts predominantly on α receptors to cause a vasoconstriction that is not significantly modulated by β_2 receptors.

Neural Control of Veins

Veins appear to be innervated by α-adrenergic fibers of the sympathetic nervous system only. It is important to recognize that the two regions in the human cardiovascular system which contain the most capacity to store volume (**high capacitance regions**) are the **splanchnic** and **cutaneous venous beds.** These venous beds are also the most richly innervated, particularly the larger veins in these regions which contain the major fraction of the total blood volume, while the smaller venules are sparsely innervated. There is evidence that active sympathetic vasoconstriction of veins participates in the regulation of ventricular filling pressure. Reflex-induced increase in venous tone in compensation for mild hemorrhage in dogs appears to account for about one-third of the reduction in venous capacitance, while another third appears to be accounted for by passive venous collapse, and another third by transcapillary fluid shifts. Such assessments have been difficult to make in human subjects, and it can only be assumed that active control of venous tone is of at least as great importance, and probably greater, given the responses required of the veins to upright posture and heat stress.

Sympathetic Cholinergic Vasodilator Fibers

There are some species, including man, in which stimulation of **sympathetic fibers** directed to vessels of skeletal muscles causes **vasodilatation** that is blocked by atropine. The responses to stimulation of this kind of fiber are transient and confined to arterioles. Although it was originally believed that such vasodilatation may momentarily prepare the muscle and the central circulation for a burst of activity, this lag is very brief and the idea has meager experimental support.

Cholinergic fibers originating in the craniosacral-parasympathetic outflow are known to supply arterioles in the brain, heart, erectile tissue of the genitalia, and various glands in the gastrointestinal tract. Although the role played by these vasodilator fibers is generally unknown, their importance in contributing to hyperemia in the engorgement of erectile tissue in the genitalia is well established. However, the parasympathetic nervous system does not appear to participate in any significant way in the major homeostatic reflexes contributing to the vascular tone.

P-type Nerves: Nonadrenergic, Noncholinergic

Nerve fibers which are neither adrenergic nor cholinergic have been found to innervate blood vessels. The term **P-type** is used to describe these fibers because the prevailing type of vesicle in these nerve fibers resembled those in the neurosecretory nerve fibers of the neurohypophysis that were known to store **peptides.** The fibers were first demonstrated in the gut. Ultrastructurally,

P-type nerve fibers differ from cholinergic and adrenergic fibers in that they contain **large** (100–200 nm diameter) electron-dense granular vesicles. Adrenergic nerve fibers, in contrast, are characterized by the presence of small (50 nm) electron-dense vesicles, and cholinergic fibers by small electron-lucent vesicles with the same diameter. Although it was originally argued that the P-type nerve fibers were **purinergic** (i.e., they release ATP as neurotransmitter), there is evidence for many other putative neurotransmitters.

Immunochemical and immunocytochemical studies have demonstrated several biologically active peptides that occur within the nerve cell bodies and nerve fibers, suggesting that these fibers are **peptidergic** rather than **purinergic**. Various neuropeptides seem to be located exclusively in the neurovesicles of specific populations of nerves. They are released into the venous plasma effluent by nerve stimulation, and in some cases their effects mimic those of nerve stimulation. The number of polypeptides which have been detected in neurons and hence are candidates for neurotransmitter function has increased rapidly in recent years. Some of these neuropeptides belong to the autonomic nervous system innervating various peripheral tissues including **vasoactive intestinal peptide (VIP), substance P, enkephalins, gastrin–cholecystokinin, pancreatic polypeptide, gastrin-releasing peptide, neuropeptide Y,** and **calcitonin gene-related peptide.** The peptidergic neurons have the same structural relationship to the wall of the blood vessel as to the classic types of perivascular autonomic nerves. At the present time, immunohistochemical distribution of these nerves is being intensely studied; however, the physiological significance of these peptidergic fibers is poorly understood.

The vasculature also has a high density of **vasodilatory dopaminergic receptors.** One of the lowest dose effects of dopamine and similar agonists is the lowering of blood pressure. Given these observations, the potential significance of a sympathetic–dopaminergic system has been the subject of recent studies. Once again, however, the functional importance of such innervation in controlling organ flow is poorly understood at this time.

Differential Vasomotor Control

The concept originally put forward by Cannon in 1915, that the entire sympathetic nervous system is activated *en masse* so as to produce uniform outflow, has been modified over the past several decades. There are significant regional variations in the responsiveness of arterioles to sympathetic activity. There are a number of factors which enable the nervous system to provide differential vasomotor control among organs. One important factor is that the density of α-adrenergic innervation varies from organ to organ. Innervation to arterioles is especially dense in vessels supplying skin, splanchnic organs, skeletal muscle, kidneys, and adipose tissue. Veins in the splanchnic and cutaneous circulation are heavily innervated, while veins deep in the limbs are sparsely innervated. Second, sensitivity of vascular smooth muscle to norepinephrine varies from region to region, in part dependent on the density of α-receptor sites. Third, there is heterogeneity of α-adrenergic receptors between organs. Fourth, neuronal reuptake of norepinephrine differs from region to region. Fifth, structure and vascular size vary between tissues and contribute to the heterogeneity of responses to changes in sympathetic stimulation. In small vessels with small junctional clefts, the actions of released norepinephrine can be more localized.

Regional variations in the responsiveness of arterioles to sympathetic activity also result from variations in regional levels of basal myogenic tone. It is well recognized that the level of myogenic tone varies among different organs, being greatest in the heart, brain, and skeletal muscle, and less in the kidneys. Vasoconstrictor sympathetic nerves raise resistance above vascular basal tone by active vasoconstriction, but can only lower vascular resistance below basal tone by so-called passive dilatation. Thus, in regions with **high basal tone** (e.g., skeletal muscle) and which receive a tonic sympathetic vasoconstrictor outflow, considerable vasodilatation can be achieved by withdrawal of resting sympathetic tone. In contrast, in regions which have **low basal tone** (e.g., kidneys), minimal vasodilatation can be achieved by withdrawal of sympathetic tone.

It is important to recognize that blood flow is closely linked to the rate of **metabolism** in active vascular beds such as skeletal muscle, cerebral and coronary. An increase in metabolic activity in these beds normally results in an autoregulatory vasodilatation of blood vessels in these beds which overrides sympathetic neural control.

Release of endogenous vasoactive substances (autacoids) such as **nitric oxide, eicosanoids, histamine, kinins, adenine nucleotides,** and locally produced vasodilator metabolites all can counteract sympathetic vasoconstriction and also contribute to regional modulations of vascular sympathetic responses.

Finally, it must be recognized that **cirulating humoral agents** can both impede and potentiate the response to neurogenic vasoconstrictor activity. For example, **angiotensin II** potentiates the effects of norepinephrine while vasodilator substances such as **atrial natriuretic peptide** impede the response to neurogenic vasoconstrictor activity. Thus, the sympathetic influence on regional circulations may also vary depending on the circulating levels as well as on regional differences in the vascular reactivity to vasoactive hormones. It is evident that all of the above factors which account for regional differences in the response to sympathetic vasoconstrictor discharge must be carefully considered when examining the contribution of sympathetic nerves in the regulation of vascular tone and regional blood flow.

References

1. Rowell LB. Human cardiovascular control. New York: Oxford University Press, 1993.
2. Lombard JH. In: Lee RMKW, ed. Blood vessel changes in hypertension: structure and function, Vol. II, Chapter 5. Boca Raton, FL: CRC Press, 1989.
3. MacKay MJ, Cheung DW. In: Lee RMKW, ed. Blood vessel changes in hypertension: structure and function, Vol. II, Chapter 6. Boca Raton, FL: CRC Press, 1989.
4. Shepherd JT, Vanhoutte PM. The human cardiovascular system. Facts and concepts. New York: Raven Press, 1979.
5. Shepherd JT, Abboud FM, volume eds. Handbook of physiology. Section 2: The cardiovascular system. Vol. 3: Peripheral circulation and organ blood flow, Part 2. Bethesda: American Physiological Society, 1983.

9
Cerebral Circulation

Donald J. Reis
Department of Neurology and Neuroscience
Cornell University Medical College
New York, New York

Eugene V. Golanov
Department of Neurology and
Neuroscience
Cornell University Medical College
New York, New York

The brain, metabolically the most active organ in the body, relentlessly utilizes oxygen and glucose to maintain its functional integrity. While the brain weighs but 1–2% of average body mass, it utilizes 20% of its oxygen consumption and 15% of the cardiac output during wakefulness and sleep. It is therefore profoundly dependent upon its circulation. Moreover, because of the complex regional anatomy and physiology of brain and spinal cord, the cerebral circulation is regionally organized to provide a sufficient supply of blood to accommodate shifting patterns of neuronal activity.

In man and most vertebrates, the brain receives its blood supply from two principal arterial sources. Internal carotid branches of the **common carotid arteries** supply cortical and subcortical territories of the forebrain while branches of the **vertebral arteries** supply cerebellum, brainstem, and posterior cerebrum through their principal branches. The anterior and posterior circulations intermingle at the Circle of Willis at the base of the brain providing a means of collateral flow. As the arteries enter the brain, they subdivide until, upon loss of their muscular coat, they penetrate the parenchyma in a complex capillary network. Cerebral capillaries are characterized by **endothelium with tight junctions** which provide a physical barrier for the free passage of molecules and form one component of the **blood–brain barrier**. The capillaries join into venules and veins which drain the parenchyma and open into the dural sinuses which drain into the large jugular and paravertebral networks.

The cerebral circulation is highly and hierarchically regulated. At the lowest level, regional cerebral blood flow (rCBF) is **autoregulated,** being maintained constant over a range of perfusion pressures (roughly equivalent to the arterial pressure, AP) from approximately 50 to 140 mm Hg. Over this range, passive elevations in AP result in increasing vascular resistance which leaves rCBF unchanged. Breakthrough at the upper level of autoregulation results in the rCBF being directly dependent upon AP which, if unchecked, may result in cerebral edema (hypertensive encephalopathy). Breakthrough in the lower range results in a reduction of rCBF paralleling reduction in AP and leading, if unchecked, to cerebral hypoxia and infarction.

The cellular basis of autoregulation is not certain. It may be **myogenic** and consist of reactive smooth muscular contraction in response to muscular stretch, it may be **metabolic** and result from variations in the clearance of vasoactive metabolites, and/or it may be **endothelially dependent** and reflect variations in production of vasoactive endothelial products released in response to shear stress.

Primer on the Autonomic Nervous System

Metabolic control is the second level of control and overrides autoregulation. Two kinds of metabolic signals are of importance: blood gases and local metabolic products of neuronal activity. Blood gases, specifically O_2 and CO_2, may profoundly influence global rCBF. The response to hypercarbia is direct and described by a continuous hyperbolic function. At midzone, with $PaCO_2$ corresponding to normal resting levels, rCBF is at its normal value. However, small changes in the $PaCO_2$ will substantially elevate (**hypoventilation**) or reduce (**hyperventilation**) rCBF. Regulation by CO_2 is vascular and results from alterations in vasoconstriction in response to changes in extracellular pH.

In contrast, the response to hypoxia is unimodal so that rCBF is not changed in the face of progressive hypoxia until PaO_2 falls below approximately 50 mm Hg. It then increases steeply as the PaO_2 falls. The response of rCBF to hypoxia is not entirely the result of direct actions upon blood vessels: it may, in part, be neurogenic and reflexive. However, it does not result from stimulation of arterial chemoreceptors but rather appears to result from direct stimulation of chemosensors on neurons in the lower brainstem, notably the **rostral ventrolateral reticular nucleus** (RVL).

A second form of metabolic regulation relates to elevations of rCBF associated with increased **neuronal activity**. The linkage of metabolism and flow overlaps topographically and forms the basis of functional mapping of the human brain by positron emission tomography (PET) or fast functional MRI. The underlying assumption for this mode of regulation is that active neurons generate metabolic products which, upon diffusion, produce local vasodilation. The vasodilator metabolites(s) responsible have yet to be definitively identified. Candidates include H^+, K^+, lactate, CO_2, nitric oxide (NO), and adenosine.

An alternative view is that the activity of a few interneurons may couple neuronal activity to flow by the release of vasoactive molecules. Theoretically, such neurons may not generate sufficient amounts of diffusible metabolites to influence rCBF but rather they increase flow by release of specific vasodilator signals.

Neurogenic regulation is a third level of regulation, in turn, superimposed on the autoregulatory and metabolic mechanisms. Two types of neurogenic control exist: **peripheral neurogenic regulation** and **intrinsic or central neurogenic regulation.**

Peripheral neurogenic regulation is mediated by neurons whose axons lie outside the CNS and directly innervate extracerebral vessels. There are three principal neuronal sources. **Sympathetic vasomotor** nerves derive from sympathetic ganglia, notably the superior cervical ganglia, and store, synthesize, and release the vasoconstrictors norepinephrine and neuropeptide Y (NPY). **Parasympathetic vasomotor** nerves arise from parasympathetic ganglia (e.g., sphenopalatine) and release the vasodilators acetylcholine and vasoactive intestinal peptide (VIP). **Trigeminal** nerves also innervate cerebral vessels through peripheral branches of bipolar neurons in the trigeminal ganglion and release the vasodilator peptides substance P (SP) and calcitonin gene-related peptide (CGRP). The release of the trigeminal vasodilators occurs largely as part of an axon reflex in response to painful or damaging stimuli. The peripheral innervation of cerebral vessels influences flow in large territories and may also contribute to trophic regulation of blood vessels.

The **intrinsic** or **central neurogenic** regulation of the cerebral circulation results from the activity of neurons whose processes are entirely contained within the CNS. The systems regulating rCBF are, for the most part, represented in brain nuclei governing the autonomic nervous system. The principal evidence for such control is that electrical or chemical stimulation of several critical brain areas, including the cerebellar fastigial nucleus, the rostral ventral medulla, the midline thalamus, the basal forebrain, and some other areas of the brainstem reticular formation, may profoundly and diffusely: (a) elevate rCBF but not metabolism (primary vasodilation); (b) increase cerebral metabolism, and secondarily, rCBF (secondary vasodilation); and (c) reduce metabolism and flow together (secondary vasoconstriction).

Primary vasodilation, which is greatest in cerebral cortex, appears dependent upon the activity of intrinsic neurons which, when activated, may generate local electrical and vascular signals. Primary vasodilation also has relevance in that, when initiated, it suspends cerebrovascular autoregulation, making rCBF dependent upon systemic blood pressure. Primary vasodilation may be part of an anticipatory system of brain which permits the cerebral circulation to prepare for increased metabolic demand before metabolism is engaged.

Interestingly, some of the networks which subserve central neurogenic vasodilation also appear to mediate a novel **central neurogenic neuroprotection.** Thus, stimulation of the cerebellar fastigial nucleus may reduce, by 50%, the volume of the focal ischemia infarction produced by occlusion of the middle cerebral artery in rat. The mechanism for the neuroprotection is not known but appears not to be the result of elevating rCBF and/or reduction of metabolism in the salvaged zone. Whether it results from transcription of neuroprotective genes molecules, suppression of expression of neurotoxic molecules, and/or modification of ion channels is not known.

References

1. Edvinsson L, MacKenzie ET, McCulloch J, eds. Cerebral blood flow and metabolism. New York: Raven Press, 1993:1–683.
2. Heistad DD. Autoregulation, hypertension and regulation of the cerebral circulation. In: Caplan LR, ed. Brain ischemia. Berlin: Springer-Verlag, 1995:237–46.
3. Reis DJ, Golanov EV. Central neurogenic regulation of regional cerebral blood flow (rCBF) and relationship to neuroprotection. In: Caplan LR, ed. Brain ischemia. Berlin: Springer-Verlag, 1995:273–88.
4. Reis DJ, Iadecola C. Intrinsic central neural regulation of cerebral blood flow and metabolism in relation to volume transmission. In: Fuxe K, Agnati L, eds. Volume transmission in the brain: new aspects of eletrical and chemical communication. New York: Raven Press, 1991:523–38.

10 High- and Low-Pressure Baroreflexes

Dwain L. Eckberg
Hunter Holmes McGuire Department of Veterans Affairs Medical Center
Medical College of Virginia
Richmond, Virginia

High- and low-pressure baroreflexes represent classic **negative feedback mechanisms.** Pressure changes alter firing of stretch–sensitive neurons located in the walls of vessels and cardiac chambers. Changes of baroreceptor input to the brain provoke changes of neural output from vagal and sympathetic motoneurons. These changes of efferent nerve activity set in motion cardiovascular adjustments which counter the pressure changes that initiated the cascade of neurological events. Thus, baroreflex mechanisms finely tune heart rate, atrioventricular node conduction, myocardial contractility and electrophysiologic properties, and peripheral resistance, on a beat-by-beat basis, and dampen the effects of environmental perturbations that arise during everyday living. This chapter focuses primarily on **arterial** baroreflexes in **healthy humans.**

Anatomy

Arterial baroreceptors are located in the adventitia of the carotid sinuses and aortic arch. Neurons thought to be baroreceptors appear in histologic sections as complex arborizations, onion–like structures, or free nerve endings. All barosensitive neurons are tethered to surrounding structures; this coupling contributes viscoelastic properties that figure importantly in baroreceptor transduction. Afferent baroreceptor impulses travel over rapidly conducting, myelinated and slowly conducting, unmyelinated nerve fibers in the carotid sinus and aortic nerves to the medulla.

The experimental literature lumps (inappropriately) a variety of heterogeneous receptors located in the walls of other intrathoracic vessels and the heart, as **cardiopulmonary baroreceptors.** These receptors are widely distributed, in the superior and inferior vena cavae; atria, ventricles, and coronary arteries; and pulmonary arteries and veins. Afferent fibers from cardiopulmonary receptors course with sympathetic nerves to the spinal cord, and with vagus nerves to the medulla. Most myelinated afferent cardiopulmonary neurons fire with periodicities related to atrial or ventricular events; most unmyelinated afferent neurons fire sporadically, without clear relation to cardiac events.

Nearly all baroreceptor neurons, cardiopulmonary and arterial, converge on the same neuron pools (and in about 15% of instances, on the same neurons) in the **nucleus tractus solitarii** (solitary tract nucleus) of the medulla. Because of its position as a way station for incoming baroreceptor information, this nucleus may be a major center for arterial and cardiopulmonary baroreflex integration (4). Incoming baroreceptor information is carried over interneurons (with many possibilities for interactions with other neural activity, including particularly, that related to respiration), to vagal motoneurons in the medulla, and, via the rostral ventrolateral medulla, to sympathetic motoneurons in the spinal cord.

Transduction

Arterial baroreceptors sense **distortion,** not pressure. However, since the degrees of pressure and distortion usually are related closely, baroreceptor transduction is discussed in terms of pressure changes. Arterial baroreceptors are extraordinarily sensitive; they respond to changes of arterial **flow** that do not provoke measurable changes of pressure. (This assertion may be true in part because the ability of laboratory devices to transduce pressure changes is crude, relative to that of baroreceptors.) Individual receptors begin firing when some **threshold** pressure is exceeded, fire in proportion (that is, nearly **linearly**) to further pressure elevations, and reach a **saturation** level, above which additional increases of pressure do not provoke increases of firing.

Recordings made from families of baroreceptor neurons document a smoothly rounded threshold region—a gradual increase, rather than the abrupt onset of firing that occurs in individual baroreceptors. This appearance results because as pressure increases, more baroreceptors are recruited, and those whose firing had already commenced fire at more rapid rates. Thus, the relation between arterial pressure and multifiber baroreceptor nerve activity is **sigmoid,** with threshold, linear, and saturation regions. In animals, and probably also in humans, resting arterial pressure (called the **operational,** or **set point**) lies on the linear portion of this relation.

The viscoelastic coupling of baroreceptors to their surroundings exerts an important influence on their function. One manifestation of this is **rate sensitivity:** rapid pressure changes elicit more rapid firing rates than slow pressure changes. Another is **adaptation:** firing rates are more rapid at the beginning of a step increase of pressure than they are at the end. A third is **hysteresis:** firing rates are greater when pressure is increasing than when pressure is returning to baseline levels.

Figure 1 illustrates firing patterns of a single rat arterial baroreceptor, during cyclic mechanical stretching, plotted as functions of the baseline degree of stretch. In each of the three insets, the top tracing is nerve firing, the middle tracing is the degree of stretch, and the bottom tracing is the instantaneous baroreceptor firing frequency. The bottom inset is particularly insightful: it depicts virtual silence of the baroreceptor at low levels of stretch, and asymmetry of firing during stretch, such that firing is more rapid on the rising than on the falling portion of each stretch.

Methods for Study of Human Baroreflexes

Although two groups have recorded human arterial baroreceptor traffic directly (during neck surgery), virtually all that is known about human baroreflex function is derived from correlations between R–R interval (or heart rate) or sympathetic nerve activity, and spontaneous or provoked changes of arterial distending pressure (2). Such correlations usually yield a baroreflex

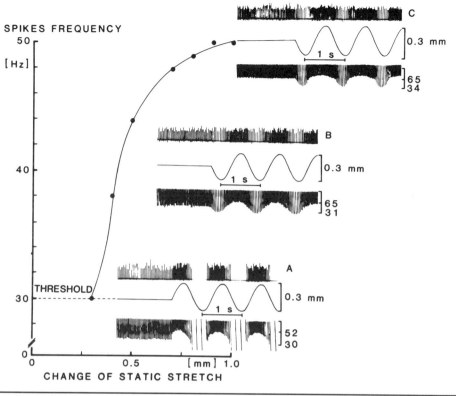

Figure 1.   Firing patterns of a single rat aortic baroreceptor to cyclic stretch. Reproduced with permission from Arndt JO, Dorrenhaus A, Wiecken H. J Physiol Lond 1975;252:59–78.

slope (or **gain**) over a very limited range of the linear portion of the sigmoid arterial pressure–vagal, or reverse sigmoid–sympathetic response relation.

More information on baroreflex responses can be obtained when pressure changes are elicited experimentally. For example substantial elevations (amounting to tens of mm Hg) can be provoked by Valsalva maneuvers (voluntary straining against a closed glottis). After release of straining, R–R interval increases can be plotted as functions of preceding arterial (usually systolic) pressures to derive baroreflex slopes and, sometimes, indications of baroreflex threshold. **Bolus injections** or **infusions** of vasoactive drugs, such as sodium **nitroprusside** or **phenylephrine** hydrochloride, can be given to provoke arterial pressure changes, and these pressure changes can be related to R–R intervals and sympathetic nerve activity. (However, it may be difficult to effect major changes of arterial pressure with vasoactive drug infusions in subjects who have very responsive baroreflexes.) **Sequential** injections of a vasodepressor followed by a vasoconstrictor agent may yield information on baroreflex thresholds, as well as slopes in the linear range.

Finally, **pressure or suction** can be applied as single or repetitive pulses to a chamber worn around the neck, to modify carotid transmural pressure. This approach has two advantages. First, activity of only one barosensitive area, the carotid baroreceptors, can be modified selectively. Second, very large pressure changes (limited primarily by subjects' tolerances) can be applied. [One method (2) employs a brief 40 mm Hg pressure increment, followed by a series of 15 mm Hg pressure decrements, to −65 mm Hg—a total change of 105 mm Hg.] Neck chamber methods have several disadvantages: Although pressure is transmitted from the chamber to internal structures in the neck reproducibly in serial applications of neck pressure or suction, it is not transmitted totally. More importantly, changes of transmural carotid pressure provoked by neck pressure or suction are opposed by reflex changes of arterial pressure sensed by aortic baroreceptors. Since all baroreceptor inputs terminate on the same solitary tract nucleus neuron pool, abrupt changes of carotid baroreceptor activity occurring simultaneously with opposing changes of aortic baroreceptor activity are discounted. For example, sustained (lasting seconds) neck pressure may alter efferent sympathetic nerve traffic for only one heart beat. (Vagal or R–R interval responses to carotid baroreceptor stimulation last longer than sympathetic responses.) Probably as a result of aortic baroreceptor opposition, baroreflex slopes measured during neck pressure changes are much less than baroreflex slopes measured during arterial pressure changes (which provoke parallel changes of firing in **all** baroreceptors).

One problem besets all methods used to estimate baroreflex gain during sustained (lasting more than 1 sec) changes of baroreceptor input: because baroreflex adjustments occur so rapidly, measured arterial pressure changes represent pressure changes driving baroreceptors, **less** baroreflex-mediated pressure adjustments.

It is unlikely that noninvasive methods can alter activity of human **cardiopulmonary** baroreceptors selectively. A genre of literature from humans and animals is based on the notion that experimental perturbations, such as infusions of "subpressor" doses of pressor agents, leg raising, mild hemorrhage or volume infusion, or lower body suction, which alter pressure measured in the cardiopulmonary region (usually in the vena cavae or right atrium), but which do not alter pressure measured in arteries, are selective for cardiopulmonary receptors. The fallacy in this thinking arises from at least two mistaken notions. The first is that the cardiovascular system can be segmented; since this system is continuous, it is theoretically unlikely that a perturbation can be applied to one segment that does not affect all segments. The second is that arterial baroreceptors sense pressure; baroreceptors sense changes of dimensions, not pressure. Therefore, absence of pressure changes cannot be taken as evidence for absence of dimension changes. (This assertion is related to the fact that arterial baroreceptors are so sensitive and efficient that they can respond to changes of dimension in baroreceptive arteries by restoring arterial pressure nearly perfectly.) Although minor levels (20 mm Hg or less) of lower body suction (the prototype of experimental interventions used in humans to perturb cardiopulmonary receptors "selectively") do not alter arterial pressure, they provoke major reduction of carotid artery and ascending aorta dimensions (6).

Integrated Baroreflex Responses

Figure 2 depicts average muscle sympathetic nerve and R–R interval responses of a group of healthy subjects to abrupt increases or decreases of

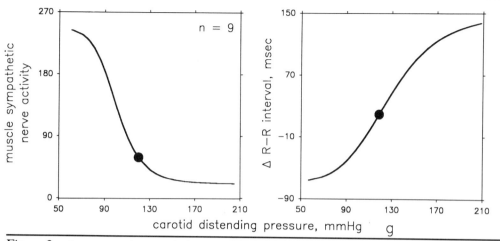

Figure 2. Average muscle sympathetic nerve and R–R interval responses of a group of healthy subjects to brief neck pressure or suction. The closed circle indicates resting arterial pressure.

carotid baroreceptor input provoked by brief neck pressure or suction. These data illustrate several important features of human baroreflex function. First, in humans as in animals, the relation between arterial distending pressure and vagal–cardiac nerve activity is sigmoid (reverse sigmoid, in the case of sympathetic nerve activity). Second, resting pressure (denoted by the closed circles) lies on the linear portion of both relations; therefore, **all** arterial pressure changes elicit sympathetic and vagal neural responses. Third, in healthy young supine subjects (as were studied to obtain these data), resting arterial pressure is only slightly below the threshold for sympathetic activation. In such subjects, baseline levels of sympathetic activity are low, and small elevations of arterial pressure above baseline levels silence muscle sympathetic motoneurons.

Figure 3 illustrates how arterial baroreceptors control vagus nerve traffic to the heart (as reflected by R–R intervals), and sympathetic nerve traffic to the large (about 40% of body mass), muscle vascular bed. During increases and decreases of arterial pressure provoked by infusions of phenylephrine and nitroprusside, sympathetic and vagal traffic varied reciprocally. At the highest pressure (top row), sympathetic "bursts" were absent and fluctuations of R–R intervals were maximal, and at the lowest pressure (bottom row), sympathetic bursts were plentiful and large, and fluctuations of R–R intervals were nearly absent.

The role of baroreceptors in setting **absolute levels** of arterial pressure is controversial. Denervation of arterial baroreceptors leads to permanent and large lability of arterial pressure, but to only transient arterial pressure elevation. However, subsequent denervation of cardiopulmonary receptors leads to sustained hypertension. This indicates that arterial, but not cardiopulmonary, baroreceptors buffer rapid fluctuations of arterial pressure, and that in the absence of arterial baroreceptors, cardiopulmonary baroreceptors can maintain arterial pressure at normal levels.

Baroreflex Resetting

Tethering of baroreceptors to surrounding structures introduces a viscoelastic element which importantly determines baroreceptor function. After the

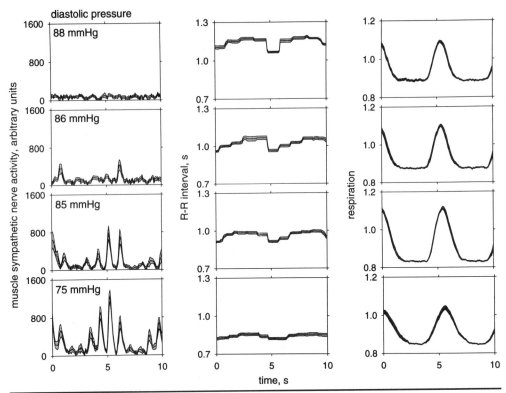

Figure 3.   Average (±SEM) muscle symapthetic nerve traffic and R–R intervals of one supine healthy subject, at different arterial pressures during infusions of phenylephrine (top row), saline (second row), and nitroprusside (bottom two rows).

beginning of abrupt distention of a baroreceptive artery, afferent baroreceptor nerve traffic decays (or **adapts**) as a power function; that is, the log of baroreceptor nerve firing, plotted as a function of the log of pressure, is linear. After an abrupt step increase of pressure, baroreceptor firing decays to about one-fourth of its peak value in less than 0.5 sec. One practical implication of this is that changes of baroreceptor nerve activity provoked by sustained stimuli, such as neck suction, are likely to decline very rapidly. (The experimental literature contains numerous examples of studies in which the tacit and erroneous assumption is made that increases of baroreceptor nerve traffic are the same at the beginning as at the end of neck suction.)

The relation between arterial pressure and efferent autonomic outflow is highly fluid. This is illustrated by Fig. 4. These sigmoid arterial pressure input–vagal-cardiac nerve output relations were measured in two supine subjects studied while awake, every 3 hr, for 24 hr. Shifts of the stimulus–response relations shown in this figure occur very rapidly (within tens of seconds) during experimentally induced arterial pressure changes, and extend the range of pressures over which baroreflexes are operative.

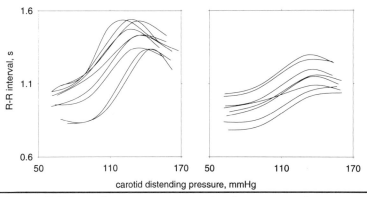

Figure 4. Average R–R interval responses to a ramped neck pressure–suction sequence of two subjects studied, while awake, over 24 hr.

Cardiopulmonary Baroreflexes

Hainsworth ably reviewed reflexes triggered by **cardiac** receptors. It seems unlikely that small changes of effective blood volume, such as those provoked by low levels of lower body suction, alter cardiopulmonary, but not arterial baroreceptor, function. Nonetheless, there are several human reflex responses that seem to be initiated by cardiopulmonary receptors. One is the human response to intracoronary injections of **radiographic contrast medium.** The simultaneous occurrence of bradycardia and hypotension suggests that during such injections, arterial baroreflex responses are overridden. (The combination of hypotension and bradycardia occurs also during inferior left ventricular ischemia.) A second is the marked diuresis that sometimes accompanies **supraventricular tachycardias,** which may represent a neurohumoral response initiated by atrial receptors.

References

1. Arndt JO, Dorrenhaus A, Wiecken H. The aortic arch baroreceptor response to static and dynamic stretches in an isolated aorta–depressor nerve preparation of cats in vitro. J Physiol Lond 1975;252:59–78.
2. Eckberg DL, Sleight P. Human baroreflexes in health and disease. Oxford: Clarendon Press, 1992.
3. Hainsworth R. Reflexes from the heart. Physiol Rev 1991;71:617–58.
4. Mifflin SW, Felder RB. Synaptic mechanisms regulating cardiovascular afferent inputs to solitary tract nucleus. Am J Physiol 1990;259:H653–61.
5. Persson P. Cardiopulmonary receptors in "neurogenic hypertension." Acta Physiol Scand 1988; 570:1–53.
6. Taylor JA, Halliwill JR, Brown TE, Hayano J, Eckberg DL. 'Nonhypotensive' hypovolaemia reduces ascending aortic dimensions in humans. J Physiol Lond 1995;483:289–298.

11

The Bezold–Jarisch Reflex

Virend K. Somers
Cardiovascular Division
Department of Medicine
The University of Iowa
Iowa City, Iowa

Allyn L. Mark
College of Medicine
The University of Iowa
Iowa City, Iowa

Introduction

The heart serves not only as a pump, but also as a sensory organ with both neural and endocrine functions. Stimulation of sensory nerve endings in the heart can induce potent reflex hemodynamic effects, primarily vasodilation and bradycardia. Activation of this reflex may contribute to **neurocardiogenic** or **vasovagal syncope** and to exertional syncope in **aortic stenosis**. The cardiac inhibitory reflex should be suspected whenever hypotension is associated with paradoxical bradycardia, such as during inferoposterior myocardial infarction.

Physiology

The afferent limb of the reflex consists of cardiac sensory nerve endings which originate in the atria and ventricles and travel via the **vagus** to the central nervous system. The sensory receptors are distributed predominantly in the ventricles and are activated by chemical agents such as **veratrum alkaloids, nicotine,** and **phenyldiguanide.** Mechanical stimulation of the ventricle, either by acute increases in left ventricular pressures and inotropism or by ventricular distortion, also elicits the reflex.

Clinical Conditions Predisposing to Activation of the Bezold–Jarisch Reflex

Afferents for the reflex are distributed preferentially in the **inferoposterior wall of the left ventricle.** Thus, in animal studies occlusion of the circumflex coronary artery (supplying the inferoposterior left ventricle) results in hypotension and bradycardia, and no reflex skeletal muscle vasoconstriction in response to the hypotension. These reflex responses are less pronounced with occlusion of the left anterior descending artery (supplying the anterior wall). Vagotomy abolishes the reflex inhibitory response to occlusion of the circumflex artery. In humans, there is an increased incidence of bradyarrhythmias and hypotension in inferior wall infarction (70%) as compared to anterior wall infarction (30%). In patients with Prinzmetal's angina, spasm of vessels supplying the inferior myocardium induces bradycardia, in contrast to tachycardia during anterior wall ischemia. Following intracoronary thrombolytic therapy, patients with

right coronary artery occlusion and reperfusion have a greater incidence of bradycardia and hypotension than those with left coronary reperfusion, in whom hypertension and tachycardia are more frequent. During coronary arteriography, bradycardia and hypotension are most marked during injections into a dominant right coronary artery, supplying the inferior wall of the heart.

The Bezold–Jarisch reflex may also be implicated in **exertional syncope** in patients with **aortic stenosis.** During exercise in normal subjects blood pressure and heart rate increase in response to stimulation of somatic afferent receptors in skeletal muscle (Fig. 1). The increased blood pressure results from increased cardiac output and vasoconstriction in viscera and in nonactive muscles. In patients with aortic stenosis, leg exercise is associated with increased left ventricular end-diastolic pressure and absence of vasoconstriction in the nonexercising (forearm) muscle. Furthermore, in patients with aortic stenosis and a history of exertional syncope, paradoxical forearm **vasodilation** occurs during leg exercise. After valve replacement, the paradoxical forearm vasodilation is replaced by forearm vasoconstriction during exercise.

Acute hypotension occurs in about 30% of patients during **hemodialysis.** Possible etiologies include pericardial effusion and tamponade or autonomic neuropathy. However, Converse *et al.* recently showed that patients with hypotension during dialysis often have intact sympathetic activity, but with reduction

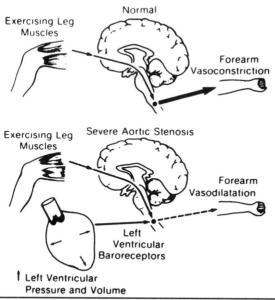

Figure 1. Schematic diagram showing effects of activation of left ventricular baroreceptors during exercise in patients with severe aortic stenosis. The upper schematic shows afferent impulses originating in exercising leg muscle, normally producing reflex vasoconstriction in the nonexercising forearm. The lower schematic shows increased left ventricular pressure with activation of left ventricular baroreceptors and consequent inhibition, and reversal, of forearm vasoconstriction. Reprinted with permission from the American College of Cardiology (J Am Col Cardiol 1983;1:90–102).

of intravascular volume develop paradoxical bradycardia, vasodilation, sympathetic inhibition and profound hypotension. In these patients, echocardiographic studies demonstrated that hemodialysis was accompanied by progressive reduction in left ventricular end systolic dimensions with virtual cavity obliteration prior to hypotensive episodes. In hypotension-resistant hemodialysis patients, arterial pressure remained stable throughout dialysis, with progressive increases in heart rate and sympathetic activity. Thus, excessive myocardial contraction around an empty chamber, with consequent deformation of ventricular mechanoreceptors, may activate the cardiac inhibitory reflex and promote hypotension and syncope in patients on hemodialysis.

There has recently been a surge of interest in the use of **upright tilt** as a diagnostic test in patients with recurrent neurocardiogenic or vasovagal syncope. In many of these patients, upright tilt results in **hypotension with paradoxical bradycardia** and syncope. Sequential AV pacing does not prevent syncope, indicating a potent vasodilator component. There is marked withdrawal of efferent sympathetic nerve activity to muscle blood vessels during vasovagal syncope in humans (Fig. 2). Prolonged upright tilt with pooling of blood in the lower extremities results in decreased cardiac filling pressure and increased myocardial contractility. This can produce activation of cardiac mechanoreceptors with consequent sympathetic withdrawal, vasodilation, bradycardia, and syncope. Release of humoral agents such as epinephrine, vasopressin, and prostaglandins potentiate this response.

Mechanisms other than the Bezold–Jarisch reflex may be implicated in **neurocardiogenic syncope.** Vasodepressor syncope has been reported during nitroprusside infusion in a patient after heart transplantation, where ventricular vagal afferent pathways are presumably denervated. A study of patients after heart transplantation revealed that 7 of 10 patients demonstrated bradycardia and hypotension during upright tilt. In 4 of these patients there was no evidence of vagal efferent reinnervation. Thus, left ventricular receptors alone may not completely explain all cases of simultaneous hypotension and bradycardia.

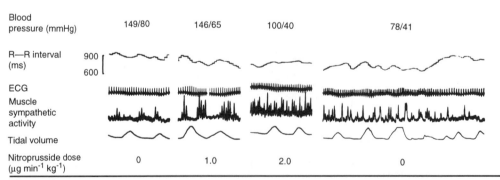

Figure 2.   Vasovagal response during sodium nitroprusside infusion in a healthy subject. Initially, as arterial blood pressure decreases, muscle sympathetic nerve activity increases. Impending vasovagal syncope is accompanied by a fall in blood pressure with simultaneous reduction in sympathetic nerve discharge [reproduced from Ref. (6) with permission].

In this regard, recent studies indicate a possible role for humoral substances such as **serotonin** and **nitric oxide** in mediating simultaneous hypotension and bradycardia. These may act at a central neural level. During severe hemorrhagic hypotension in rats, paradoxical bradycardia and sympathetic withdrawal are accompanied by increased sympathetic activity to the adrenal gland. This increased adrenal nerve activity is prevented by inhibitors of serotonin synthesis. Serotonin administration into cerebral ventricles can induce hypotension, inhibition of renal sympathetic activity, and increased adrenal sympathetic activity. Thus, **serotonin** may act centrally to **inhibit reflex sympathetic activation** and serotonin antagonists may be effective in preventing vasodepressor syncope. **Nitric oxide** has also been reported to act as a central neurotransmitter which might **inhibit sympathetic nerve activity** and promote bradycardia and hypotension. The role of serotonin and nitric oxide in reflex control and the pathogenesis of neurocardiogenic syncope in humans is unclear.

References

1. Mark, AL. The Bezold–Jarisch reflex revisited: clinical implications of inhibitory reflexes originating in the heart. J Am Coll Cardiol 1983;1:90–102.
2. Converse RL, Jr., Jacobsen TN, Jost CMT, Toto RD, Grayburn PA, Obregon TM, Fouad–Tarazi F, Victor RG. Paradoxical withdrawal of reflex vasoconstriction as a cause of hemodialysis-induced hypotension. J Clin Invest 1992;90:1657–65.
3. Sra JS, Jazayeri MR, Avitall B, Dhala A, Deshpande S, Blanck Z, Akhtar, M. Comparison of cardiac pacing with drug therpay in the treatment of neurocardiogenic (vasovagal) syncope with bradycardia or asystole. N Engl J Med 1993;328:1085–90.
4. Wallin BG, Sundlof G. Sympathetic outflow to muscles during vasovagal syncope. J Auton Nerv Syst 1982;6:287–91.
5. Fitzpatrick AP, Banner NA, Cheng A, Yacoub M, Sutton R. Vasovagal reactions may occur after orthotopic heart transplantation. J Am Coll Cardiol 1993;21:1132–37.
6. Eckberg DL, Sleight P. In: Human baroreflexes in health and disease, Oxford, New York: Clarendon Press, 1992:153–215.

12   *Other Cardiovascular Reflexes*

Michael J. Joyner
Department of Anesthesiology
Mayo Clinic
Rochester, Minnesota

Overview

The discussion of cardiovascular reflexes generally focuses on those reflexes that sense changes in arterial blood pressure and central blood volume. However, several important mechanisms play a key role in regulating the cardiovascular and autonomic responses to stresses such as exercise and the upright posture, and in regulating complex autonomic responses to mental stress. Four general mechanisms that govern some of the autonomic responses to these common physiologic events deserve attention: (1) **Muscle chemoreflexes.** Muscle chemoreflexes are subserved by fine afferents located within skeletal muscles. These afferents are activated by metabolites, from contracting skeletal muscles, and evoke reflex increases in arterial pressure when activated. (2) **Central command** is a mechanism that provides immediate "feed forward" adjustments of heart rate, blood pressure, respiration, and potentially blood flow during the preparation for the initiation of exercise. This mechanism is thought to govern the rapid increases in these variables that occur during the onset of exercise. (3) **Veno–arteriolar axon reflex.** This is a mechanism that causes local vasoconstriction during periods of venous distention. It may account for up to 40% of the vasoconstriction observed in limbs during assumption of the upright posture. (4) **Mental stress.** There are complex autonomic responses during mental or emotional stress including a marked, neurally mediated muscle vasodilation.

Muscle Chemoreflexes and Central Command

Skeletal muscles are innervated by thinly myelinated group III afferents and unmyelinated group IV afferents. These afferents synapse in the dorsal root ganglia and stimulate spinal neurons that travel centrally and activate the brainstem cardiovascular centers (1, 2). These afferents are sensitive to various mechanical and chemical stimuli. The first clear demonstration of the potential importance of these afferents in the autonomic adjustments to exercise was made in the 1930s when the heart rate and blood pressure responses to handgrip exercise were observed during conditions of unrestricted blood flow to the contracting forearm muscles and also when an arm cuff was inflated to above systolic blood pressure to render the muscles ischemic. Under ischemic conditions the rise in blood pressure with contractions was markedly augmented (1). Additionally, when forearm ischemia was maintained in the absence of exercise (postexercise ischemia) the blood pressure remained at the high level observed during exercise. By contrast, during exercise without arm ischemia or when arm ischemia stopped at the end of exercise, the rise in pressure observed during exercise returned rapidly toward control values. It was hypothesized that the afferents located within the skeletal muscle sensitive to the metabolic by products of contractions stimulated the marked rise in arterial pressure. In a subsequent study, made in a patient with selective sensory denervation in one leg but normal motor strength, postexercise ischemia was not associated with increased blood pressure after contractions ceased (Fig. 1).

At rest, and during mild exercise, group III afferents are primarily mechanosensitive and group IV afferents are primarily chemosensitive, responding to a variety of metabolic stimuli including K^+, hydrogen ion, phosphate, and adenosine. Additionally, the group III afferents can become sensitized during exercise so that they also respond to chemical stimuli (1, 2).

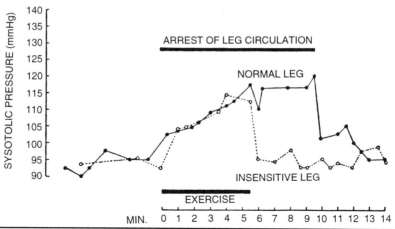

Figure 1. Original figure from Alam and Smirk (Clin Sci 1938;3:247–252) demonstrating that when sensory nerves from muscles are interrupted, postexercise ischemia fails to maintain the increase in arterial pressure after exercise stops. This experiment confirmed the existence of a "muscle chemoreflex" that depended on afferents from skeletal muscles. Of note is the similarity of the pressure responses during exercise which suggest either that the chemosensitive afferents do not contribute to the rise in pressure during exercise, or that when their input is eliminated, other blood pressure-regulating signals, such as central command, operate to increase arterial pressure (figure used with permission).

What is the function of the rise in pressure? Several investigators have hypothesized that the purpose of the afferents is to sense a mismatch between blood flow and metabolism in the active muscles. Such a flow/metabolism mismatch would lead to the build–up of "ischemic" metabolites. These metabolites would then stimulate the fine afferents and evoke a reflex increase in arterial pressure (1, 2). This increase in pressure would then improve perfusion of the active muscles and reduce or eliminate the flow metabolism mismatch. There is evidence in exercising animals to suggest this scheme occurs. By contrast, it is unclear in humans if these afferents play an important role in matching blood flow and metabolism in the active muscles (1, 2).

Observations over many years have demonstrated that there was an instantaneous rise in heart rate and respiration at the onset of **exercise.** Additionally these adaptations occur at a speed that cannot be accounted for on the basis of reflexes (1, 2). In this context, a neural signal proportional to the central motor drive is thought to activate the brainstem cardiovascular centers. Several lines of evidence favor the existence of a **central command** signal. First, the heart rate and blood pressure responses to exercise are greater in humans who have been partially paralyzed with curare (2). Second, stimulation of key locomotor centers in anesthetized animals can also evoke increases in heart rate and respiration. Observations similar to these form the experimental basis supporting the concept of central command.

Several important points would be made about **central command** and **muscle chemoreflex** mechanisms. First, the signals are primarily involved with autonomic regulation during exercise. There are a host of physiologic mechanisms in addition to these two which can undoubtedly contribute to the physiological adjustments in exercise. In this context, experimental maneuvers which reduce or eliminate the role of central command or muscle chemoreflexes can have very little overall effect on the autonomic responses to exercise (1, 2). Such observations do not lessen the potential importance of these mechanisms during exercise in intact subjects, but merely point out that they are not essential to observe the normal exercise response and also that physiologic adjustments to exercise are under the influence of multiple redundant control and regulatory mechanisms. The second important point that should be made about these two mechanisms is that in addition to their primary functions, they also appear to **reset arterial baroreflexes.** In these circumstances the set point of arterial baroreflexes increases and normal regulation of heart rate and blood pressure occurs around an elevated baseline. This resetting of arterial baroreflexes is thought to permit the rise in arterial pressure seen both during muscle chemoreflex activation and when central command is engaged. Finally, under normal physiologic conditions these two mechanisms operate together to regulate the autonomic responses to exercise.

Veno-arteriolar Axon Reflex

The **upright posture** also represents an important physiologic challenge that humans routinely respond to on a daily basis. As a result of the upright posture there is a shift in blood volume from the thorax to the lower extremities, a reduction of venous return, and the need to activate peripheral vasoconstrictor mechanisms to maintain arterial pressure in the face of lower venous return and cardiac output. An important and underappreciated reflex that contributes to this peripheral vasoconstrictor response is the **veno-arteriolar axon reflex** (3). This reflex is a **local reflex** that does not require integration at the level of spinal cord or brain. When a limb is lowered below heart level there is **venous distention** in the limb under observation. This venous distention appears to evoke, via local mechanisms, **vasoconstriction** in the blood vessels perfusing that limb.

Henriksen, in a series of studies, has demonstrated the presence of this reflex in patients with spinal cord lesions and also in patients undergoing spinal anesthesia (3). These observations confirm the local nature of this reflex. Additionally, he has calculated that up to 40% of the increase in vascular resistance observed upon standing can be accounted for on the basis of the veno–arteriolar axon reflex. Finally, this reflex appears to occur in skin adipose tissue and skeletal muscle of the limbs.

Physiologic Responses to Emotional Stress

Emotional or mental stress is one of the most frequent stresses encountered during everyday life (4). Emotional stress can cause marked alterations in cardiac output, blood pressure, heart rate, sweating, and gastrointestinal function. It is also well known that severe emotional stress can cause marked vasodilation in forearm skeletal muscle. The increases in forearm blood flow during emotional stress can be as marked as those seen during heavy forearm exercise. Such vasodilation may also contribute to emotional fainting.

L–NMMA

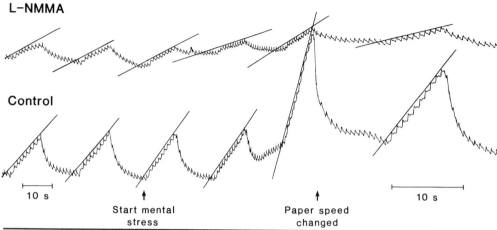

Control

10 s   ↑   ↑   10 s

Start mental   Paper speed
stress   changed

Figure 2.   Original plethysmographic record of the forearm blood flow (FBF) responses to mental stress. FBF is proportional to the slope and was measured using venous occlusion plethysmography. An increase in slope means that FBF rose. The top tracing shows the response in the forearm treated with the NO synthase blocker L–NMMA. The bottom tracing shows the control forearm. Baseline FBF was lower in the forearm treated with L–NMMA. The marked rise in FBF that commenced in the control forearm about 40 sec after the onset of mental stress was absent in the forearm treated with L–NMMA. This demonstrates the key role NO can play during neurogenic vasodilation in the forearm during mental stress. The recorder speed was increased after the dramatic rise in flow to facilitate analysis of the tracing. Figure from Ref. (5) (used with permission).

It is known that intact innervation of the upper extremity is required to observe this forearm vasodilation and roughly 50% of this vasodilation can be blocked by selective administration of atropine to one forearm muscle (4, 5). Recent observations indicate that up to 70% of the vasodilation observed in the forearm during mental stress can be blocked by the **nitric oxide synthase inhibitor** monomethyl arginine (L–NMMA) (see Fig. 2 and Ref. (5)). These observations suggest that forearm skeletal muscles are innervated with **cholinergic vasodilator fibers** and that these fibers may also either release **nitric oxide** (NO) or stimulate the vascular endothelium to release nitric oxide. These observations are some of the first to suggest that neurally mediated release of the vasodilating substance NO may play a key role in regulating autonomic function in conscious humans. Responses to mental stress also show that there can be fight or flight vasodilation in humans similar to the defense reaction seen during brain stimulation in animal models.

References

1. Joyner MJ. Muscle chemoreflexes and exercise in humans. Clin Auton Res 1992;2:201–8.
2. Rowell LB, O'Leary DS. Reflex control of the circulation during exercise: chemoreflexes and mechanoreflexes. J Appl Physiol 1990;69:407–18.
3. Henriksen O. Local sympathetic reflex mechanism in regulation of blood flow in human subcutaneous adipose tissue. Acta Physiol Scand 1977;101(Suppl. 450):1–48.
4. Roddie IC. Human responses to emotional stress. Ir J Med Sci 1977;146:395–417.
5. Dietz NM, Rivera JM, Eggener SE, Fix RT, Warner DO, Joyner MJ. Nitric oxide contributes to the rise in forearm blood flow during mental stress in humans. J Physiol (Lond) 1994;480:361–8.

13

Autonomic Control of the Pupil

H. Stanley Thompson
The University of Iowa
Iowa City, Iowa

The **iris** hangs in a bath of **aqueous humor.** The actions of the sphincter and dilator muscles on the size of the pupil are not impeded by bulky tissue, and they are in plain view (Fig. 1). It is not surprising that 80 to 100 years ago, at the very beginning of autonomic pharmacology, the pupil was frequently used as an indicator of drug action. In those years it was shown that parasympathetic and sympathetic neural impulses to the iris muscles could be modified by drugs at the synapses and at the effector sites because it was at these locations that the transmission of the impulse depended on chemical mediators. In the following paragraphs these well-known, autonomically active drugs are grouped according to the site and mechanism of their action.

A few general cautionary words should first be said about **the interpretation of pupillary responses** to topically instilled drugs. There are large **interindividual differences** in the responsiveness of the iris to typical drugs, and this becomes most evident when weak concentrations are used. For example, 0.25% **pilocarpine** will produce a minimal constriction in some patients and an intense miosis in others. This means that the most secure clinical judgments stem from comparisons with the action of the drug on the other, normal eye.

The general status of the patient will also influence the size of the pupils. If the patient becomes uncomfortable or anxious while waiting for the drug to act, both pupils may dilate. If the patient becomes drowsy, both pupils will constrict. Thus, if a judgment is to be made about the dilation or contraction of the pupil in response to a drug placed in the conjunctival sac, one pupil should be used as a control whenever possible.

Parasympatholytic (Anticholinergic) Drugs

The **belladonna alkaloids** occur naturally. They can be found in various proportions in deadly nightshade (*Atropa belladonna*), henbane (*Hyoscyamus niger*), and jimsonweed (*Datura stramonium*). Potions made from these plants were the tools of professional poisoners in ancient times. The word "belladonna" ("beautiful lady") was derived from the cosmetic use of these substances as mydriatics in sixteenth-century Venice. The mischief caused by the ubiquitous jimsonweed is typical of this group of plants. **Jimsonweed** has been used as a poison, has been taken as a hallucinogen, and has caused accidental illness and death, and it can cause an alarming accidental mydriasis. These solanaceous plants, which are related to the tomato, potato, and eggplant, are still cultivated for medical purposes.

Atropine and **scopolamine** block parasympathetic activity by competing with acetylcholine at the effector cells of the iris sphincter and ciliary muscle, thus preventing depolarization. After conjunctival instillation of atropine (1%),

mydriasis begins within about 10 min and is fully developed at 35 to 45 min; **cycloplegia** is complete within 1 hr. The pupil may stay dilated for several days, but accommodation usually returns in 48 hr. Scopolamine (0.2%) causes mydriasis that lasts, in an uninflamed eye, for about 2 days; it is a less effective cycloplegic than atropine.

Tropicamide and **cyclopentolate** are synthetic parasympatholytics with a relatively short duraton of action. Tropicamide (1%) is an effective, short-acting mydriatic (3 to 6 hr), which results in only a very transient paresis of accommodation. Compared with tropicamide, cyclopentolate (1%) seems to be a more effective cycloplegic and a slightly less effective mydriatic, especially in dark eye; accommodation takes about half a day to return and the pupil still may not be working perfectly after more than 24 hr.

Botulinum toxin blocks the release of acetylcholine, and **hemicholinium** interferes with the synthesis of acetylcholine both at the preganglionic and at the postganglionic nerve endings, thus interrupting the parasympathetic pathway in two places. The outflow of sympathetic impulses is also interrupted by systemic doses of these drugs, since the chemical mediator in sympathetic ganglia is also acetylcholine.

Parasympathomimetic (Cholinergic) Drugs

Pilocarpine and **methacholine** are structurally similar to acetylcholine and are capable of depolarizing the effector cell, thus causing miosis and spasm of accommodation. Methacholine sometimes is still used in a weak (2.5%) solution to test for cholinergic supersensitivity of the sphincter muscle in autonomic failure. It is being replaced by weak pilocarpine (0.1%).

Arecoline is a naturally occurring substance with an action similar to that of pilocarpine and methacholine; its chief advantage is that it acts quickly; a 0.025% solution produces a full miosis in 15 min (compared to 30 min for 1% pilocarpine).

Carbachol acts chiefly at the postganglionic cholinergic nerve ending to release the stores of acetylcholine. There is also some direct action of carbachol on the effector cell. A 1.5% solution causes intense miosis, but the drug does not penetrate the cornea easily and is therefore usually mixed with a wetting agent (1:3500 benzalkonium chloride).

Acetylcholine is liberated at the cholinergic nerve endings by the neural action potential and is promptly hydrolyzed and inactivated by cholinesterase. Cholinesterase, in turn, can be inactivated by any one of the many anticholinesterase drugs. These drugs either block the action of cholinesterase or deplete the stores of the enzyme in the tissue. They do not act on the effector cell directly, they just potentiate the action of the chemical mediator by preventing its destruction by cholinesterase. It follows from their mode of action that these drugs will lose their cholinergic activity once the innervation has been completely destroyed.

Physostigmine (eserine) is the classic **anticholinesterase**. Along the Calabar coast of West Africa the native tribes once conducted trials "by ordeal" using a poison prepared from the bean of the plant *Physostigma venenosum*. The local name for this big bean was the "esere nut." The **organic phosphate esters**

[echothiophate (Phospholine), isoflurophate (diisopropyl fluorophosphate—DFP), tetraethyl pyrophosphate, hexaethyltetraphosphate, parathion], many of which are in widespread use as insecticides, cause a much longer-lasting miosis than the other anticholinesterases, but even this potent effect, thought to be due to interference with cholinesterase synthesis, can be reversed by pralidoxime chloride.

Sympathomimetic (Adrenergic) Drugs

Epinephrine stimulates the receptor sites of the dilator muscle cells directly. When applied to the conjunctiva, the 1:1000 solution does not penetrate into the normal eye in sufficient quantity to have an obvious mydriatic effect. If, however, the receptors have been made supersensitive by previous denervation, or if the corneal epithelium has been damaged, allowing more of the drug to get into the eye, then this concentration of epinephrine will dilate the pupil.

Phenylephrine in the 10% solution has a powerful mydriatic effect. Its action is almost exclusively a direct alpha stimulation of the effector cell. The pupil recovers in 8 hr and shows a **rebound miosis** lasting several days. A 2.5% solution is now commonly used for mydriasis. **Ephedrine** acts chiefly by releasing endogenous norepinephrine from the nerve ending, but it also has a definite direct stimulation effect on the dilator cells.

Tyramine (5%) and **hydroxyamphetamine** (1%) have an indirect adrenergic action; they release norepinephrine from the stores in the postganglionic nerve endings; as far as is known this is their only effective mechanism of action.

Cocaine (5 to 10%) is applied to the conjunctiva as a topical anesthetic, a mydriatic, and a test for **Horner's syndrome.** Its mydriatic effect is the result of an accumulation of norepinephrine at the receptor sites of the dilator cells. The transmitter substance builds up at the neuroeffector junction because cocaine prevents the reuptake of the norepinephrine back into the cytoplasm of the nerve ending. Cocaine itself has no direct action on the effector cell nor does it serve to release norepinephrine from the nerve ending, and it does not retard the physiologic release of norepinephrine form the stores in the nerve ending. Its action is indirect, it interferes with the mechanism for prompt disposition of the chemical mediator, and in this respect its action is analogous to that of the anticholinesterases at the cholinergic junction. If the nerve action potentials along the sympathetic pathway are interrupted, as in Horner's syndrome, the transmitter substance will not accumulate and the pupil will not

Figure 1.   **The innervation of the iris muscles,** showing the pathways and the terminology in general use. Note that an alerting stimulus dilates the pupil in two ways—it inhibits the iris sphincter nucleus and, at the same time sends a message down to the cervical cord and out along the cervical sympathetic pathway. This arrives at the iris about half a second after the sphincter–relaxing message and causes the radial dilator muscle to tighten—widening the pupil. Reprinted with permission from Thompson HS *Alder's Pathology of the Eye* St. Louis: Mosby-Year Book, 1992:429.

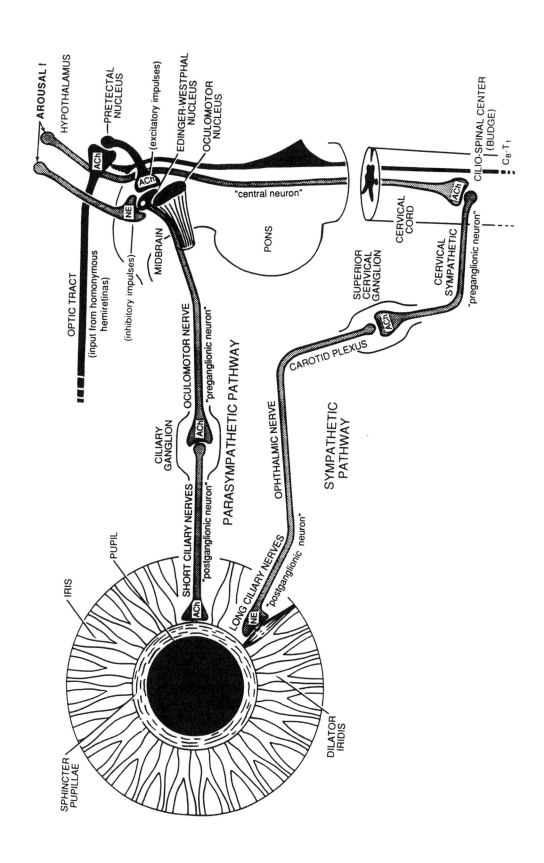

dilate. The duration of cocaine mydriasis is quite variable; it may last more than 4 hr. It does not show rebound miosis.

Sympatholytic Drugs (Adrenergic Blockers)

Thymoxamine (0.5%) and dapiprazole (0.5%) are α-adrenergic blockers that will reverse phenylephrine mydriasis by taking over the α-receptor sites on the iris dilator muscle.

Other Agents

Substance P affects the sphincter fibers directly, and will constrict the pupil of a completely atropinized eye.

The chief pupillary action of morphine is to cut off cortical inhibition of the iris sphincter nucleus in the midbrain, with resultant miosis. Topical morphine, however, even in strong solutions (5%), has a minimal miotic effect on the pupil.

Nalorphine and levallorphan are antinarcotic drugs that, given parenterally, reverse the miotic action of morphine.

Intravenous heroin seems to produce miosis in proportion to its euphoric effect. The pupils of habituated heroin users apparently constrict less to the same dose of heroin. Given the plasma drug concentration and the size of the pupil in darkness it should be possible to come up with a measure of the degree of physical dependence in a given individual.

During the induction of anesthesia the patient may be in an excited state and the pupils are often dilated. As the anesthesia deepens, supranuclear inhibition of the sphincter nuclei is cut off and the pupils become small. If the anesthesia becomes dangerously deep and begins to shut down the midbrain, the pupils become dilated and fail to react to light.

The concentration of calcium and magnesium ions in the blood may affect the pupil. Calcium facilitates the release of acetylcholine, and when calcium levels are abnormally low, the amount of acetylcholine liberated by each nerve impulse drops below the level needed to produce a postsynaptic potential, thus effectively blocking synaptic transmission. Magnesium has an opposite effect: a high concentration of magnesium can block transmission and this may dilate the pupil.

Iris Pigment and Pupillary Response to Drugs

In general, the more pigment in the iris, the more slowly the drug takes effect and the longer its action lingers. This is probably due to the drug being bound to iris melanin and then slowly released. It should be noted that there are wide individual differences in pupillary responses to topical drugs. There is probably a greater range of responses among blue eyes than there is between the average response of blue eyes and the average response of dark brown eyes. Some of these individual differences are due to corneal penetration of the drug.

References

1. Loewenfeld IE. The pupil: anatomy, physiology and clinical applications. Ames: Iowa State University Press, 1993:797–826, 1255–1558.
2. Thompson HS. The pupil. In: Hart WM, ed. Alder's physiology of the eye, Chapter 12, 9th edition. St. Louis: Mosby–Year Book, 1992:429.

14

Aging and the Autonomic Nervous System

Lewis A. Lipsitz
Harvard Medical School
Hebrew Rehabilitation Center for the Aged
Boston, Massachusetts

Healthy aging is associated with several abnormalities in autonomic nervous system function that can impair an elderly individual's adaptation to stress. However, aging alone should not be considered a state of autonomic failure, since many compensatory mechanisms remain intact, enabling older persons to respond to the usual demands of everyday life.

Two of the most common age-associated manifestations of autonomic nervous system impairment are **orthostatic** and **postprandial hypotension,** defined as a decline 20 mm Hg or greater in systolic blood pressure upon assumption of the upright posture, or within 1 hr of eating a meal, respectively. These are two distinct conditions which may or may not occur together in the same patient. Both are related to inadequate baroreflex compensation for reduced venous blood return to the heart, due to blood pooling in the lower extremities or splanchnic circulation. Orthostatic hypotension is observed in less than 7% of healthy normotensive elderly people, and in as many as 30% of those over age 75 with multiple pathological conditions. The epidemiology of postprandial hypotension is unknown, but it is particularly common in the nursing home population, and in elderly patients with unexplained syncope. Both conditions are more common in people with hypertension.

Several of the physiologic abnormalities that predispose normal elderly people to hypotension are summarized in Table 1. The onset of disease in old age, such as diabetes, cerebrovascular disease, Parkinson's Disease, malignancy, and amyloidosis, as well as the medications used to treat them, may have additional adverse effects on autonomic function. The following sections will address the effect of normal aging on autonomic function. These effects are most obvious in the cardiovascular system where they have received the most rigorous investigation.

Table 1. Age-Related Physiologic Changes Predisposing to Hypotension

1. Decreased baroreflex sensitivity
   (a) Diminished heart rate response to hypotensive stimuli
   (b) Impaired α–adrenergic vascular responsiveness
2. Impaired defense of intravascular volume
   (a) Reduced secretion of renin, angiotensin, and aldosterone
   (b) Increased atrial natriuretic peptide, supine and upright
   (c) Decreased plasma vasopressin response to orthostasis
   (d) Reduced thirst after water deprivation
3. Impaired early cardiac ventricular filling (diastolic dysfunction)

Baroreflex Function

Normal human aging is associated with an impairment in baroreflex sensitivity. Baroreflex function is further impaired by age-associated elevations in blood pressure. A decline in baroreflex sensitivity is evident in the blunted cardioacceleratory response to stimuli such as upright posture, nitroprusside infusions, and lower-body negative pressure which lower blood pressure, as well as reduced bradycardic response to drugs such as phenylephrine which elevate blood pressure. Furthermore, it is manifest by greater blood pressure reduction during hypotensive stresses such as upright posture or meal ingestion.

The baroreflex may be impaired at any of multiple sites along its arc, including carotid and cardiopulmonary pressure receptors, afferent neuronal pathways, the brainstem (nucleus tractus solitarii) and higher regulatory centers, efferent sympathetic and parasympathetic neurons, postsynaptic cardiac β receptors, or intracellular signal transduction pathways. Several lines of evidence discussed below localize the defect to the β-receptor and signal transduction proteins within the myocardium.

Sympathetic Activity

Studies of sympathetic nervous system activity in healthy human subjects demonstrate **an age-related increase in resting plasma norepinephrine levels and muscle sympathetic nerve activity,** as well as the plasma norepinephrine response to upright posture and exercise. The elevation in plasma norepinephrine is due primarily to an increase in norepinephrine spillover at sympathetic nerve endings and secondarily to a decrease in clearance. Despite apparent elevations in sympathetic nervous system activity with aging, cardiac and vascular responsiveness is diminished. Infusions of β-adrenergic agonists result in smaller increases in heart rate, left ventricular ejection fraction, cardiac output, and vasodilation in older compared to younger men.

Parasympathetic Activity

Previous studies demonstrating age- related reductions in heart rate (HR) variability in response to respiration, cough, and the Valsalva maneuver suggest that aging is associated with impaired vagal control of HR. Elderly patients with unexplained syncope have even greater impairments in HR responses to cough and deep breathing than healthy age-matched subjects without syncope.

Although loss of the **respiratory sinus arrhythmia** and attenuation of the HR response to vagal maneuvers suggest **impaired parasympathetic control of HR,** these measures cannot distinguish sympathetic from parasympathetic influences on HR variablitiy. Furthermore, the reflex responses to respiratory maneuvers are dependent on the extent of BP change, and therefore may vary from one individual to the next depending on the performance of the test and associated BP response. Recently, **HR spectral analysis** has been used to quantify the relative contributions of sympathetic and parasympathetic nervous systems to HR variability. The HR power spectrum produced by this technique can be divided into low- and high-frequency components. Previous pharmacologic blocking studies using beta-blockade and/or atropine have suggested that the low frequency oscillations (0.6–0.1 Hz) represent baroreflex-mediated sympathetic and parasympathetic influences on heart rate variability, while the high-frequency portions of the heart rate power spectrum (0.15–0.5 Hz) represent the respiratory sinus arrhythmia and are under parasympathetic control. Spectral analysis techniques have confirmed that healthy aging is associated with reductions in both baroreflex and parasympathetic modulation of heart rate, with a relatively greater loss of the high-frequency parasympathetic component.

Neurotransmitters and Receptors

As noted above, plasma norepinephrine levels increase with advancing age, in large part due to increased spillover at adrenergic nerve terminals, and to a smaller extent due to decreased plasma clearance. Likewise, any change in the level of a neurotransmitter must be interpreted with regard to changes in production and clearance. Other catecholamines, as well as serotonin and acetylcholine neurotransmitters which influence autonomic nervous system functions have received much less attention in humans. In the brain, a decline in dopamine and norepinephrine is related to a loss of dopaminergic and noradrenergic neurons in the substantia nigra and locus ceruleus. The clinical implications of these changes are not fully understood.

The enzymes **choline acetyltransferase** (CAT) and **acetylcholinesterase** (AChE) which are responsible for synthesis and degradation of acetylcholine, respectively, decrease in the cerebral cortex with aging. Furthermore, **muscarinic and nicotinic receptors** have been reported to decrease in cortical structures. These findings provide indirect evidence for a decrease in central cholinergic neurotransmission with normal aging.

Cardiac β–Adrenergic Receptors

The age-related decrease in chronotropic response to sympathetic stimulation has been attributed to multiple molecular and biochemical changes in β-receptor-coupling and postreceptor events. The number of β receptors in cardiac myocytes is unchanged with advancing age, but the affinity of receptors for agonists is reduced. Postreceptor changes with aging include a decrease in the activity of G_s protein and the adenylate cyclase catalytic unit, and a decrease in cAMP– dependent phosphokinase–induced protein phosphorylation. As a result of these changes, **G protein-mediated signal transduction is impaired.**

The decrease in cardiac contractile response to sympathetic stimulation has been studied in rat ventricular myocytes where it appears to be related to decreased influx of calcium ions via sarcolemmal calcium channels, and a reduction in the amplitude of the cytosolic calcium transient after β-adrenergic stimulation. These changes are similar to those seen in receptor desensitization due to prolonged exposure of myocardial tissue to β-adrenergic agonists. Thus, age-associated alterations in β-adrenergic response may be due to desensitization of the adenylate cyclase system in response to chronic elevations of plasma catecholamine levels.

Vascular Adrenergic Receptors

The vascular response to sympathetic stimulation has received less attention, but also appears to be altered by aging. The vasorelaxation response of both arteries and veins to infusions of the β-adrenergic agonist isoproterenol is attenuated in elderly people. Arterial α-adrenergic responses to norepinephrine infusion also appear to be reduced in healthy elderly subjects. However, this **impairment is reversible** by suppression of sympathetic nervous system activity with guanadrel. This remarkable observation suggests that the abnormality in α-adrenergic response also represents receptor desensitization due to heightened sympathetic nervous system activity. It also indicates that some of the physiologic changes associated with aging may be reversible.

Volume Regulation

Aging is associated with a progressive decline in **plasma renin, angiotensin II,** and **aldosterone levels,** and elevations in atrial natriuretic peptide, all of which promote salt wasting by the kidney. In many healthy, elderly individuals there is also **a defective plasma vasopressin response to upright posture.** These physiologic changes predispose elderly people to volume contraction and hypotension. Furthermore, healthy elderly individuals do not experience the same sense of thirst as younger subjects when they become hyperosmolar during water deprivation or hypertonic saline infusion. Consequently, dehydration may develop rapidly during conditions such as an acute illness, preparation for a medical procedure, diuretic therapy, or exposure to a warm climate when fluid losses are increased and/or access to oral fluids is limited.

Due to an **age-related stiffening of the heart** and an associated impairment in early ventricular diastolic filling, the heart becomes more dependent on preload in order to generate an adequate cardiac output. Conditions that reduce preload, such as upright posture, meal digestion, or volume contraction, may therefore threaten cardiac output. In the absence of appropriate baroreflex-mediated cardioacceleration, cardiac output will fall and hypotension will ensue.

References

1. Lipsitz LA. Orthostatic hypotension in the elderly. N Engl J Med 1989;321:952–7.
2. Lipsitz LA, Nyquist RP, Wei JY, Rowe JW. Postprandial reduction in blood pressure in the elderly. N Engl J Med 1983;309:81–3.
3. Lakatta EG. Deficient neuroendocrine regulation of the cardiovascular system with advancing age in healthy humans. Circulation 1993;87:631–6.
4. Lipsitz LA, Mietus J, Moody GB, Goldberger AL. Spectral characteristics of heart rate variability before and during postural tilt: relations to aging and risk of syncope. Circulation 1990;81:1803–10.
5. Hogikyan RV, Supiano MA. Arterial α-adrenergic responsiveness is decreased and sympathetic nervous system activity is increased in older humans. Am J Physiol 1994;266(Endocrinol Metab 29):E717–24.
6. Davis KM, Minaker KL. Disorders of fluid balance: dehydration and hyponatremia. In: Hazzard WE *et al.*, eds. Principles of geriatric medicine and gerontology, 3rd edition. New York: McGraw–Hill, 1994:1183–90.

PART III

Pharmacology

15 Dopaminergic Neurotransmission

Irwin J. Kopin
Clinical Neuroscience Branch
CNP, DIR, NINDS
Bethesda, Maryland

Dopamine (DA), **norepinephrine** (NE), and **epinephrine** (EPI) are the three catecholamines found in animals. About 100 years ago, EPI was identified as the excitatory hormone released from the adrenal medulla. It was thought also to be released from sympathetic nerve terminals, and remained the focus of attention for the next half century. When, in 1951, NE was established as the sympathetic neurotransmitter and was found to be differentially distributed in brain, it became the subject of intense interest. The effects of antidepressants on NE metabolism and inactivation led to hypotheses regarding the role of NE in neuropsychiatric disorders. At that time, DA was recognized mainly as an intermediate in the biosyntheses of EPI and NE. The discovery of very high concentrations of DA in the **striatum** and the striking DA deficiency in brains of **Parkinson's disease** patients drew attention to the importance of DA in brain motor function. When antipsychotic drugs were found to produce parkinsonian symptoms and to antagonize the effects of DA, excess dopaminergic activity was implicated in psychiatric disorders. Opposing neuroendocrine side effects of antipsychotics and drugs effective in treating Parkinson's disease suggested that DA also played an important role in **endocrine function.** In addition to its actions in **brain** and **pituitary,** DA has effects in peripheral tissues, including the retina, kidney, cardiovascular system, lungs, and gastrointestinal tract. Thus DA appears to have neurotransmitter/modulator/humoral effects.

Localization of DA Neurons and Their Projections

With the development of fluorescence and immunohistochemistry, it has become possible to identify catecholaminergic neurons and their axonal projections. Dopaminergic neurons could be distinguished from other catecholaminergic neurons by absence of **dopamine-β-hydroxylase** as well as by biochemical analyses of specific brain regions. Such studies, combined with anterograde autoradiographic and retrograde HRP (horseradish peroxidase) techniques for tracing axonal pathways, as well as with neurophysiological methods to monitor neuronal activity, established the neuroanatomical pathways and function of dopaminergic neurons. With radioisotopically labeled drugs that bind specifically to **DA receptors or transporters,** the anatomical distribution, as well as the kinetic properties of the binding or transport sites, could be examined. The most recent development in defining dopaminergic systems has been the application of molecular genetic approaches to demonstrate the expression of mRNA encoding the proteins that constitute the enzymes, transporters, and receptors involved in the formation, uptake, and storage and actions of DA. Such studies have demonstrated the heterogeneity of dopaminergic systems in the peripheral tissues as well as in brain and provide a basis for understanding the difference in effects of various drugs that stimulate or block subtypes of the receptors.

Brain Dopaminergic Systems

Three major dopaminergic systems have been described in the brain. At first, attention was focused on the **nigrostriatal pathway**, i.e., projections of DA-containing neurons from the **substantia nigra compacta** (SNc) to the **caudate nucleus and putamen** (**striatum**), particularly because of the clinical relevance to Parkinson's disease and its relatively successful treatment with the precursor of DA, levodopa (1). The neuroendocrine and antipsychotic effects of drugs such as **reserpine**, which depletes brain amines, and **phenothiazines**, which block DA receptors, were explained by the two other brain dopaminergic systems, the **tuberoinfundibular** and the **mesocorticolimbic** systems. The dopaminergic neurons of the tuberoinfundibular pathway are located in the median eminence of the hypothalamus and project to the hypophyseal portal veins where they release DA directly into the portal veins that carry blood to the pituitary. DA is the primary **prolactin secretion inhibitory factor** and regulates secretion of other pituitary hormones. Blockade of pituitary DA receptors, or depletion of neuronal DA with drugs such as resepine, elevates prolactin levels and causes gynecomastia. At this site, DA functions as a neurohormone.

The dopaminergic neurons of the mesocorticolimbic system are in areas contiguous to and not clearly demarcated from the SNc (A8 and A10) and project to the cortex and limbic systems. These neurons have been implicated in psychiatric disorders, particularly **schizophrenia, cocaine addiction,** and **stress responses,** and are thought to modulate the effects of a variety of peptide neurotransmitters.

DA in Peripheral Tissues

DA and its receptors are present in cardiovascular tissues, lungs, kidney, gastrointestinal tract, and endocrine organs. The physiological role of endogenous dopamine on peripheral organ function has not been as clearly delineated as in the brain, but pharmacological actions and therapeutic benefits of drugs that act on some peripheral DA receptors have been clearly demonstrated (5–7).

DA Receptor Subtypes

The first distinction between DA receptor subtypes was based on the ability of one subtype (D_1) to activate adenylcyclase and thereby stimulate **cyclic AMP production,** whereas the other receptor subtype (D_2) failed to affect adenylcyclase or even diminished cyclic AMP formation. Subsequent demonstration of specific binding sites for radioactively labeled DA agonists and antagonists of the two classes of responses further supported the division of DA

Table 1. Dopamine Receptor Subtypes

	D₁-like		D₂-like		
Subtype:	D₁	D₅	D₂	D₃	D₄
Adenylcyclase:	Activates	Activates	Inhibits		
Channel:	Ca^{2+}		$K+$		?
Brain regions, olfact. tub., amygdala	Striatum accumbens	Hippocampus, hypothalamus, olfact. tub., s. nigra	Striatum, accumbens, amygdala	Olfact. tub., hypothalamus, mesolimbic	Frontal cortex, medulla
Peripheral tissues:	Parathyroid	Kidney	Pituitary		Heart
Agonists:	SKF 38393 SKF 82526 (fenoldopam)		Ergolines (Bromocriptine, Pergolide, Lisuride), aporphines (Apomorphine)		
Antagonist	N-CH₃-7-Halo-SKF-38393 Sch 33390		Butyrophenones (Spiperone), benzamides (Sulpiride, Raclopride)		
(Specific):	None		Haloperidol	AJ76, UH232	Clozapine

receptors into at least two subtypes. The synthesis of agonists and antagonists specific for the two subtypes further supported this distinction. In brains of most species, including humans, **D$_1$ receptor** density is greater than that of **D$_2$ receptors.** Cloning and characterization of the molecular structures of the D$_1$ and D$_2$ receptors not only validated their pharmacological distinction but led to the discovery of other types of DA receptors. Three additional DA receptors have been cloned and characterized. D$_3$ and D$_4$ receptors are pharmacologically similar to the D$_2$ receptor; the D$_5$ receptor resembles the D$_1$ subtype, but appears neuron-specific and has a fivefold higher affinity for DA. Using *in situ* hybridization to locate mRNAs encoding these receptors, the regions with the highest density of DA receptors are the caudate, putamen, nucleus accumbens, and olfactory tubercle. The major characteristics and distribution of DA receptor subtypes are summarized in Table 1. There are **alternative transcripts** of the D$_3$ receptor, but their functional significance, if any, has not been determined. The **D$_4$** receptor, although highly homologous with the D$_2$ and D$_4$ receptor genes, has an order of magnitude higher affinity for **clozapine,** an "atypical" neuroleptic that does not produce parkinsonian side effects. Five genetically determined variants of the D$_4$ receptor have been distinguished in humans, differing in the number (2, 3, 4, 5, or 7) of repeats of a 48-base pair sequence encoding the amino acids in the third cytoplasmic loop of the receptor. Such structural differences could be a basis for individual differences in response to endogenous transmitters or to therapeutic agents. The availability of methods to quantify receptor mRNA in postmortem human brain has spurred studies of the density of these receptors in neuropsychiatric disorders. Elevated levels of both D$_3$ and D$_4$ receptors have been reported in basal ganglia or forebrain of schizophrenic patients. Recently, transgenic mice in which D$_1$ receptors have been "knocked out" have become available; it is likely that analogous mutants with deficits in other dopamine receptors, alone or in combination with other genetically engineered receptors, will be available soon. The variety and distribution of these multiple dopamine receptor subtypes holds promise that more specific therapeutic agents may be developed to treat a number of psychiatric and neurological disorders while limiting undesirable side effects.

Dopamine transport and storage are other functions that can now be studied using molecular biological techniques and are the subject of intense study (5).

References

1. Hornykiewicz O. Mechanisms of neuronal loss in Parkinson's disease: a neuroanatomical-biochemical approach. Clin Neurol Neurosurg 1992;94 (Suppl): S9.
2. Kuhar MJ. Molecular pharmacology of cocaine: a dopamine hypothesis and its implications. Ciba Found Symp 1992;166:81–9.
3. Seeman P, Van Tol HH. Dopamine receptor pharmacology. Trends Pharmacol Sci 1994;15:264–70.
4. Civelli O, Bunzow JR, Grandy DK. Molecular diversity of the dopamine receptors. Ann Rev Pharmacol Toxicol 1993;32:281–307.
5. Amara SG, Kuhar MJ. Neurotransmitter transporters: recent progress. Ann Rev Neurosci 1993;16:73–93.

16 Noradrenergic Neurotransmission

David S. Goldstein
Clinical Neurochemistry Section
Clinical Neuroscience Branch
National Institute of Neurological Disorders and Stroke
National Institutes of Health
10/6N252
Bethesda, Maryland

The chemical transmitter at sympathetic nerve endings is **norepinephrine** (NE). Sympathetic stimulation releases NE, and noradrenergic binding to adrenoceptors on cardiovascular smooth muscle cells causes the cells to contract. Sympathoneural NE therefore satisfies the main criteria defining a **neurotransmitter**—a chemical released from nerve terminals by electrical action potentials that interacts with specific receptors on nearby structures to produce specific physiological responses.

Different stressors can elicit **different patterns of sympathoneural responses,** and therefore differential NE release, in the various vascular beds. This redistributes blood flows. Local sympathoneural release of NE also markedly affects cardiac function and glandular activity. The adjustments usually are not sensed, and the organism usually does not feel distressed. Examples of situations associated with prominent changes in sympathoneural outflows include orthostasis, mild exercise, postprandial hemodynamic changes, mild changes in environmental temperature, and performance of nondistressing locomotor tasks.

In contrast, in response to perceived global, metabolic threats, whether from external or internal stimuli, increased neural outflow to the adrenal medulla elicits catecholamine secretion into the adrenal venous drainage. In humans, the predominant catecholamine in the adrenal venous drainage is **epinephrine** (EPI). EPI rapidly reaches all cells of the body (with the exception of most of the brain), producing a wide variety of hormonal effects at low blood concentrations. One can comprehend all the many effects of EPI in terms of countering acute threats to survival that mammals perennially have faced, such as sudden lack of metabolic fuels, trauma with hemorrhage, intravascular volume depletion and hypotension, and fight-or-flight confrontations. Thus, even mild **hypoglycemia** elicits marked increases in plasma levels of EPI, in contrast with small increases in plasma levels of NE. **Distress** accompanies all these situations, the experience undoubtedly fostering the long-term survival of the individual and the species by motivating avoidance learning and producing signs universally understood among other members of the species.

Noradrenergic Innervation of the Cardiovascular System

Sympathetic nerves to the ventricles travel through the ansae subclaviae, branches of the left and right **stellate ganglia.** The fibers in the ansae subclaviae pass along the dorsal surface of the pulmonary artery into the plexus that supplies the left main coronary artery. In primates, cardiac sympathetic nerves originate about equally from the superior, middle, and inferior cervical (stellate) ganglia.

Individual cardiac nerves supply relatively localized regions of myocardium, with the **right sympathetic chain** generally projecting to the **anterior left ventricle** and the left to the posterior left ventricle. Sympathetic innervation of the sinus and atrioventricular nodes also has a degree of sidedness, the right sympathetics projecting more to the sinus node and the left to the atrioventricular node. Thus, left stellate stimulation produces relatively little sinus tachycardia.

Epicardial sympathetic nerves provide the main source of noradrenergic terminals in the myocardium. Sympathetic nerves travel with the coronary arteries in the epicardium before penetrating into the myocardium, whereas vagal nerves penetrate the myocardium after crossing the atrioventricular groove and then continue in the subendocardium. Postganglionic noradrenergic fibers reach all parts of the heart. The sinus and atrioventricular nodes and the atria receive the densest innervation, the ventricles less dense innervation, and the Purkinje fibers the least. Sympathetic and vagal afferents follow intracardiac routes similar to those of the efferents.

The heart contains high concentrations of NE, compared with concentrations in other body organs. Atrial myocardium possesses the highest concentrations. In humans, ventricular myocardial NE levels range from 3.5 to 14 nmol/ g. Myocardial cells do not store NE; instead, myocardial NE is localized to vesicles in sympathetic nerves.

Although the coronary arteries also possess sympathetic noradrenergic innervation, assessing the regulation and physiological role of this innervation has proven difficult, because several other factors complicate neural control of the coronary vasculature. Alterations in myocardial metabolism and systemic hemodynamics change coronary blood flow, coronary vasomotion in response to sympathetic stimulation depends on the functional integrity of the endothelium, and coronary arteries appear to receive less dense innervation than do other arteries.

The body's myriad **arterioles** largely determine **total resistance** to blood flow and therefore contribute significantly to **blood pressure.** Sympathetic nerves enmesh blood vessels in lattice-like networks in the adventitial outer surface that extends inward to the **adventitial-medial border,** with the concentration of sympathetic nerves increasing as arterial caliber decreases, so that small arteries and arterioles, the smallest nutrient vessels possessing smooth muscle cells, possess the most intense innervation. The unique architectural association between sympathetic nerves and the vessels that determine peripheral resistance has enticed cardiovascular researchers, particularly in the area of autonomic regulation, for many years. Sympathetic vascular innervation varies widely among vascular beds, with dense innervation of resistance vessels in the gut, kidney, skeletal muscle, and skin. Sympathetic stimulation in these beds produces profound vasoconstriction, whereas stimulation in the coronary, cerebral, and bronchial beds elicits weaker constrictor responses, consistent teleologically with the "goal" of preserving blood flow to vital organs during stress. NE released from the sympathetic nerve terminal acts mainly locally, with only a small proportion of released NE reaching the bloodstream. One must therefore keep in mind the indirect and distant relationship between plasma NE levels and sympathetic nerve activity in interpreting plasma NE responses to stressors, pathophysiologic situations, and drugs.

Norepinephrine Synthesis

Enzymatic steps in NE synthesis have been characterized in more detail than those for any other neurotransmitter. Catecholamine biosynthesis begins with uptake of the amino acid **tyrosine** (TYR) into the cytoplasm of sympathetic neurons, adrenomedullary cells, possibly paraaortic enterochromaffin cells, and specific centers in the brain. Other neutral L-amino acids compete with TYR for transport into the brain and presumably into sympathetic terminals.

Tyrosine hydroxylase (TH) catalyzes the conversion of TYR to dihydroxyphenylalanine (DOPA, dopa). This is the enzymatic rate-limiting step in catecholamine synthesis. The enzyme is almost saturated under normal conditions. Thus, although alterations in dietary TYR intake normally should not affect the rate of catecholamine biosyntheses under baseline conditions, after prolonged rapid turnover of catecholamines, TYR availability may become a limiting factor. The enzyme is stereospecific. Concentrations of **tetrahydrobiopterin**, Fe^{2+}, and molecular oxygen regulate TH activity. Dihydropteridine reductase (DHPR) catalyzes the reduction of **dihydropterin,** produced during the hydroxylation of TYR. Since the reduced pteridine, tetrahydrobiopterin, is a key cofactor for TH, **DHPR deficiency** decreases the amount of TYR hydroxylation for a given amount of TH enzyme. Both phenylalanine hydroxylase and TH require tetrahydrobiopterin as a cofactor. DHPR deficiency therefore also inhibits phenylalanine metabolism and presents clinically as an atypical form of **phenylketonuria.**

Catecholamines and dopa feedback-inhibit TH, and α-methyl-para-TYR inhibits the enzyme competitively. Conversely, exposure to stressors that increase sympathoadrenal outflows augments the synthesis and concentration of TH in sympathetic ganglia, sympathetically innervated organs, the adrenal gland, and the locus ceruleus of the pons. Multiple and complex mechanisms contribute to TH activation during sympathoadrenal stimulation. **Short-term mechanisms** include feedback inhibition and phosphorylation of the enzyme, the latter depending on membrane depolarization, contractile elements, and receptors. **Long-term mechanisms** include changes in TH synthesis, probably determined by as yet poorly understood mechanisms of transsynaptic induction and retrograde transport. During stress-induced sympathetic stimulation, acceleration of catecholamine synthesis in sympathetic nerves helps to maintain tissue stores of NE. Even with diminished stores after prolonged sympathoneural activation, increased nerve traffic can maintain extracellular fluid levels of the transmitter.

L-aromatic amino acid decarboxylase (L–AADC, also called **dopa decarboxylase,** DDC) in the neuronal cytoplasm catalyzes the rapid conversion of dopa to DA. Many types of tissues contain the enzyme—especially the kidneys, gut, liver, and brain. Activity of the enzyme depends on pyridoxal phosphate. Although DDC metabolizes most of the dopa formed in catecholamine-synthesizing tissues, some of the dopa enters the circulation unchanged. This provides the basis for using plasma dopa levels to examine catecholamine synthesis. α-Methyldopa, an effective drug in the treatment of high blood pressure, inhibits DDC and therefore NE synthesis. This inhibition does not explain the antihypertensive action of the drug; rather, α-methylNE, formed from α-methyldopa in catecholamine-synthesizing tissues, stimulates α_2 adrenoceptors in the brain and thereby inhibits sympathetic outflow. Other DDC inhibitors include **carbidopa** and **benserazide.** These catechols do not readily penetrate the blood–brain barrier, and by inhibiting conversion of dopa to DA in the periphery, they enhance the efficacy of L-dopa treatment of Parkinson's disease. DDC blockade increases dopa levels and decreases levels of dihydroxyphenylacetic acid (DOPAC), a DA metabolite. The rates of increase in extracellular fluid dopa levels and of decrease in DOPAC levels after acute DDC inhibition provide *in vivo* indices of TH activity.

Dopamine-β-hydroxylase (DBH) catalyzes the conversion of DA to NE. Like TH, DBH is localized to tissues that synthesize catecholamines, such as noradrenergic neurons and chromaffin cells. Unlike TH, which is present in the cytoplasm, DBH is confined to the vesicles. Thus, treatment with **reserpine,** which blocks the translocation of amines from the axonal cytoplasm into vesicles, prevents the conversion of DA to NE in sympathetic nerves. DBH contains, and its activity depends on, copper. Because of this dependence, children with **Menkes' disease,** a rare, X-linked recessive inherited disorder of **copper** metabolism, have neurochemical evidence of concurrently increased catecholamine biosynthesis and decreased conversion of DA to NE, with high plasma and cerebrospinal fluid ratios of dopa: dihydroxyphenylglycol (DHPG, the neuronal NE metabolite). Patients with congenital absence of DBH have virtually undetectable levels of both NE and DHPG and high levels of DA and DOPAC. DBH activity also requires ascorbic acid, which provides electrons for the hydroxylation. Each molecule of NE synthesized consumes a molecule of intragranular ascorbic acid; loss of granular ascorbic acid stops NE synthesis.

Phenylethanolamine-*N*-methyltransferase (PNMT) catalyzes the conversion of NE to EPI in the cytoplasm of chromaffin cells.

Storage

Varicosities in sympathetic nerves contain two types of cytoplasmic vesicles: **small dense-core** (diameter 40–60 nm) and **large dense-core** (diameter 80–120 nm). Vesicles generated near the **Golgi apparatus** of the cell bodies travel by **axonal transport** in the axons to the nerve terminal. Noradrenergic vesicles may also form by **endocytosis** within the axons. Since reserpine eliminates the electron-dense cores of the small but not the large vesicles, the cores of the small vesicles may represent NE, whereas the electron-dense cores of the large vesicles may represent additional components.

Cores of both types of vesicles contain **adenosine triphosphate** (ATP). The NE:ATP ratio averages about 1:4. The vesicles also contain at least three types of polypeptides: **chromogranin A,** an acidic glycoprotein; **enkephalins;** and **neuropeptide Y** (NPY). Extracellular fluid levels of each of these compounds have been considered as indices of **exocytosis.** Vesicles in sympathetic nerves actively remove and trap axoplasmic amines. Vesicular uptake favors L- over D-NE, Mg^{2+} and ATP accelerate the uptake, and reserpine effectively and irreversibly blocks it. The vesicular uptake carrier protein resembles the neuronal uptake carriers. In the brain, mRNA for the vesicular transporter is expressed in monoamine-containing cells of the **locus ceruleus, substantia nigra,** and **raphe nucleus,** corresponding to **noradrenergic, dopaminergic,** and **serotonergic** centers. Neurotransmitter specificity therefore appears to depend on different transporters in the cell membrane, rather than on different vesicular transporters.

Release

Adrenomedullary chromaffin cells, much easier to study than sympathetic nerves, have provided the most commonly used model for studying mechanisms of catecholamine release. Agonist occupation of **nicotinic acetylcholine receptors** release catecholamines from cells. Since nicotinic receptors mediate ganglionic neurotransmission, researchers have presumed that the results obtained in adrenomedullary cells probably apply to postganglionic sympathoneural cells.

The **exocytotic theory of NE release** includes the following features: **acetylcholine** depolarizes the terminal membranes by **increasing membrane permeability to sodium.** The increased intracellular sodium levels directly or indirectly enhance **transmembrane influx of calcium,** via voltage-gated calcium channels. The increased cytoplasmic calcium concentration evokes a cascade of as yet incompletely defined biomechanical events resulting in **fusion** of the vesicular and axoplasmic membranes. The interior of the vesicle exchanges briefly with the extracellular compartment, and the soluble contents of the vesicles diffuse into the extracellular space. As predicated from this model, manipulations besides application of acetylcholine that depolarize the cell, such as electrical stimulation or increased K$^+$ concentration in the extracellular fluid, also activate the **voltage-gated calcium channels** and trigger exocytosis. During cellular activation, simultaneous, stoichiometric release of soluble vesicular contents— ATP, enkephalins, chromogranins, and DBH—without similar release of cytoplasmic macromolecules, has provided biochemical support for the exocytosis theory. Electron micrographs occasionally have shown an **omega sign,** with an apparent gap in the cell membrane at the site of fusion of vesicle with the axoplasmic membrane. Ultrastructural evidence has suggested release of the contents of large as well as small dense-core vesicles by exocytosis. Exactly how increased intracellular Ca^{2+} concentration evokes exocytosis in sympathetic nerves is unknown.

At least **two storage pools** of NE may exist in sympathetic nerve terminals—a small, readily releasable pool of newly synthesized NE and a large reserve pool in long-term storage. The relationship between the two pools of NE and the two forms of vesicles, large and small dense-core, has not been established.

Sympathetic nerve endings can also release NE by calcium-independent, nonexocytotic mechanisms. One such mechanism probably is reverse transport through the neuronal uptake carrier. The indirectly acting sympathomimetic amin **tyramine** releases NE nonexocytotically, since tyramine releases NE independently of calcium and does not release DBH. As predicted from the ionic requirements for neuronal reuptake, increases in intracellular Na^+ concentrations, such as produced by **ouabain,** enhance carrier-mediated efflux of NE. Myocardial ischemic hypoxia evokes calcium–independent release of NE. The **hydrophilic nature** of catecholamines and their ionization at physiological pH probably prevent NE efflux by simple diffusion.

As noted above, sympathetic stimulation releases other compounds besides NE. Some of these compounds may function as neurotransmitters. ATP, adenosine, NPY, acetylcholine, and EPI have received the most attention.

Pharmacological stimulation of a large variety of receptors on noradrenergic terminals affects the amount of NE released during cellular activation. Compounds **inhibiting NE release** include acetylcholine, gamma-amino butyric acid, prostaglandins of the E series, opioids, adenosine, and NE itself. Compounds **enhancing NE release** include angiotensin II, acetylcholine (at nicotinic receptors), ACTH, GABA (at $GABA_A$ receptors), and EPI (via stimulation of presynaptic β_2-adrenoceptors). In general, whether these compounds at physiological concentrations exert modulatory effects on endogenous NE release remains unproven, especially in humans. Substantial evidence, however, does support inhibitory presynaptic modulation by NE itself, via autoreceptors on sympathetic nerves. This modulatory action appears to vary with the vascular bed under study, being prominent in skeletal muscle beds such as the forearm, relatively weak in the kidney, and virtually absent in the adrenals.

In addition to local feedback control of NE release, **reflexive "long-distance" feedback pathways,** via high- and low-pressure baroreceptors, elicit reflexive changes in sympathoneural impulse activity. Alterations in receptor numbers or of intracellular biomechanical events after receptor activation also affect responses to agonists. These factors may therefore regulate NE release by transsynaptic local and reflexive long-distance mechanisms.

Disposition

Unlike acetylcholine, which is inactivated mainly by extracellular enzymes, NE is inactivated mainly by **uptake into cells,** with subsequent intracellular metabolism or storage. Reuptake into nerve terminals (**uptake-1**) is the predominant means of terminating the actions of released NE. Uptake-1 is energy-requiring and carrier-mediated. The carrier can transport catecholamines against large concentration gradients. The only common structural feature of all known substrates for uptake-1 is an aromatic amine, with the ionizable nitrogen moiety not incorporated in the aromatic system. Uptake-1 does not require a catechol nucleus. Alkylation of the primary amino group decreases the effectiveness of the transport, explaining why sympathetic nerves take up NE more efficiently than they do EPI and why they do not take up **isoproterenol,** an extensively alkylated catecholamine, at all. Methylation of the phenolic hydroxyl groups also markedly decreases susceptibility to uptake-1, and so sympathetic nerves do not take up **O-methylated catecholamine metabolites** such as **normetanephrine.**

Neuronal uptake by dopaminergic neurons differs from that by noradrenergic neurons, since the former take up DA more avidly than they take up NE, whereas the latter take up both catecholamines about equally well.

Desipramine and **other tricyclic antidepressants** block uptake by noradrenergic neurons more effectively than they block uptake by dopaminergic neurons. These pharmacological differences imply **distinct transporters** for NE and DA. Recent molecular genetic studies have confirmed this distinction. The human NE transporter protein includes 12 or 13 hydrophobic and therefore probably membrane-spanning domains. This structure differs substantially from that of adrenoceptors and other receptors coupled with G-proteins but is very similar to that of the DA, GABA, serotonin, and vesicular transporters, suggesting a family of neurotransmitter transporter proteins.

Neuronal uptake absolutely requires intracellular K^+ and extracellular Na^+ and functions most efficiently when Cl^- accompanies Na^+. Transport does not directly require ATP; however, maintaining ionic gradients across cell membranes depends on ATP, and the carrier uses the energy expended in maintaining the transmembrane Na^+ gradient to cotransport amines with Na^+. Many drugs or *in vitro* conditions inhibit uptake-1, including **cocaine, tricyclic antidepressants,** low extracellular Na^+, Li^+, ouabain, and nitrogen mustards such as **phenoxybenzamine.**

NE taken up into the axoplasm by the uptake-1 transporter is subject to two fates: translocation into storage vesicles and deamination by monoamine oxidase. The combination of enzymatic breakdown and vesicular uptake constitute an intraneuronal "sink", keeping cytoplasmic concentrations of NE very low. Reserpine effectively blocks the vesicular transport of amines from the axoplasm into the vesicles. This not only shuts down conversion of DA to NE but also prevents the conservative recycling of NE. Reserpine therefore rapidly depletes NE stores. After reserpine injection, plasma DHPG levels increase rapidly, reflecting marked net leakage of NE from vesicular stores, and then decline to very low levels, reflecting the abolition of vesicular uptake and of β-hydroxylation of DA.

Neural and nonneural tissues contain **monoamine oxidase** (MAO), which catalyzes the oxidative deamination of DA to form DOPAC and of NE to form DHPG. Because of the efficient uptake of catecholamines into the axoplasm of catecholaminergic neurons, and because of the rapid exchange of amines between the vesicles and axoplasm, the neuronal pool of MAO, located in the **outer mitochondrial membrane,** figures prominently in the overall function of catecholaminergic systems. Two isozymes of MAO, MAO-A and MAO-B, have been described, based mainly on pharmacological characteristics: **clorgyline** blocks MAO-A, and **selegiline** and **pargyline** block MAO-B. MAO-A predominates in neural tissue, whereas both subtypes exist in nonneuronal tissue. Thus, inhibitors of MAO-A potentiate the pressor effects of tyramine, whereas inhibitors of MAO-B do not. NE and EPI are substrates for MAO-A, and DA is a substrate for both MAO-A and MAO-B. The deaminated products are short-lived aldeydes. For DA, the aldehyde intermediate is converted rapidly to DOPAC by aldehyde dehydrogenase; for NE, the aldehyde intermediate is converted mainly to DHPG by an **aldehyde reductase.** The formation of the aldehydes reduces a **flavine** component of the enzyme. The reduced enzyme reacts with molecular oxygen, regenerating the enzyme but also producing **hydrogen peroxide,** which may be toxic to cells, because the peroxidation releases **free radicals.** MAO-B inhibitors may delay neurological degeneration in patients with Parkinson's disease, possibly by limiting oxidative injury.

Since **catechol-O-methyltransferase** (COMT) in nonneuronal cells catalyzes the O-methylation of DHPG to form **methoxyhydroxyphenylglycol** (MHPG) and of DOPAC to form **homovanillic acid** (HVA), plasma levels of DHPG and DOPAC probably reflect mainly neuronal metabolism of NE and DA.

MAO inhibitors are effective antidepressants. A phenomenon known as the **cheese effect** limits their clinical use. In patients taking MAO inhibitors, administration of sympathomimetic amines such as in many nonprescription decongestants, or ingestion of foods such as aged cheese, wine, or meat, which contain tyramine, can produce **paroxysmal hypertension.** Since tyramine and other sympathomimetic amines displace NE from sympathetic vesicles into the axoplasm, blockade of MAO in this setting causes axoplasmic NE to accumulate, and outward transport of the NE, perhaps via the uptake-1 carrier, stimulates cardiovascular smooth muscle cells, producing intense vasoconstriction and hypertension. When given alone, MAO inhibitors usually decrease blood pressure and produce orthostatic hypotension, by unknown mechanisms.

Nonneuronal cells remove NE actively by a process called **uptake-2,** characterized by the ability to transport **isoproterenol,** susceptibility to blockade by O-methylated catecholamines, **corticosteroids,** and β-haloalkylamines, and an absence of susceptibility to blockade uptake-1 blocker cocaine and desipramine. In contrast with uptake-1, uptake-2 functions independently of extracellular Na^+. The uptake-2 carrier has little if any stereoselectivity and has low affinity and specificity for catecholamines. For instance, extraneuronal cells remove **imidazolines** such as **clonidine** by uptake-2. Thus, during infusion of a catecholamine at a high rate, the catecholamine can accumulate in extraneuronal cells, with reentry of the catecholamine into the extracellular fluid via the uptake-2 carrier after the infusion ends.

COMT catalyzes the conversion of NE to **normetanephrine** (NMN) and EPI to **metanephrine** (MN). Uptake-2 and COMT probably act in series to remove and degrade circulating catecholamines. The methyl group donor for the reaction is S-adenosyl methionine. Immunohistochemical studies have indicated exclusively extraneuronal localization of COMT, which exists at high concentration in the liver and kidney. O-Methylation of NE therefore requires extraneuronal uptake. In the cardiovascular system, myocardial and vascular endothelial and smooth muscle cells probably constitute the main sites of O-methylation of catecholamines. Because of the extraneuronal localization of COMT, recently introduced assay methods for metanephrines have enabled refined assessments of extraneuronal metabolism of catecholamines. **Vanillylmandelic acid** (VMA) and MHPG, the products of the combined O-methylation and deamination of NE, are the **two main end-products of NE metabolism,** with VMA probably formed mainly in the liver.

Reference

1. Goldstein DS. Stress, catecholamines, and cardiovascular disease. New York: Oxford University Press, 1995.

17

Purinergic Neurotransmission

Geoffrey Burnstock
Department of Anatomy and Developmental Biology
University College London
London, United Kingdom

There have been major changes in our understanding of autonomic control mechanisms. There is now compelling evidence that there is a multiplicity of autonomic neurotransmitters and that some, if not all, nerve cells store and release **more than one transmitter.** Systematic studies reveal specific combinations of transmitter substances (**chemical coding**) for different neuron types which project to particular effector structures and have defined central connections.

A **neuromodulator** is defined as a substance that modifies the process of neurotransmission. It may act as a **prejunctional modulator** by decreasing or increasing the amount of neurotransmitter released by a nerve varicosity, or it may act as a **postjunctional modulator** by altering the time course or extent of action of a transmitter (Fig. 1). There are many reports of both pre- and postjunctional modulation occurring at the autonomic neuromuscular junction. Neuromodulators may be circulating hormones, local agents such as prostaglandin, histamine, or bradykinin, or neurotransmitters released from other nerves nearby, or even from the same nerve varicosity.

ATP in Autonomic Transmission and Roles of Purinoceptors

In the early 1960s, nonadrenergic, noncholinergic (**NANC**) nerves were shown to be strongly represented in the gastrointestinal tract of a wide range of vertebrate species and were also identified in a variety of other organs, including lung, bladder, seminal vesicles, esophagus, uterus, eye, trachea, and parts of the cardiovascular system. It was proposed that the principal active substance released from these nerves, at least those in the intestine and bladder, was the purine nucleotide **ATP;** these NANC nerves were termed **purinergic.**

In 1978 a basis for distinguishing two types of purinergic receptor (P_1 and P_2) was proposed which relied largely on an analysis of the voluminous literature about the actions of purine nucleotides and nucleosides on a wide variety of tissues. P_1 **purinoceptors** are more responsive to **adenosine** and **AMP** than to ATP and **ADP; methylxanthines** such as **theophylline** and **caffeine** are selective competitive antagonists with respect to these receptors, and occupation of these receptors leads to inhibition or activation of an adenylate cyclase system with resultant changes in levels of intracellular cAMP. P_2 **purinoceptors** are more responsive to ATP and ADP; these receptors are not antagonized by methylxanthines and do not act via an adenylate cyclase system, and their occupation may lead to **prostaglandin synthesis.**

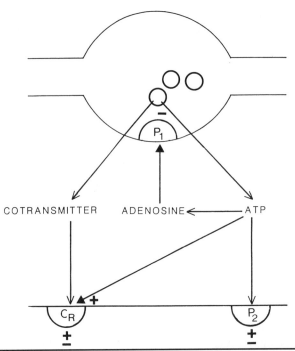

Figure 1. Purinergic cotransmission and modulation. Schematic diagram showing ATP release together with a cotransmitter (such as acetylcholine, norepinephrine, nitric oxide, or glutamate) to act on P_2 purinoceptors mediating responses (excitatory (+) or inhibitory (−)) which are synergistic with the responses mediated by the receptor for the cotransmitter (C_R). ATP is broken down rapidly by ectoenzymes (Ca/Mg-activated ATPase, 5′-nucleotidase) to adenosine which acts as a *prejunctional* modulator of cotransmitter release, while ATP acts as a *postjunctional* modulator to enhance cotransmitter action.

Purinoceptor Classification

Following the introduction of P_1 and P_2 subclasses of purinoceptors, partly on the basis of the relative potencies of purine analogs and partly on the basis of transduction mechanisms, P_1 purinoceptors were divided into A_1 and A_2 subclasses and later P_2 purinoceptors were divided into P_{2X} and P_{2Y} purinoceptors. Currently, with the additional information provided by molecular biology, P_1 purinoceptors have been classified into A_1, A_{2a}, A_{2b}, and A_3 subclasses (Table 1).

Concerns have been expressed about the recent additions to **P_2 purinoceptor subclasses** representing an "apparent random walk through the alphabet" with the introduction of P_{2U}, P_{2D}, P_{2S} purinoceptors in addition to P_{2X}, P_{2Y}, P_{2Z}, and P_{2T} purinoceptors. This background has motivated Abbracchio and Burnstock to propose a new broad framework for P_2 purinoceptor subclassification which will allow a more rational development as more subtypes and molecular structures are recognized. Essentially, they have suggested that P_2 purinoceptors should be divided into two main families: **P2X purinoceptors** mediating **fast** responses via **ligand-gated ion channels** and **P2Y purinoceptors** mediating **slower** responses via **G proteins.** Further subdivisions in each of these two major families is sug-

Table 1.

Major subclasses		Agonist	Antagonist	Distribution	Major roles in transmission
P_1 (adenosine)	A_1	PA	CPX[a]	Brain Peripheral nerve endings	Mainly acts as a prejunctional modulator of transmitter release in both CNS and PNS
	A_2 A2a and A2b Subclasses	NECA	XAC	Brain Gastrointestinal and vascular muscle	Relaxation
	A_3	APNEA	BW-A522	Testis	
P2 (ATP/ADP)	P2X family (ligand-gated ion channels)	$\alpha\beta$mATP UTP/ATP 2hexylthioATP ATPγS $A_{P5}A$	Suramin $\alpha\beta$mATP desensitization PPADS	Vas deferens Bladder Vascular smooth muscle	Fast synaptic transmission in ganglia and CNS Fast neuromuscular transmission Control of secretion Slow junctional transmission
	P2X$_1$ → P2X$_5$ Subclasses			Brain	
	P2Y family (G-proteins)	2mSATP UTP/ATP $A_{P3}A$	Suramin Reactive blue 2	Endothelial cells Hepatocytes Pancreatic β cells	
	P2Y$_1$ → P2Y$_7$ subclasses			Osteoclasts Platelets Intestinal smooth muscle Chromaffin cells	
	P2Z Family	ATP^{4-}	Suramin Hexamethylene amiloride	Mast cells Lymphocytes Macrophages	

[a]CPA, N^6-cyclopentyladenosine; NECA, 5'-N-ethyl-carboxamidoadenosine; APNEA, M-[2-(4-aminophenyl) ethyl]adenosine; CPX, 1,3-dipropyl-8-cylopentylxanthine; XAC, xanthine amine cogener; $\alpha\beta$mATP, α,β-methylene ATP; ATPγS, adenosine 5'-O-(3-thio)triphosphate; 2mSATP, 2-methylthio-ATP; PPADS, pyridoxalphosphate-6-azophenyl-2', 4'-disulfonic acid; $A_{P3}A$, P^1,P^3-bis(adenosyl)triphosphate(diadenosine triphosphate); $A_{P5}A$, P^1,P^5-(adenosyl)pentaphosphate(diadenosine pentaphosphate).

gested on the basis of cloned receptors and the recent development of new selective agonists (Table 1). This basic framework of fast and slow receptors is in accordance with that developed for other neurotransmitters including acetylcholine (nicotinic and muscarinic receptors), GABA (GABA$_A$ and GABA$_B$), and glutamate (ionotropic and metabotropic receptors) (see Table 1). The precise identification and numbering of the subclasses within these two major P2 purinoceptor families is likely to be debated in the coming period.

Sympathetic Cotransmission

There is a substantial body of evidence to show that norepinephrine (NE) and ATP act as cotransmitters, being released from sympathetic nerves in variable proportions depending on the tissue and species. Many of the early and more detailed studies were made on the vas deferens. Evidence for purinergic cotransmission includes: block of the prazosin-resistant component of the response to sympathetic nerve stimulation by the **ATP antagonists** arylazido amino-proprionyl-ATP (ANAPP$_3$), suramin, or the **selective desensitizer of the P$_{2X}$ purinoceptor**, α,β-methylene ATP; release of ATP during nerve stimulation, which is abolished by 6-hydroxydopamine, but is unaffected by selective depletion of NE by **reserpine**; selective block by ATP antagonists of **excitatory junction potentials (ejps)** in response to sympathetic nerve stimulation and mimicry of ejps by ATP, but not by NE.

Studies of sympathetic cotransmission involving ATP and NE have now also been carried out on a number of different isolated blood vessels and in whole animals. In rabbit coronary vessels, in contrast to most other vessels where NE and ATP cause synergistic constriction via α_1 adrenoceptors and P$_{2X}$ purinoceptors, respectively, the predominant effect of ATP is vasodilatation via P$_{2Y}$ purinoceptors. Since in this vessel the predominant effect of NE is vasodilatation via β-adrenoceptors, this is consistent with the synergism that appears to be characteristic of cotransmission.

While early studies established adenosine as the principal modulator of transmitter release from sympathetic nerves via prejunctional P$_1$ purinoceptors, several authors have also identified **prejunctional P$_2$ purinoceptors** on autonomic nerve terminals in various tissues. In the rat vas deferens and iris it has been suggested that these prejunctional ATP receptors are probably P$_{2Y}$ purinoceptors. Recent experiments suggest that receptors for naturally occurring dinucleotides on nerve terminals in the brain can also modulate release of transmitters.

Parasympathetic Cotransmission

Acetylcholine (ACh) and ATP appear to be cotransmitters in parasympathetic neurons in the bladder. It has been shown recently that there is plasticity in expression of cotransmitters in parasympathetic nerves supplying the human urinary bladder, in that the ratio of purinergic to cholinergic components of excitatory transmission is much increased in interstitial cystitis. There is also indirect evidence for ATP being colocalized with ACh and the peptides neuropeptide Y (NPY) or somatostatin, in subpopulations of intrinsic neurons in the heart and airways that project to small blood vessels in these organs.

Sensory–Motor Cotransmission

Subpopulations of sensory nerves have been suggested to utilize ATP as well as substance P (SP) and calcitonin gene-related peptide (CGRP). By analogy with other systems, it seems likely that ATP coexists in different proportions with these two peptides, perhaps cooperating in **axon reflex** activity. Since the role of these nerves during axon reflexes to many organs is motor rather than sensory they have been termed **sensory–motor nerves** to distinguish them from the other subpopulation of afferent fibers which have a pure sensory role and whose terminals contain few vesicles and a predominance of mitochondria.

Nonadrenergic, Noncholinergic Inhibitory Cotransmission in the Gut

Evidence that ATP was the NANC inhibitory transmitter in nerves supplying the guinea pig taenia coli was first presented in 1970. In the late 1970s evidence for **vasoactive intestinal polypeptide** (VIP) as a slow NANC inhibitory transmitter in various regions of the gastrointestinal tract was presented, and recently it has been proposed that **nitric oxide** (NO) is also a NANC inhibitory transmitter in the gut. The current consensus of opinion is that ATP, VIP, and NO are probably cotransmitters mediating responses with different time courses in NANC inhibitory nerves, but that they vary considerably in proportion in different regions of the gut.

Somatic Neuromuscular Transmission

There are many reports of coexistence and release of ATP with ACh at somatic motor nerve endings. ATP acts as a neuromodulator of both the release (via adenosine) and action of ACh. There is little information available to date to support a cotransmitter role for ATP at these junctions of mature adults, but patch-clamp studies have shown that micromolar concentrations of ATP, as well as ACh, activate channels in the membrane of cultured myoblasts and myotubes.

Nerve–Nerve Synaptic Transmission in Autonomic Ganglia and Central Nervous System

There is recent, compelling evidence for purinergic synaptic transmission in both the coeliac ganglion and the medial habenula in the brain. Excitatory postjunctional potentials (EPSPs) have been recorded that are blocked by P_{2X} purinoceptor antagonists and mimicked by ATP.

References

1. Abbracchio M, Burnstock G. Purinoceptors: are there families of P2X and P2Y purinoceptors? Pharmacol Ther, 1994;64:445–75.
2. Burnstock G. Purinergic nerves. Pharmacol Rev 1972;24:509–81.
3. Burnstock G. A basis for distinguishing two types of purinergic receptor. In: Straub RW, Bolis L, eds. Cell membrane receptors for drugs and hormones: a multidisciplinary approach. New York: Raven Press, 1978:107–18.

4. Burnstock G. Co-transmission. The fifth Heymans lecture—Ghent, February 17, 1990. Arch Int Pharmacodyn Ther 1990;304:7–33.
5. Burnstock G. Physiological and pathological roles of purines: an update. Drug Dev Res 1993;28:195–206.

18   Amino Acid Neurotransmission

William T. Talman
Neurology and Neuroscience
The University of Iowa
and Neurology Service
Veterans Affairs Medical Center
Iowa City, Iowa

As detailed in earlier chapters, the autonomic nervous system is highly organized from its peripheral receptors to the terminals of visceral efferents. Afferent nerve fibers from mechano– and chemoreceptors originate in neurons of autonomic ganglia. Those cells project into the central nervous system where signals are processed and, through actions of converging peripheral and central inputs, are integrated into meaningful autonomic responses to simple and complex stimuli. **Amino acids** acting as putative **neurotransmitters** may play a role in signal transduction at each level of this system.

This section will briefly outline participation of three representative amino acids, the excitatory amino acid **glutamate** and inhibitory amino acids **GABA** and **glycine**, in transmitting signals that modulate sympathetic output of one well-defined cardiovascular reflex, the baroreceptor reflex. Depending on the brain region under consideration, evidence for this involvement varies considerably. In no region can it be said that all criteria have been met to establish any one of these amino acids as a transmitter at a particular synapse, but significant data have developed over the past decade to suggest that each agent may contribute to varying degrees at different sites.

Although none of the three amino acids has been implicated in mechano- or chemoreceptor transduction at the level of the peripheral receptor, some evidence suggests that glutamate transmission may be involved in the periphery. Specifically, **glutamate binding sites** are transported from the **nodose ganglion** toward the **aortic arch.** Thus, both receptors that bind glutamate and aortic baroreceptors may be found in close proximity. In addition, neurons within the nodose ganglion are activated by introduction of glutamate and its analogs.

Each of the three putative transmitters is present in the nodose ganglion, but neurochemical evidence suggests that only GABA and glutamate may be released from **baroreceptor afferent fibers** in the **nucleus tractus solitarii** (NTS), the primary site of termination of those and other visceral afferent fibers. At this important site, each amino acid potentially may modulate cardiovascular activity. However, an agonist's actions alone are not sufficient evidence to support a role for the agent as a transmitter at a specific synapse. Another important criterion is the ability of selective antagonists to block effects of natural activation of that synapse. In the NTS, glutamate has met this criterion.

Numerous studies have confirmed that the baroreceptor reflex may be blocked by **antagonists to glutamate receptors** in the NTS. Thus, although glutamate and other agents, including glycine, may produce cardiovascular responses like those of baroreceptor reflex activation, **only blockade of glutamate receptors leads to nearly total blockade of the baroreceptor reflex** itself. It would seem then that glutamate, whose receptors are found in the NTS, may be a transmitter of primary afferents in the reflex. That it may also be involved in other cardiovascular reflexes is suggested by pressor responses produced by injecting it into some very discrete regions of the NTS of anesthetized animals or into larger regions of NTS in unanesthetized animals. Evidence from such studies supports a role for the amino acid in transmission of **chemoreceptor** reflexes as well as **baroreceptor** reflexes at the level of NTS. Attenuation of the chemoreceptor reflex by injection of glutamate antagonists into the NTS further supports its participation in the reflex.

GABA, on the other hand, may also be released from **vagal**, possibly baroreceptor, afferents, but its release into NTS does not produce a cardiovascular effect like that of baroreceptor reflex activation. Instead, it may inhibit baroreceptor reflex neurons in the NTS. Whether directly involved in cardiovascular reflex transmission, GABA, and glycine as well, have been shown to participate in integration of signals coming into NTS. It is possible that the former is derived from peripheral afferents as well as from projections of other central nuclei, while glycine, which apparently is not released from vagal afferents, **may arise from local interneurons.** Like GABA, it participates in modulating responses of neurons in NTS to multiple incoming signals. In addition, glycine also indirectly activates local neurons by initiating release of the excitatory agent acetylcholine from cholinergic terminals in NTS.

The baroreceptor reflex pathway continues beyond NTS with projections that pass rostrally and caudally to different cardiovascular nuclei in the ventral medulla. More rostrally axons project directly to a region, the **rostral ventrolateral medulla** (RVLM), that plays an important role in tonic maintenance of blood pressure. With activation of those fibers, there is sympathoexcitation due, apparently, to release of glutamate into the RVLM. Activation of the more caudal projection also apparently leads to release of glutamate but, in this case, the excitatory effect is manifest on GABAergic neurons that project from the **caudal ventrolateral medulla** to the RVLM. Thus, their activation reduces blood pressure by inhibiting sympathoexcitatory cells upon which they terminate. The mechanisms that favor activation of one pathway that is sympathoexcitatory vs another that is sympathoinhibitory are not known, but clearly other input to the RVLM may also integrate function in that nucleus during well-defined behaviors.

For example, activation of the **lateral hypothalamus,** which may elicit a behavioral response, leads to activation of glutamate receptors on neurons in the RVLM. Resulting increased sympathetic nerve activity tends to increase blood pressure. This glutamatergic input to the rostral ventrolateral medulla provides an important integrative function by overriding the inhibitory influence of baroreceptor reflex activation that would otherwise occur with elevated blood pressure associated with the behavior.

Well before any role had been found for either GABA or glutamate in the RVLM, potential involvement of **glycinergic transmission** had already been suggested. Initially, glycine was applied to the ventral surface of the medulla where it elicited reductions in blood pressure. Thus, a depressor function was ascribed to it within the general region of the rostral ventral medulla. However, it may elicit either depressor or pressor responses depending upon the site at which it is injected into the rostral ventral medulla. The origin of glycine terminals in the region and the mechanism of its differing actions is still not known.

Completing the central portion of the sympathetic limb of the baroreceptor reflex, neurons in the RVLM project to the **intermediolateral column** of the spinal cord where sympathetic preganglionic fibers originate. At this site too, **glutamate** may play an important role. Released from descending fibers from the medulla, it affects maintenance of sympathetic tone or increases sympathetic activity in response to stimuli. GABA and glycine, likewise, may participate in modulating sympathetic activity at the level of the intermediolateral column and may be colocalized with each other or with other more classic neurotransmitters in terminals within the region.

Clearly each of these amino acids may contribute to regulation of cardiovascular function in normal animals, but they may also be part of derangements that lead to hypertension in experimental animals. Their importance is supported by shifts in sensitivity to GABA and glutamate injected into central nuclei in the spontaneously hypertensive rat model of genetic hypertension.

References

1. Gordon FJ, Talman, WT. Role of excitatory amino acids and their receptors in bulbospinal control of cardiovascular function. In: Kunos G, Ciriello J, eds. Central neural mechanisms in cardiovascular regulation, Vol. 2. New York: Birkhauser, 1992:209–25.
2. Lewis SJ, Cincotta M, Verberne AJM, Jarrott B, Lodge D, Beart PM. Receptor autoradiography with [3H] L-glutamate reveals the presence and axonal transport of glutamate receptors in vagal afferent neurons of the rat. Eur J Pharmacol 1987;144:413–5.
3. Machado BH, Bonagamba LGH. Microinjection of L-glutamate into the nucleus tractus solitarii increases arterial pressure in conscious rats. Brain Res 1992;576:131–8.
4. Sun MK, Guyenet PG. Hypothalamic glutamatergic input to medullary sympathetoexcitatory neurons in rats. Am J Physiol 1986;251:R798–810.
5. Talman WT, Wellendorf L, Martinez D, Ellison S, Li X, Cassell MD, Ohta H. Glycine elicits release of acetylcholine from the nucleus tractus solitarii in rat. Brain Res 1994;650:253–9.

19 Imidazoline Receptors and Their Native Ligands

Donald J. Reis
Department of Neurology and Neuroscience
Cornell University Medical College
New York, New York

S. Regunathan
Department of Neurology and Neuroscience
Cornell University Medical College
New York, New York

Imidazoline (I) **receptors** are nonadrenergic binding sites recognizing clonidine and allied agents. The concept of I receptors arose from observations that the central hypotensive actions of clonidine did not relate solely to the drug's actions as an α_2-adrenergic agonist but also to its structure as an imidazol(in)e.

Ligand binding has confirmed the existence of I receptors as nonadrenergic binding sites for clonidine, idazoxan, and allied agents. I receptors exist in multiple forms which differ in affinities for ligands, and in the regional cellular and subcellular distributions. The I_1 **receptor**, relatively uncommon, binds clonidine and idazoxan with approximately equal affinities and is localized to brainstem, kidney, and several other organs and tissues. Its subcellular distribution and signal transduction processes have yet to be defined. Functionally, I_1 receptors may mediate, at least in part, the central hypotensive actions of clonidine and related drugs (e.g., rilmenidine or moxonidine).

I_2 **receptors** are more prevalent. They have a greater affinity for idazoxan than for clonidine and are expressed in a number of cells/tissues including basolateral membranes of kidney, liver, brain (particularly astrocytes), adipocytes, urethra, platelets, pancreatic β-cells, placenta, and adrenal chromaffin cells. I_2 receptors are largely, if not entirely, expressed on mitochondrial membranes, are not coupled to G proteins, and appear linked in some manner with ion channels, possibly for K^+ and/or Ca^{2+}.

While all known ligands binding to I receptors also bind to α_2-adrenergic receptors, there is substantial biochemical, biological, and pharmacological evidence that the two receptors differ structurally. However, proof of difference will be established once I receptors have been cloned.

Endogenous ligands for I receptors are probably multiple. One is a substance of low molecular weight ($\sim$588 Da), purportedly neither a catecholamine nor a peptide, and partially purified from brain. It has been named **clonidine displacing substance** (CDS). CDS competitively displaces, with high affinity, clonidine and idazoxan from α_2–adrenergic, I_1, and I_2 receptors. Partially purified CDS is bioactive, having actions attributable to interactions with α_2 receptors (inhibition of contraction of vas deferens and platelet aggregation) and with nonadrenergic sites, probably I receptors (contraction of rat gastric fundus).

Purification of CDS-like material from rat brain has also yielded one defined molecule which binds to α_2 (but not other adrenergic receptors),

I_1, and I_2 receptors. This substance is **agmatine,** an amine which is the product of decarboxylation of the amino acid arginine by arginine decarboxylase (ADC). Agmatine and ADC are prevalent in bacteria, plants, and other lower forms, but was not previously believed to be widely distributed in mammalian tissue. Agmatine, however, has a lower molecular weight than "classical" CDS, does not share comparable bioactivity, and is presumably a different molecule.

The observations that agmatine is regionally stored and synthesized in brain, is stored in part in dense core vesicles, is present in appropriate concentrations, and has receptors suggest that it may be a novel neurotransmitter/modulator. It is also of interest that in bacteria agmatine is a precursor of putrescine and other polyamines through a pathway other than the decarboxylation of ornithine by ornithine decarboxylase. Whether agmatine is a precursor of polyamine biosynthesis in mammals by this alternative pathway is not known.

Another substance which may or may not be classic CDS has been identified by antibodies generated against several drugs which interact with I receptors including clonidine and idazoxan. The regional distribution of immunoreactive CDS (ir-CDS) correlates with the bioactivity of CDS-like material and does not appear to be agmatine.

In summary, the concept of I receptors, while new, is now widely accepted. However, it should be recognized that the term is imprecise. Some agents which are not imidazolines bind to the receptor, including some guanidiniums (e.g., guanabenz) and oxazoles (e.g., rilmenidine). Also, no clear functional responses specifically associated with the receptor have been identified. Hence, the characterization of the I receptor as a "receptor" has yet to meet the criterion of function. Finally, while receptors are usually named in relationship to their endogenous ligand, it is not clear whether agmatine is the only and most relevant one. However, the wide distribution in mammalian tissues of I receptors, agmatine, and ir-CDS, and the potency of drugs which bind to the I-receptor, suggests that the system may be of potential importance in biology, therapeutics, and disease.

Reference

1. Reis DJ, Bousquet P, Parini A. The imidazoline receptor: pharmacology, functions, ligands, and relevance to biology and medicine. Ann NY Acad Sci 763, 1995.

PART IV

Clinical Evaluation of Autonomic Function

Clinical Assessment of Autonomic Failure

David Robertson
Medicine, Pharmacology and Neurology
Vanderbilt University
Nashville, Tennessee

There are more **tests** of the autonomic nervous system than of any other neurological system. Many of these tests are readily applied at the bedside. Unfortunately although these bedside autonomic tests are **easy to perform,** they may be **difficult to interpret** in an individual patient. Most physicians who routinely follow patients with autonomic disorders develop a small armamentarium of tests they feel comfortable with and rely upon. For the **neurologist,** tests of peripheral sudomotor function may form the organizing nucleus of autonomic evaluation; for the **cardiologist** it may be tests of blood pressure and heart rate; for the **endocrinologist,** it may be circulating catecholamines and renin (Chapters 16 and 21); for the **ophtalmologist,** it may be pupillary tests (Chapter 13); and for the **pharmacologist,** it may be drug tests for evidence of stimulatable autonomic function or hypersensitivity. In spite of such dramatically divergent diagnostic approaches, it is remarkable how much concensus is often achieved in terms of the actual diagnosis and therapy of an individual patient.

A carefully taken **history** is obviously the single most valuable diagnostic resource. A brief listing of important points in questioning patients is shown in Table 1. More detailed discussions of some of these may be found in Chapters 47, 51 and 59, as well as in the Low text (1). Key features for evaluation in the physical exam are shown in Table 2.

In this section, attention will be given to highly informative autonomic tests. A listing of widely employed tests is shown in Table 4. Because many of these tests provide redundant information, most of them are unnecessary outside a research environment.

Orthostatic Test

Orthostatic symptoms are usually the most debilitating aspect of autonomic dysfunction readily amenable to therapy, and for this reason the blood pressure and heart rate response to upright posture should be the starting point of any autonomic laboratory evaluation. In healthy human subjects, the cardiovascular effect of upright posture has been carefully defined. When assumption of the upright posture is **active (standing),** the vigorous contraction of large muscles leads to a transient muscle vasodilatation and minor fall in arterial pressure for which the reflexes are not immediately able to completely compensate, but this short-lived depressor phase is not usually seen with **passive (tilt table)**

Table 1.   **Key Features in the Autonomic History**

Orthostatic intolerance or hypotension
 Dizziness or lightheadedness
 Visual changes
 Neck, shoulder discomfort
 Weakness
 Confusion
 Slurred speech
 Presyncope or syncope
 Postprandial angina pectoris
 Nausea
 Palpitations
 Tremulousness
 Flushing sensation
 Nocturia
 Worsening by
  Bedrest
  Food ingestion
  Alcohol
  Fever
  Hot weather/environment
  Hot bath
  Environmental heat
  Exercise
  Hyperventilation
Hypohidrosis
 Dry skin
 Dry socks and feet
 Reduced skin wrinkling
 Excessive sweating in intact regions
Genitourinary Dysautonomia
 Impotence
 Nocturia
 Urinary retention
 Urinary incontinence
 Recurrent urinary tract infection

Gastrointestinal dysautonomia
 Constipation
 Postprandial fullness
 Anorexia
 Diarrhea
 Fecal urgency and incontinence
 Weight loss
Poorly characterized dysautonomia features
 Early transient autonomic hyperfunction
 Anemia
 Ptosis
 Supine nasal stuffiness
 Supine hypertension and diuresis
 Fatigue
Nonautonomic features in multiple system atrophy
 Problems with balance/movement
 Loud respirations/snoring
 Episodic gasping respirations
 Sleep apnea
 Brief crying spells
 Emotional lability
 Leg pain
 Altered libido
 Hypnogogic leg jerking
 Hallucinations
 Difficulty swallowing
 Aspiration pneumonia
 Drooling
 Other cerebellar and extrapyramidal symptoms

upright posture. Immediately after 90° head-up tilt, about 500 ml of blood move into the veins of the legs and about 250 ml into the buttocks and pelvic area. There is a rapid, vagally mediated increase in heart rate followed by a sympathetically mediated further increase. As right ventricular stroke volume declines, there is depletion of blood from the pulmonary reservoir and central blood volume falls. Stroke volume falls and cardiac output decreases about 20%. With this decline in cardiac output, blood pressure is maintained by vasoconstriction that reduces splanchnic, renal, and skeletal muscle blood flow especially, but other circulations as well.

In the orthostatic test, **mild autonomic impairment** usually leads to a dramatic tachycardia with relatively little change in blood pressure (Table 3). In the presence of a still functioning **baroreflex**, the increased heart rate can compensate for the mild peripheral denervation, thus preventing significant decrement in blood pressure. With **moderate autonomic neuropathy**, the tachycardia may still be present, but may be unable to compensate completely, and

Table 2. Key Features in the Autonomic Physical Exam

Skin
  Dryness
  Dry socks and feet
  Reduced hand wrinkling
  Absent pilomotor reaction
  Pallor
Eyes
  Impaired pupillary motor function
  Dryness of eyes (redness, itching)
  Ptosis
Cardiovascular
  Low standing blood pressure ± tachycardia
  Unchanging pulse rate on standing
  Elevated supine blood pressure
  Loss of respiratory arrhythmia
Gastrointestinal
  Reduced salivation
  Stomach fullness
  Reduced transit time
  Impaired anal tone

Genitourinary
  Impaired morning erection
  Retrograde ejaculation
  Urgency
  Sphincter weakness
  Atonic bladder
Other
  Abnormal temperature regulation
  Reduced metabolic rate
Nonautonomic features in multiple
  system atrophy
  Extrapyramidal signs
    (rigidity > tremor)
  Cerebellar signs
  Impaired ocular movements
  Slurred speech
  Laryngeal paralysis
  Muscle wasting

Table 3. Hemodynamics
of Autonomic Failure (AF)
on Standing

	ΔBP	ΔHR
Normal	—	↑
Mild AF	—	↑ ↑ ↑
Moderate AF	↓ ↓	↑ ↑
Severe AF	↓ ↓ ↓	—

Table 4A. Tests of Baroreflex Function

Test	Afferent	Integration	Efferent	Response
Orthostasis	IX, X, CNS	Medulla	Autonomic	↑ HR
Deep breathing	X	Medulla	X	↑ HR (inspiration)
Valsalva	IX, X, CNC	Medulla	Autonomic	↑ HR then ↓ HR
Cuff occlusion	IX, X	Medulla	Autonomic	↓ BP, ↑ HR
Saline infusion	IX, X	Medulla	Autonomic	↑ BP, ↓ HR
Barocuff (suction)	IX	Medulla	X	↓ HR
Barocuff (pressure)	IX	Medulla	X	↑ HR
LBNP	IX, X	Medulla	Autonomic	↑ HR
Carotid massage	IX	Medulla	Autonomic	↓ HR, ↓ BP
Phenylephrine	IX, X	Medulla	Autonomic	↓ HR
Nitroprusside	IX, X	Medulla	Autonomic	↑ HR

Abbreviations: IX, glossopharyngeal; X, vagus; CNS, central nervous system; HR, heart rate; BP, blood pressure; LBNP, lower body negative pressure.

Table 4B.   Tests of Neurotransmitter Receptor Responsiveness

Name	Administration	Receptor	Response
1. Agonists			
Phenylephrine	IV, eye	α_1	Pressor; pupillary dilatation
Clonidine	Oral	α_2, I	Depressor (central); MSNA
Isoproterenol	IV	β_1	Increased HR
Isoproterenol	IV local	β_2	Depressor; vascular resistance
Acetylcholine	IV local	Muscarinic	Decreased vascular resistance
Methacholine	Eye	Muscarinic	Pupillary constriction
Nicotine	IV	Nicotinic	Increased HR
2. Antagonists			
Phentolamine	IV	α_1,α_2	Depressor
Yohimbine	IV	α_2	Increased BP, plasma NE
Propranolol	IV	β_1	Reduced HR
Propranolol	IV local	β_2	Increased vascular resistance
Atropine	IV	Muscarinic	Increased HR
Trimethaphan	IV	Nicotinic	Depressor; MSNA
3. Neurotransmitter-releasing agents			
Tyramine	IV	α, β	Increased BP; plasma NE
Hydroxyamphetamine	Eye	α_1	Pupillary dilatation
4. Pheochromocytoma-provoking agents			
Histamine	IV	α_1, β	Increased BP; plasma NE
Glucagon	IV	α_1, β	Increased BP; plasma NE

Abbreviations: I, imidazoline; IV, intravenous; MSNA, muscle sympathetic nerve activity; NE, norepinephrine; BP, blood pressure; HR, heart rate.

mild orthostatic hypotension may occur. As the neuropathy becomes more severe, the orthostatic fall in blood pressure becomes greater and greater and the ability of the efferent autonomic system to manifest a tachycardia is progressively attenuated. In **severe autonomic failure,** the fall in blood pressure may be more than 100 mm Hg and yet the heart rate may not rise at all.

Orthostatic tolerance is challenged by a number of factors. Important among them are food ingestion, high environmental temperature, hyperventilation, endogenous vasodilators, and many pharmacological agents. If no abnormality in orthostatic blood pressure or heart rate is detected in the hour after ingestion of a large meal, autonomic neuropathy of sufficient severity to cause cardiovascular instability is effectively ruled out.

An important aspect of evaluation of responses to orthostasis is the rapid **reduction in total blood volume** which occurs. It is not unusual for a 12% fall in total blood volume to occur within 10 min of assumption of the upright posture as fluid goes from the vascular compartment into the extravascular space. This accounts for the delay in appearance of symptoms in patients with mild autonomic impairment for some minutes after the actual assumption of upright posture. Therefore, the **long stand** (30 min) **test** is a much more severe orthostatic stress than the **short stand** (5 min) **test** commonly employed.

Table 4C. Other Autonomic Tests

Test	Afferent	Integration	Efferent	Response
Cold pressor	Pain fibers	CNS	Sympathoadrenal	↑ BP
Handgrip	Muscle afferents	CNS	Autonomic	↑ BP, ↑ HR
Mental arithmetic	CNS	CNS	Sympathoadrenal	↑ BP
Startle	Auditory	CNS	Sympathoadrenal	↑ BP, ↑ HR
Face immersion	V	Medulla	Autonomic	↓ HR
Pupil cycle time	Optic nerve	Edinger–Westphall	III	Dilate/constrict
Venous response (inspiratory gasp)	Spinal nerve	Cord	Sympathetic	Venoconstriction
Venarteriolar reflex	Noradrenergic axon	Neuron	Noradrenergic axon	Vasoconstriction
Reflex heating	Spinothalamic	Hypothalamus	Sympathetic	Vasodilatation
Thermoregulatory	Temp. receptors	Hypothalamus	Sympathetic	Sweating
QSART	Sympathetic cholinergic axon	Neuron	Sympathetic cholinergic axon	Sweating

Abbreviations: CNS, central nervous system; BP, blood pressure; V, trigeminal nerve; III, oculomotor nerve; OSART, quantitative sudomotor axon reflex test.

Tilt-table Testing

Many investigators prefer the use of **upright tilt** to the **orthostatic test** in the evaluation of the variables. In general, analogous but not identical results are obtained. The use of upright tilt is described in detail in Chapter 33. While there is no proof that upright tilt offers any diagnostic advantage over carefully obtained upright blood pressure data, many investigators use tilt because of its convenience, its capacity to calibrate the gravity stimulus, and its safety to the patient.

Pharmacological Tests

Information about prevailing sympathetic and parasympathetic activation as well as denervation hypersensitivity can be achieved by use of **muscarinic** and **adrenergic** agonists and antagonists. References (1) and (3) provide instructive examples of how **biochemical** and **physiological** tests may be combined to make novel diagnostic discoveries.

References

1. Low PA. Laboratory evaluation of autonomic function. Chapter 14 in Clinical autonomic disorders. Boston: Little, Brown, 1993:169–96.
2. Eckberg DL. Parasympathetic cardiovascular control in human disease: a critical review of methods and results. Am J Physiol 1980;239:H581–93.
3. Robertson D, Goldberg MR, Hollister AS, Onrot J, Wiley R, Thompson JG, Robertson RM. Isolated failure of autonomic noradrenergic neurotransmission: evidence for impaired beta-hydroxylation of dopamine. N Engl J Med 1986;314:1494–7.
4. Goldstein DS, Kopin IJ. In: Laragh JH, Brenner B, eds. Hypertension: pathophysiology, diagnosis, and management, Chapter 47, 1st edition. New York: Raven Press, 1990:711–32.
5. Robertson D. Assessment of autonomic function. In: Baughman Kl, ed. Clinical diagnostic manual for the house officer, Chapter 9. Baltimore: Williams & Wilkins, 1981:86–101.

21 Biochemical Assessment of Sympathetic Activity

Joseph L. Izzo, Jr.
Department of Medicine
Millard Fillmore Hospitals and
Clinical Pharmacology
State University of New York at Buffalo
Buffalo, New York

The extraordinary dynamic range of whole-body and organ-specific sympathoadrenal response has necessitated the development of a wide variety of techniques to study this pervasive integrative and regulatory system. **It is important to understand that no single technique can be used in all studies and that the information gained from using several diverse approaches is often complementary.** This chapter presents the biochemical techniques that have been developed over the last 40 years, largely in order of historical appearance.

Urinary Excretion of Catecholamines and Metabolites

Elevated **vanillylmandelic acid (VMA)** to greater than 7 mg/day (by the Pisano assay) has historically been considered diagnostic of pheochromocytoma. Although VMA is the major end-product of combined oxidation and transmethylation of NE and epinephrine, it is quite insensitive to physiologic variations in sympathetic output. Better diagnostic sensitivity of urinary metanephrines and plasma catecholamines has reduced clinical usefulness of urinary VMA.

Free Catecholamines

Total or fractionated urinary catecholamines are still used in the determination of 24-hr sympathetic nervous activity and in the diagnosis of pheochromocytoma. Under usual conditions, the majority of urinary NE is derived from circulatory rather than renal sources. Normal values are usually less than 115 μg/day.

Metanephrines

Metanephrines are the primary O-methylated metabolites of catecholamines. Although urinary metanephrines have had limited usefulness in the physiologic assessment of sympathetic tone, they are the preferred screening test for pheochromocytoma. Total 24-hr metanephrine excretion of less than 150 μg/day is considered normal.

Methoxyhydroxyphenyl Glycol (MHPG or MOPEG)

MHPG is produced in two steps: (1) oxidative metabolism in neural tissue and (2) O-methylation by the liver or kidney. MHPG can also be further metabolized to VMA. MHPG excretion was originally thought to represent CNS sympathetic output but is now known to be principally derived from peripheral sympathetic neuronal NE metabolism.

Plasma Catecholamines, Metabolites, and Enzymes

Plasma norepinephrine (NE), despite repeated attacks by some investigators, remains the most durable and reliable biochemical index to assess physiologic and pathologic increases in sympathoadrenal activity. NE found in plasma is derived both from adrenal and peripheral neuronal sources. Forearm venous plasma NE is closely related to the corresponding muscle sympathetic activity (Fig. 1).

Although the sensitivity of venous plasma NE to detect small changes in sympathetic activity is less than direct nerve traffic studies, the latter technique has limited applicability in clinical studies. The difficulty of comparing data between individuals or within individuals on different study days, the technical inability to perform adequate studies in as many as a third of subjects, the need to maintain subjects in an uncomfortable motionless position for relatively long periods of time, and the expense of the procedure are some of the problems

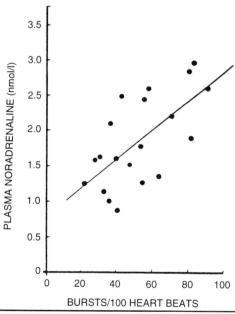

Figure 1.   Relationship between mean level of MSA (expressed as bursts/100 heart beats) and plasma concentration of noradrenaline. Each point represents one subject. $r = 0.65$, $P < 0.01$. Reprinted with permission from Wallin BG et al. Acta Physiol Scand 1981;111:69–73.

with microneurography that help justify the use of plasma catecholamines in many studies. Limitations in the use of kinetic studies (see *Catecholamine kinetic (turnover) studies* below) also support the use of plasma NE.

In general, venous plasma NE concentrations are about 30% higher than corresponding arterial values. Detractors of venous plasma NE usage argue that unequal organ sympathetic innervation causes different organs to produce NE at different rates and that assessment of whole-body sympathoadrenal activity requires use of arterial rather than venous NE. Yet further analysis reveals that this stance can also be problematic, largely due to the fact that the lung also metabolizes catecholamines. As a reasonable compromise, it may be wise to measure arteriovenous differences across the organ of interest, particularly if regional blood flow is also measured and the Fick equation is employed. For the most part, however, venous NE values are reasonable indices of vascular catecholamine production and have been found to correlate reasonably well with systemic hemodynamics in a variety of conditions and species.

Plasma catecholamines are useful in the diagnosis of **pheochromocytoma.** One caveat to their use in pheochromocytoma is that the normal range reported by most commercial laboratories is derived from young volunteers, not from appropriately controlled "at risk" patients; venous catecholamines less than 1000 pg/ml are highly unusual in established pheochromocytomas.

Dihydroxyphenyl Glycol (DHPG or DOPEG)

The primary neuronal metabolite of NE can be quantitated in plasma and has been shown to correlate closely with plasma NE and with neuronal NE turnover.

Epinephrine

In contrast to NE, epinephrine in plasma simply reflects adrenal output. In general, venous values are slightly lower than corresponding arterial values due to peripheral uptake. There is thus a slight advantage to the measurement of arterial rather than venous epinephrine but the difficulty of arterial sampling probably justifies use of venous values in many studies.

Dopamine

Free plasma dopamine normally circulates in very low concentrations (less than 50 pg/ml, which is often the limit of assay sensitivity) and has no direct relationship to other indices of sympathoadrenal activity or to well-accepted clinical syndromes. Thus it is disturbing that many clinical laboratories report plasma dopamine values as part of a "fractionated catecholamine" profile. Approximately 20 times as much dopamine circulates in the sulfoconjugated form than in the form of free dopamine.

Sulfoconjugates

In contrast to dopamine, sulfoconjugated NE and epinephrine circulate in concentrations only about three times higher than their respective free catecholamines. Acute changes in plasma catecholamines do not necessarily affect sulfoconjugate concentrations.

Dopamine Beta Hydroxylase (DBH) and Chromogranin A (CGA)

Both DBH, the enzyme responsible for the conversion of dopamine into NE in storage granules, and CGA, the major intravesicular storage protein that preserves NE, are released with catecholamines following nerve stimulation. These enzymes appear subsequently in plasma and changes in their plasma concentrations can be used in certain circumstances to reflect acute NE release.

Neuropeptide Y and Adrenomedullin

These peptides are also stored and released by sympathetic nerve terminals. Both are thought to be vasoactive, generally mimicking the actions of catecholamines. Their physiologic and diagnostic significance is currently under investigation.

Cerebrospinal Fluid Catecholamines and Metabolites

Free catecholamines and glycolic metabolites have been quantitated in cerebrospinal fluid and exist in concentrations similar to those observed in plasma. In most circumstances, little is offered by collection of CSF compared to other fluids.

Tissue Catecholamines

Catecholamine turnover in neural and peripheral tissues can be reliably assessed by the measurement of total tissue content, which is usually expressed in concentration per milligram of tissue. Peripheral tissue catecholamine content is inversely proportional to sympathetic nerve traffic because as catecholamine release increases, tissue stores are depleted. Tissue concentrations have been used most widely in the brain and heart, in both animal and human experiments.

Platelet catecholamine content has been utilized as a global integrated index of sympathetic function and in the diagnosis of pheochromocytoma. In platelets, nonspecific uptake (uptake 2) causes platelet catecholamine content to increase in parallel with systemic sympathoadrenal activity.

Catecholamine Kinetic (Turnover) Studies

The principal champions of the use of modified clearance techniques to estimate sympathetic nervous activity believe that wide interindividual or inter-organ variations in catecholamine metabolism seriously impair the use of free plasma catecholamines as indices of whole-body or organ-specific sympathetic nervous activity. Yet there is actually little evidence that the kinetic techniques themselves offer major advantages over simpler methods such as arteriovenous differences or even venous catecholamine concentrations in most studies. In fact, they may introduce their own artifacts.

The clearance of a given substance can be calculated from its steady-state infusion or delivery rate into the circulation and its steady-state plasma concentration:

$$\text{Clearance of X } (C_x, \text{ ml/min}) = \frac{\text{infusion rate of X (mg/min)}}{\text{steady-state plasma X (mg/ml)}}.$$

If the infused substance is identical to a native substance, it is also necessary to measure the basal plasma X concentration prior to infusion and to subtract this value from the plateau concentration of X achieved during the steady-state infusion. Given the plateau plasma X value (corrected if necessary) and the corresponding clearance rate of X from the circulation, a basal plasma appearance rate of X can be calculated:

$$\text{Appearance of X (mg/min)} = [\text{basal plasma X (mg/ml)}] \times [C_x \text{ (ml/min)}].$$

These formulas have been applied to the infusion of exogenous NE; when X is NE, the basal NE appearance rate is a measure of sympathetic nervous activity. In the case of NE, the appearance rate is often termed the **NE spillover rate** in reference to the fact that the majority of NE released by peripheral noradrenergic nerves undergoes immediate reuptake by the nerve terminals (**uptake 1**) or is metabolized (**uptake 2**). It must be remembered that as much as 80% of neuronally released NE is removed from the synapses by these mechanisms. The remainder (about 20%) that escapes these mechanisms becomes spillover. As long as the activities of the uptake mechanisms remain constant, the NE spillover rate (or plasma appearance rate) is a reasonable index of neuronal NE release and sympathetic nervous activity.

Radiotracer Infusions

Certain objections have arisen to the use of unlabeled NE infusions, largely on the theoretical grounds that the infused catecholamines could alter sympathoadrenal activity. As a result, tritiated NE infusions were developed by Esler and others to quantitate the amount of nerve traffic via the measurement of the rate of spillover of NE from synaptic clefts into plasma according to the formula

$$\text{Regional NE spillover} = [(C_v - C_a) + C_a * E] * PF,$$

where C = concentration, a = arterial, v = venous, E = extraction, PF = plasma flow. Central to the validity of this technique are the assumptions that true steady-state tritiated-NE concentrations are achieved across all compartments and that the release of tritiated NE into plasma after neuronal uptake is insignificant. Recent experiments by Zelis and coworkers (personal communication) suggest that an equilibrium period of 90–120 minutes is required before reaching steady-state in all compartments; all previous work used 45-min. equilibration periods. For example, using older whole-body kinetics, the lung has been calculated to be the major production site of NE, a finding that does not conform to known lung NE content or innervation density.

Despite these peculiarities, kinetic techniques have revealed that different organ beds can respond differently to systemic sympathoadrenal stimulation and that plasma catecholamines are not always adequately sensitive to detect differences between groups. For example, the kidney may experience sympathetic inhibition while muscle beds are stimulated. Similarly, using spillover methodology, hypertensives have been found to release more NE than normotensives in response to mental stress, whereas plasma NE responses did not differ between the two groups. There remain, however, significant limitations to the use of kinetic techniques. Perhaps the biggest drawback is the reluctance of many institutional review boards to approve the use of radiotracers for this purpose in humans. Another major drawback is the expense. Finally, the recommendation to infuse the tracer through a fluoroscopically placed central venous catheter is another significant barrier.

Analytical Methods for Catecholamines

There are two major methods of catecholamine detection in current use: **high-pressure liquid chromatography (HPLC)** and **radioenzymatic methods.** The two have a high degree of agreement but have different spectra of applications. The most widely used radioenzymatic method depends on **catechol-O-methyl transferase** activity to cause quantitative incorporation of a radioactive methyl group onto epinephrine or NE, thereby producing metanephrine and normetanephrine, which are analyzed after chromatographic separation and oxidation. Alternatively, NE can be quantitated by N-methylation to form epinephrine. Radioenzymatic methods for catecholamines are extremely sensitive (usually to 1 pg/sample) and are capable of detecting femtomolar quantities reliably. Unfortunately, they are also extremely expensive. The use of these methods is particularly justified if reliable quantitation of plasma epinephrine is desired, if repeated blood sampling is necessary, or if the work is to be carried out in small animals.

HPLC is the method of choice for urine and tissue samples where the concentrations of catecholamines are relatively high and the amount available for analysis is at least 50 pg per sample. Plasma NE values have been consistently measured by several laboratories using these techniques. Normal **resting plasma epinephrine values** (often less than 25 pg/ml) often challenge **the assay's sensitivity limits,** however. Difficulties with the assay include the problems of consistency of alumina extraction and the adequate maintenance of the electrochemical detection system required. Most laboratories that remain consistently productive maintain more than one HPLC system for catecholamine analysis.

References

1. Landsberg L, Young JB. Catecholamines and the adrenal medulla. In: Wilson JD, Foster DW, eds. Williams' textbook of endocrinology, Chapter 10, 8th ed. Philadelphia: W. B. Saunders, 1992: 637–40.
2. Goldstein DS, Kopin IJ. In: Laragh JH, Brenner B, eds. Hypertension: pathophysiology, diagnosis, and management, Chapter 47, 1st edition. New York: Raven Press, 1990: 711–732.

3. Wallin BG, Sundlof G, Eriksson BM, Dominiak P, Grobecker H, Lindblad LE. Plasma noradrenaline correlates to muscle sympathetic nerve activity in man. Acta Physiol Scand 1981;111: 69–73.

4. Esler M. Clinical application of noradrenaline spillover methodology: delineation of regional human sympathetic nervous responses. Pharmacol Toxicol 1993;73:243–53.

5. Goldstein DS, Eisenhofer G, Garty M, Folio CJ, Stull R, Brush JE Jr., Sax FL, Keiser HR, Kopin IJ. Implications of plasma levels of catechols in the evaluation of sympathoadrenomedullary function. Am J Hypertens 2:S133–9, 1989.

PART V

Environmental and Physical Stresses

22 Exercise and the Autonomic Nervous System

Vernon S. Bishop
Department of Physiology
The University of Texas Health Science Center
San Antonio, Texas

The autonomic nervous system plays a key role in the regulation of the cardiovascular response during **exercise.** The general concept is that at the onset of exercise, the central nervous system generates a **cardiorespiratory pattern (central command)** appropriate to the somatomotor signal. The central command then initiates a withdrawal of parasympathetic activity to the heart and an increase in ventilation rate, and is also probably involved in the resetting of the arterial baroreflex toward higher pressures. Although we know very little about the central neural connections involved in initiating the changes in parasympathetic and sympathetic outflow in the exercised state, we do know that central command and the arterial baroreflexes are critical to the sympathoexcitatory response at the onset of exercise (Fig. 1).

At the **onset of exercise,** it is generally accepted that heart rate (HR) is increased primarily by central command (**decrease in vagal activity to the heart**). As exercise continues or its level increases, further elevations in HR may occur as a result of increases in sympathetic outflow to the heart. If the resulting increase in cardiac output is inadequate to elevate the arterial pressure to the level required by the new operating point of the arterial baroreflex, then sympathetic outflow to the peripheral circulation will increase. The net effect of this increase in sympathetic outflow is to increase vascular resistance in regions not involved in the exercised response. Upward resetting of the operating point of the **arterial baroreflex** appears to be the major factor responsible for the sympathoexcitatory response to exercise (Fig. 1). As a result of this upward resetting, an error signal is created between the actual arterial pressure and the pressure of the new operating point. In order to minimize the error, sympathetic outflow is increased. It is important to note that once the error signal is corrected and the system is operating on the new baroreflex curve, not only the systemic pressure is elevated but also the level of sympathetic outflow relative to the pressure is elevated. This resetting of the operating point of the reflex provides an effective means of increasing sympathetic outflow and arterial pressures. In addition to the sympathoexcitatory response resulting from the resetting of the arterial baroreflexes, reflexes initiated from **muscle mechanosensitive and chemosensitive receptors,** as well as from **cardiac vagal afferents,** contribute to the regulation of sympathetic activity to the peripheral circulation.

Mechanosensitive and chemosensitive receptors located in the muscle provide important afferent signals relative to the activity and perfusion of exercising

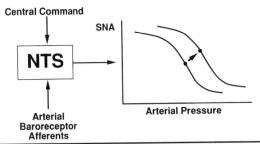

Figure 1. A schematic illustration of the role of central command and arterial baroreceptor afferents on the sympathetic component of the arterial baroreflex. Studies from DiCarlo and Bishop (2) indicate that central command and baroreceptor afferents are required for the upward resetting of the baroreflex. [Adapted from (1)].

muscles. In general, we assume that mechanical activation of the muscle receptor signals muscle activity and that the resulting afferent activity contributes to central command. Activation of the chemosensitive receptors by metabolites released during muscle contraction is probably involved when a mismatch between vascular resistance and cardiac output occurs. Increased activity from these receptors results in an increase in sympathetic activity to both active and inactive muscles.

In most animal models and humans, there is a **redistribution of cardiac output** to the exercising muscle. Basically, this involves an increase in sympathetic outflow to the visceral organs which results in an increase in vascular resistance in these regions. On the other hand, the resistance to the exercising muscle is diminished. The increased resistance to the nonexercising regions is initially the result of the upward resetting of the arterial baroreflex. As the exercise continues an additional increase in vascular resistance may occur due to activation of chemosensitive muscle afferents (1, 3).

In addition to the arterial baroreflexes and chemosensitive reflexes from the exercising muscle, cardiac vagal afferents also contribute to the redistribution of cardiac output during exercise. In rabbits, renal and mesenteric vascular resistances increase during running while systemic resistance decreases. Blockade of cardiac vagal afferents by intrapericardial injections of procainamide results in further increases in renal and mesenteric vascular resistance. However, it does not significantly affect systemic vascular resistance (Fig. 2A). This observation suggests that cardiac afferents modulate the magnitude of the sympathetic-mediated vasoconstriction of the visceral organs. Furthermore, when the tonic influence of the cardiac vagal afferents is increased by exercise training, the role of the cardiac vagal afferents in modulating vascular resistance of the visceral organs is also increased. Note that in the exercised endurance-trained state, the increase in renal and mesenteric vascular resistance is substantially less than in the untrained state (Figs. 2A and 2B). However, in the exercise-trained rabbit, blockade of the cardiac vagal afferents causes a greater increase in renal and mesenteric vascular resistance than in the untrained exercising rabbit. These findings

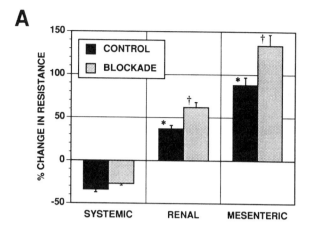

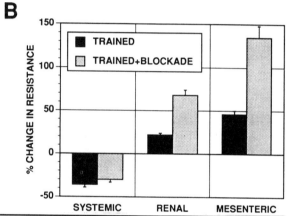

Figure 2. (A) Change in systemic, renal, and mesenteric resistance during exercise with cardiac afferents intact (control) and when cardiac afferents are blocked with procainamide (blockade). (B) Influence of cardiac afferents on systemic, renal, and mesenteric resistance during exercise in rabbits following endurance exercise training. Trained: response to exercise in endurance-trained rabbits with cardiac afferents intact. Trained plus blockade: response of the endurance-trained rabbits with cardiac afferents blocked with procainamide.

suggest that cardiac vagal afferents may be involved in determining the cardiovascular responses to a given workload.

In conclusion, one must realize that the role of neural mechanisms in the exercise response varies depending upon many factors. These include the type of exercise, the number of muscle groups involved, the duration of the exercise, and the level of endurance training.

References

1. Rowell LB, O'Leary DS. Reflex control of the circulation during exercise: chemoreflexes and mechanoreflexes. J Appl Physiol 1990;69(2):407–18.
2. DiCarlo SE, Bishop VS. Onset of exercise shifts operating point of arterial baroreflex to higher pressures. Am J Physiol 1992;262(31):H303–7.

3. DiCarlo SE, Bishop VS. Regional vascular resistance during exercise: role of cardiac afferents and exercise training. Am J Physiol 1990;258(27):H842–7.
4. DiCarlo SE, Bishop VS. Exercise training enhances cardiac afferent inhibition of baroreflex function. Am J Physiol 1990;258(27):H212–20.
5. DiCarlo SE, Bishop VS. Exercise training attenuates baroreflex regulation of nerve activity in rabbits. Am J Physiol 1988;255(24):H974–9.

23

Hypothermia

Bruce C. Paton
University of Colorado
Denver, Colorado

Hypothermia is defined as a core body temperature of <35°C. It may range from mild (32–35°C) to profound (<30°C). Several types of hypothermia exist.

Induced hypothermia protects organs in cardiac and transplantation surgery, and preserves isolated tissues such as blood and skin. Profound cold (cryotherapy) is used to destroy tissues and preserve cells such as sperm. **Accidental hypothermia** occurs if heat loss exceeds heat production or maintenance. **Incidental hypothermia** develops in neurologic, metabolic, and dermatologic diseases that interfere with body temperature control: hypothyroidism, diabetes, stroke, and brain tumors affecting the hypothalamus. Gram-negative sepsis is frequently associated with hypothermia.

Etiology

Heat is lost by four modes—conduction, convection, evaporation, and radiation. Pathophysiologic responses depend on speed of hypothermia development and duration. Immersion in very cold water induces hypothermia quickly with only minor changes in physiologic balance. Prolonged exposure to hypothermia may cause severe changes in metabolism and electrolyte and acid–base balance.

General Response to Heat Loss

The hypothalamus controls responses based on signals received from the periphery (skin) and the central nervous system (blood temperature). **Shivering** increases metabolism and vasoconstriction restricts further heat loss. Changes in skin temperature trigger shivering that can increase heat production fivefold, at the expense of increased oxygen consumption. Oxygen consumption falls 7% per degree Celsius, and there is slowing or reduction of many physiologic functions.

Specific Systematic Changes

Heart rate diminishes progressively. Below 30°C blood pressure may be difficult to measure by usual means because of stiff arteries and low blood pressure. Below 29°C arrhythmias are likely; **atrial fibrillation** is the most common. Below 27°C **ventricular fibrillation** or bradycardia may lead to **asystole** and death. Vasoconstriction shunts blood to core structures, maintains blood pressure, and reduces peripheral heat loss.

Respiratory rate falls; ventilation becomes shallow, partly because of increasing stiffness of the chest wall muscles. Respiration may cease below 29°C, but occasionally continues below 20°C. Tracheal and bronchial ciliary function stops; the cough reflex is suppressed and pneumonia is a common complication. Pulmonary edema is frequent in prolonged hypothermia.

Between 32 and 35°C cognitive functions deteriorate with **disorientation,** confusion, and character changes; **unconsciousness** occurs at 25–28°C. Reflexes slow, then cease. Pupils dilate and become fixed, simulating death. Diminished oxygen demand protects the CNS, permitting prolonged submersion or cessation of blood flow without residual damage. The spinal cord is similarly protected from prolonged ischemia.

Gastrointestinal motility decreases; **stress ulcers** may occur; **pancreatitis** is found after prolonged exposure to hypothermia. Serum sodium falls and potassium rises; glucose levels are variable. **Metabolic acidosis** is common if hypothermia is prolonged. The hematocrit and viscosity increase; the coagulation cascade slows without a specific abnormality; disseminated intravascular coagulation (DIC) occurs occasionally; thrombotic complications are common in fatal cases.

There is no correlation between TSH and temperature: thyroid hormone levels are normal unless the patient is hypothyroid; adrenal corticosteroids are usually normal, but may be reduced in prolonged exposure with adrenocortical exhaustion. **Cortisol** levels may rise during rewarming. Endogenous insulin levels remain normal. Exogenous insulin is not effective if body temperature is below 31°C. Thermoregulation is impaired with age. There is diminished perception of ambient temperature with lower body temperature, metabolic rate, and peripheral blood flow.

Diagnosis

Core temperature (rectal, esophageal, tympanic bladder) is essential for correct diagnosis. Hypothermia is possible in: (a) healthy victims of exposure or drowning, (b) otherwise healthy persons intoxicated by drugs or alcohol, (c) individuals with predisposing diseases such as hypothyroidism, hypopituitarism, malnutrition, muscular dysfunction and inactivity, hypoglycemia, or ketoacidosis, and (d) elderly individuals, without serious illness, who are exposed to mild cold.

Physical findings include slurred speech, impaired coordination, shivering, cold trunk skin, pale color (bright pink if vasodilated), diminished or absent reflexes, dilated and fixed pupils, slow respirations, slow heart rate, imperceptible pulse, blood pressure not measurable, no bowel sounds. Sometimes patients initially appear dead.

Clinical management consists of assessing consciousness, cardiorespiratory function, temperature, associated diseases and/or injuries, etiology, and duration of hypothermia. **Lab evaluation** should include a complete blood-screening biochemistry including BUN, sugar, and electrolytes, and in severe cases, a coagulation screen, acid–base measurement. A chest x-ray should also be obtained. Severely affected patients should be treated in intensive care with full physiologic monitoring (temperature, arterial and venous pressures, fluid balance, cardiac output); endotracheal intubation may be necessary (risk of inducing ventricular fibrillation is very small).

Treatment includes correction of physiological abnormalities with rewarming. Rewarming methods are: (a) remove cold wet clothing, place in warm dry environment, allow spontaneous rewarming; (b) active–external: hot water tub, hot water bottles, hydraulic or warm air blankets; (c) active–internal: hot food and drink, warmed intravenous fluids, warmed humidified air, lavage (gastric, thoracic, peritoneal, hemodialysis, extracorporeal circulation). The method chosen should be appropriate to severity. The patient should be rewarmed as rapidly as possible with full control. Permit access to the patient for resuscitation in case of need. Mortality (0–80%) depends on severity, duration, associated diseases, and injuries. Serum potassium greater than 10 mEq/liter and or need for CPR may predict fatal outcome.

References

1. Lloyd EL. Hypothermia and cold stress. Rockville, MD: Aspen Publications, 1956.
2. Paton BC. Accidental hypothermia. In: Schonbaum and Lomax, eds. Thermoregulation. New York: Pergamon Press, 1991.
3. Danzl D. Accidental hypothermia. In: Auerbach and Geehr, eds. Management of Wilderness and Environmental Emergencies, 3rd edition. St. Louis: Mosby, 1994.

24   *Environmental Hyperthermia*

Timothy J. Ingall
Department of Neurology
Mayo Clinic Scottsdale
Scottsdale, Arizona

The normal **core body temperature** (CBT) in man is near 37°C (98.6°F). This temperature is maintained independently of external conditions, by the interaction of a number of different thermoregulatory systems. Mild elevations of body temperature may occur in normal individuals who exercise in a hot environment. When this occurs, a number of physiologic responses are seen, including increases in plasma volume and heart rate and a decrease in stroke volume. The human body can tolerate increases in CBT up to approximately 40.5°C (104.9°F). The brain, and other body tissues, are at risk of thermal damage if the CBT exceeds 40.5°C.

There are two groups in the population who are at great risk for heat stress disorders related to environmental heat exposure. The first group is **young, healthy individuals** who undertake **prolonged exertion in a hot environment.** Heat stress disorders have been seen in football players, marathon runners, armed forces personnel on maneuvers, and laborers undertaking strenuous activity. Dehydration, the presence of infection, ingestion of alcohol or other drugs (Table 1), and possibly a prior history of heatstroke are factors which predispose young persons to heat stress disorders. The second, and largest, group at risk of heat stress disorders is **the elderly.** Those at particular risk include the lower socioeconomic groups, and those with systemic illnesses such as congestive heart failure, diabetes mellitus, malnutrition, alcoholism, dementia, and medications that impair thermoregulation. Physiologic factors contributing to hyperthermia in the elderly include reduced perception of environmental temperature changes, decreased vasodilatation, and reduced sweating. Heat stress disorders induced by exposure to environmental heat include heat rash, heat syncope, heat edema, heat cramps, heat exhaustion, and heatstroke.

Heat Rash

Affected individuals develop pruritic, glistening vesicles on a red base in an area of skin which is typically anhidrotic. Thermoregulation is maintained.

Heat Syncope

Postural hypotension, or syncope, can be seen in heat stress. These symptoms are thought to result from thermogenic vasodilatation, with associated orthostatic pooling of blood and diminished venous return.

Table 1. **Drugs Associated with Hyperthermia**

Alcohol
Amphetamines
Atropine
Benztropine mesylate
Beta blockers
Butyrophenones
Cannabinoids
Cocaine
Diuretics
LSD
Methyldopa
Monoamine oxidase inhibitors
Opiates
Phenothiazines
Tricyclic antidepressants
Vasoconstrictors

Heat Edema

Unacclimatized individuals may develop mild dependent edema when first exposed to a hot environment. This resolves with acclimatization.

Heat Cramps

Exertion in a hot environment can lead to skeletal muscle cramps. This may be caused by hyponatremia.

Heat Exhaustion

Heat exhaustion is the most common heat stress disorder. It is thought to be due to a combination of **dehydration** and **salt depletion.** The CBT is mildly elevated [<40.5°C (104.9°F)] and the individual is dehydrated and oliguric. Symptoms include cramps, thirst, weakness, and fatigue. Affected individuals are frequently agitated, and delirium may develop. Untreated heat exhaustion may progress to heatstroke.

Heatstroke

Classic heatstroke is defined as heatstroke that develops in individuals undertaking normal activities during prolonged exposure to high environmental temperatures. **Exertional heatstroke** is an extreme form of exertional hyperthermia which is seen most commonly in young adults who undertake strenuous activity in a hot environment. Three criteria define heatstroke.

1. Core body temperature above 41°C (105.8°F).
2. Hot, dry skin which may be pink or ashen.
3. Disturbances of the central nervous system.

Significant systemic complications can occur with heatstroke (Table 2). Early manifestations include **headache, drowsiness, confusion,** and **hyperventilation.** This is accompanied by metabolic changes including hypocalcemia, hypokalemia, hypoglycemia, and a primary respiratory alkalosis. Cerebellar signs and hemiplegia may develop, followed by coma and seizures. In severe cases, congestive heart failure, adult respiratory distress syndrome, pancreatitis, melena, and **disseminated intravascular coagulation** may occur. **Rhabdomyolysis** and **renal failure** are common in exertional heatstroke, but occur infrequently in classic heatstroke. The exact mechanisms producing tissue damage in heatstroke are unknown. Hyperthermia is thought to be the major cause of tissue injury. Other factors, such as metabolic acidosis, disseminated intravascular coagulation, circulatory failure, hypoxia, and myoglobinuria are also thought to contribute to tissue damage associated with hyperthermia.

Treatment of Heatstroke

Heatstroke is a **medical emergency** necessitating prompt management to reduce CBT. Initial treatment includes removing the patient from the hot

Table 2. **Complications of Heatstroke**

Central nervous system
  Agitation, confusion, and eventually coma
  Flaccidity
  Hemiplegia
  Cerebellar dysfunction
  Papilledema
  Seizures
Skeletal muscle
  Elevated creatine kinase levels which may be associated with
    rhabdomyolysis
Kidneys
  Renal failure in 5% of classic heatstroke cases and 25% of
    exertional heatstroke cases
Cardiovascular system
  Low cardiac output
  Low diastolic pressure
  High pulse pressure
  Cardiac failure
  Inverted T waves on EKG
  Conduction disturbances
Gastrointestinal system
  Diarrhea
  Vomiting
  Pancreatitis
  Hematemesis and melena
Pulmonary system
  Hyperventilation and respiratory alkalosis
  Pulmonary edema
  Adult respiratory distress syndrome
Hemostasis
  Disseminated intravascular coagulation (severe cases)
Laboratory findings
  Elevated transaminase levels
  Low prothrombin levels
  Hypoglycemia
  Hypocalcemia (early), hypercalcemia (late)
  Hypokalemia and hypophosphatemia (early), hyperkalemia (late)
  Lactic acidosis (severe cases)
  Leukocytosis up to 30,000 per milliliter
  Thrombocytopenia

environment, removing constricting clothing, dousing the patient with water, and fanning the patient to increase heat dissipation. Once the patient is at a medical facility, they can be immersed in an ice-water bath while other measures are taken as needed to protect the airway and provide hemodynamic support. A rectal thermistor probe should be used to monitor CBT. Complications, such as intravascular coagulation, rhabdomyolysis, renal failure, **lactic acidosis,** and other metabolic abnormalities may develop. If these occur, they should be treated with established medical protocols. **Seizures** may occur as the CBT falls. These should be treated with **intravenous diazepam.** While ice-water immersion is the standard treatment to reduce CBT, other measures are available, including immersion in tap water, warm air spray, and iced peritoneal lavage. Heatstroke is associated with significant mortality. Mortality rates as high as 52% have been reported. Early recognition and appropriate treatment can keep mortality as low as 5 to 10%. Longer duration of hyperthermia, prolonged coma, oliguric renal failure, hyperkalemia, and high levels of transaminases are associated with poor outcome. Survival from heatstroke is usually associated with good recovery, although some patients may have **residual cerebellar dysfunction or peripheral neuropathy.**

References

1. Ingall TJ. Hyperthermia and hypothermia. In: Low PA, editor. Clinical autonomic disorders: evaluation and management. Boston: Little, Brown and Company, 1993:713–29.
2. Knochel JP. Heat stroke and related heat stress disorders. Disease-a-Month 1989;35:301–78.
3. Simon HB. Hyperthermia. N Engl J Med 1993;329:483–7.
4. Harchelroad F. Acute thermoregulatory disorders. Clin Geriatr Med 1993;9:621–39.

25   *Neuroleptic Malignant Syndrome*

P. David Charles
Division of Movement Disorders
Department of Neurology
Vanderbilt University
Nashville, Tennessee

Thomas L. Davis
Division of Movement Disorders
Vanderbilt University
Nashville, Tennessee

The **neuroleptic malignant syndrome** (NMS) is a rare and potentially fatal syndrome of hyperthermia, rigidity, autonomic instability, and mental status derangement (1). It is an idiosyncratic reaction to drugs that alter the **dopaminergic pathways** of the central nervous system. **Neuroleptics** are the usual inciting agents. These are dopamine antagonists commonly prescribed for the treatment of psychiatric disorders. The incidence of NMS is estimated to be 0.1 to 1.4% of patients treated with neuroleptics. A similar syndrome can be caused by the sudden **withdrawal of dopamine agonists** used in the treatment of **Parkinson's disease.**

The clinical features of NMS are distinctive but the four cardinal findings need not occur in every patient. The considerable list of potential symptoms (Table 1) can be grouped into the four general areas of **hyperthermia, muscular rigidity, mental status changes,** and **autonomic dysfunction.**

Hyperthermia is present in virtually all cases and often exceeds 103.0°F. **Muscular rigidity** is severe and can be associated with tremor and bradykinesia;

all three features are caused by **extrapyramidal dysfunction.** Passive movement of the limbs in all directions (**lead pipe rigidity**) is resisted. **Mental status changes** include confusion, delirium, speech disorders, and decreased states of consciousness. **Autonomic dysfunction** is usually characterized by rapid fluctuations between hypertension associated with hypotension and tachycardia. Other autonomic features include sialorrhea, incontinence, and dysphagia. Tachypnea is probably caused by a combination of autonomic instability, muscular rigidity of the chest wall, and aspiration.

The laboratory findings of NMS are useful in establishing the diagnosis. The sustained muscular contraction of rigidity causes **muscle fiber necrosis** and the blood concentration of creatine kinase (CK) may exceed 10,000 IU. Other less specific features are a leukocytosis and elevated serum concentrations of transaminases, lactic acid dehydrogenase, and aldolase.

The main **morbidity and mortality** in patients with NMS are irreversible brain injury from hyperthermia and myoglobinuria and renal failure from rigidity-induced skeletal muscle necrosis. Other conditions contributing to morbidity and mortality are aspiration pneumonia, myocardial infarction, disseminated intravascular coagulation, and metabolic and electrolyte derangements.

Levenson divided the clinical features into major and minor categories. The major features are hyperthermia, rigidity, and a markedly elevated blood

Table 1. Clinical Findings in Neuroleptic Malignant Syndrome

Hyperthermia
  Often >103°F
Rigidity
  Lead pipe in nature
  Other extrapyramidal findings
    Tremor
    Bradykinesia
    Dystonic posturing
Mental status changes
  Confusion
  Obtundation
  Mutism
Autonomic instability
  Blood pressure lability
  Tachycardia
  Tachypnea
  Sialorrhea
  Incontinence
  Diaphoresis
Laboratory
  CPK often >10,000
  Leukocytosis
  Lactic acid dehydrogenase elevation
  Aldolase elevation
  Transaminase elevation

concentration of CK. The minor features are mainly related to autonomic instability and include labile blood pressure, tachycardia, tachypnea, diaphoresis, and confusion. The diagnosis is established by the occurrence of all three major features, or two major and four minor features.

Neuroleptics are among the most commonly prescribed drugs in the United States. **Phenothiazines, thiothixine,** and **butyrophenones** are the agents most common implicated in causing NMS. **Haloperidol** is the single most common drug associated with the NMS. The expanding list of implicated drugs now includes amoxapine, tetrabenazine, reserpine, metoclopramide, clozapine, monoamine oxidase inhibitors, and tricyclic antidepressants (Table 2). Dopamine antagonism in the central nervous system is the common factor shared by all of these agents; some are more potent dopamine antagonists than others. Intramuscular injection of depot preparations of neuroleptics may increase the risk of NMS and definitely prolong recovery because prompt drug withdrawal is not possible.

Individuals at increased risk for NMS cannot be identified prior to initiating therapy. The onset of symptoms is most often within the first 30 days of starting treatment. Rapid dose escalation, dehydration, psychomotor agitation, and underlying organic brain disease probably increase the frequency of NMS in at-risk individuals. Depot preparations of neuroleptics administered without concurrent use of antiparkinsonian agents also increases the risk of NMS. **NMS recurs in one-third of patients** when neuroleptics are reintroduced after recovery from the initial episode. In situations where the need for neuroleptic therapy outweighs the risk, the chance of a second NMS episode can be reduced by waiting at least 2 weeks after resolution of symptoms and then using the lowest possible dose of a low-potency agent.

The differential diagnosis of NMS includes other syndromes with hyperthermia as a prominent feature, fever complicating Parkinson's disease or other extrapyramidal syndromes, and lethal catatonia. **Malignant hyperther-**

Table 2.   Potential Precipitants: Neuroleptic Malignant Syndrome

Precipitants	Examples
Typical neuroleptics	
Phenothiazines	Fluphenazine, chlorpromazine, thioridazine promethazine, prochlorperazine, trifluoperazine
Dibenzoxazepines	Pimozide
Butyrophenones	Halperidol
Dihydroindolones	Molindone
Thioxanthenes	Thiothixene
Dibenzoapines	Loxapine
Atypical neuroleptics	Clozapine, risperidone
Antiemetics	Metoclopramide
Tricyclic antidepressants	Amitriptyline, imipramine, etc.
Benzodiazepines (in overdose and in pharmacy)	Diazepam, lorazepam, etc.
Withdrawal of dopamine agonist	L-DOPA, pergolide, bromocriptine, etc.
Polypharmacy (in combination with neuroleptics)	Alcohol, lithium, cimetidine

mia and NMS have similar clinical features, but are distinguishable because malignant hyperthermia is inherited as an autosomal dominant gene and is only triggered by the administration of anaesthetic agents. **Heat stroke** shares some features with NMS but **lacks rigidity.** Neuroleptics increase the risk of heat stroke; this may confuse diagnosis in individuals whose history is compatible with both disorders. The clinical features of NMS can be mimicked in patients with Parkinson's disease whose rigidity worsens at the time of concurrent fever or infection. The same is true for other neurodegenerative disorders of the extrapyramidal system. Common infectious and metabolic disorders must be ruled out prior to making the diagnosis of NMS. **Lethal catatonia** is a rare disorder of psychotic patients known years before the development of neuroleptics. Its clinical features are identical to those of NMS and the two conditions are only distinguished by the prior use of neuroleptics.

The precise **pathogenesis** of NMS is not established. Disruption of the dopaminergic pathways of the hypothalamus and basal ganglia leads to hyperthermia and rigidity. The experimental infusion of a **dopamine agonist** on the **thermoregulatory center** of the hypothalamus causes a dose-dependent **decrease in body temperature.** Basal ganglia dysfunction commonly produces tremor and other extrapyramidal symptoms in addition to rigidity. The autonomic instability of the nervous system combined with sustained muscle contraction exacerbates hyperthermia. **Augmentation of serotonergic pathways** may also have a role in the pathogenesis of NMS. The cerebrospinal fluid of patients with NMS shows a persistent **reduction of homovanillic acid,** a metabolite of dopamine, and **5-hydroxyindoleacetic acid,** a metabolite of serotonin. Other factors must be involved in the pathogenesis of NMS because its occurrence is rare, while the drugs known to induce the syndrome are prescribed to millions of patients each year. Furthermore, the reintroduction of neuroleptic agents in patients with a history of NMS does not always cause a recurrence.

Patients with NMS should be treated in an intensive care unit. Treatment begins with the immediate **withdrawal of the offending neuroleptic** or the **reintroduction of the antiparkinson agent** that was discontinued. The average time for recovery from NMS is 10 days and this is prolonged when depot preparations of neuroleptics were used. Therapy with **bromocriptine,** a dopamine agonist, reduces the recovery time of NMS. It acts primarily by restoring the dopaminergic balance in the preoptic area of the hypothalamus and basal ganglia. **Dantrolene,** a skeletal muscle relaxant, reduces the muscle rigidity of malignant hyperthermia and is also useful in NMS. Benzodiazepines are useful to treat the agitated mental confusion and the rigidity.

Prompt supportive measures in combination with drug therapy have significantly reduced the mortality from NMS. Cooling blankets are effective in combating hyperthermia and vigorous fluid replacement is essential to prevent dehydration. Aspiration is a common complication of NMS because of decreased chest wall compliance and depressed level of consciousness. Therefore, mechanical ventilation when indicated, combined with aggressive pulmonary toilet and appropriate antibiotic therapy in the event of pneumonia, is helpful. Renal failure, resulting from muscle breakdown, is the most common and severe complication of NMS. Fluid replacement and hemodialysis are the primary treatment modalities. The mortality from NMS increases to 50% if renal failure develops.

Electroconvulsive therapy (ECT) is a last resort when **lethal catatonia** enters the differential diagnosis. The two syndromes are clinically indistinguishable and lethal catatonia would not respond to the recommended treatment of NMS.

References

1. Delay J, Deniker P. Drug-induced extrapyramidal syndromes. In: Vinken PJ, Bruyn GW, eds. Handbook of clinical neurology. Disease of the basal ganglia. Amsterdam: North-Holland, 1968:248–66.
2. Caroff SN, Stephan CM. Neuroleptic malignant syndrome. Med Clin North Am 1993; 77(1):185–202.
3. Rodnitzky RL, Keyser DL. Neurologic complications of drugs. Psych Clin North Am 1992; 15(4):498–503.
4. Levenson JL. Neuroleptic malignant syndrome. Am J Psychiatry 1985;142:1137–45.
5. Guze BH, Baxter LR. Neuroleptic malignant syndrome. N Eng J Med 1985;313(3):163–6.
6. Schneider SM. Neuroleptic malignant syndrome: controversies in treatment. Am J Emer Med 1991;9(4):360–2.

26

Malignant Hyperthermia

Beverley A. Britt
Department of Anaesthesia and Pharmacology
The Toronto Hospital
Toronto General Hospital
Toronto, Ontario, Canada

Malignant hyperthermia (MH) is an autosomal dominant trait of humans and pigs due to a defect in the **ryanodine** (RYR1) gene. So far eight single-point mutations have been detected in human MH patients covering 20% of families so far studied and one single-point mutation has been found in pigs. MH is closely related to **central core disease** (CCD) since four single-point mutations cause both MH and CCD. Lesser degrees of relationship have been found to other muscle disorders such as **muscular dystrophy, myotonic dystrophy,** and **myotonia congenita.**

MH reactions are triggered by **a prolonged opening of the ryanodine pores** with, therefore, a sudden release of CA^{2+} from the sarcoplasmic reticulum to the cytoplasm through a defective ryanodine receptor. There is, consequently, increased heat, water, CO_2, and lactic acid production and increased O_2 and ATP consumption.

For reactions to occur **environmental triggers,** in addition to the abnormal gene, need to be present. The best known triggers are anaesthetic agents such as **succinylcholine, halothane, isoflurane,** and **enflurane.** Reactions, particularly those beginning with **masseter muscle rigidity** (MMR), are more likely to occur if halothane administration has preceded succinylcholine infusion. Other lesser known triggers, which can exacerbate an anaesthetic-induced reaction, or can even rarely trigger a reaction, include: **workplace chemical, street drugs, x-ray contrast dyes, violent exercise,** muscle trauma, elevated CO_2, fever, infection, pain, shivering, and agitation.

Males are more commonly affected than females. MH is rare before 3 years of age but then the incidence rises rapidly until 30, when it declines to being almost unknown by age 75.

Very mild or **abortive MH reactions** may consist of only isolated MMR or fever. **Fulminant MH reactions** are characterized by a rising CO_2, MMR advancing to generalized rigidity, tachycardia, ventricular arrhythmias, unstable blood pressure, tachypnea, mottled cyanosis, and fever. **Laboratory changes** include hypoxia, hypercarbia, and metabolic acidosis; early elevations and late reductions in serum calcium and potassium, elevations of serum PO_4, Mg^{2+}, blood glucose, and lactic acid; and late elevations of CPK, LDH, AST, ALT, and myoglobin. About 20% of patients never manifest any rigidity. Occasionally reactions may begin only in the recovery room, or even after return to the ward. **Potentially fatal complications** comprise ventricular fibrillations, pulmonary edema, acute disseminated intravascular coagulopathy, obstruction of the renal tubules with myoglobin, and brain death secondary to hypoxia. Postoperatively the patient may complain of muscle pain and fatigue for considerable periods of time.

Survival has risen from less than 20% in the first half of the century to nearly 98% today. MH must be differentiated from other conditions that increase heat production or reduce heat loss.

Some, but by no means all, MH patients suffer from **muscle pains or cramps,** either continuously or episodically; acute exercise and/or heat-induced reactions; short thick-muscle bellies, sometimes with intervening areas of atrophy; King–Denborough syndrome; joint hypermobility; and hernias. The serum CK and the 24-hr urine creatine may be elevated. Phosphate/phosphocreatine ratios are increased and pHs are reduced during exercise on NMR examination. Platelet calcium permeability may be impaired. Red blood cell membranes may exhibit a slightly increased vulnerability to hemolysis. In lymphocytes, **halothane** may stimulate increased calcium release form storage sites into the cytoplasm. A few MH patients exhibit **electromyogram** (EMG) **abnormalities** such as increased and/or short-duration polyphasic action potentials.

Certain diagnosis of the **MH trait** can only be made by the **caffeine halothane contracture test,** which measures the effect of halothane or caffeine on contractures of isolated skeletal muscle fascicles. In North America the parameters measured are the amplitude of contractures in the presence of 3% halothane (normal: <0.5–0.7 g), the amplitude of contractures in the presence of 2 mM caffeine (normal: <0.2–0.3 mM), and the dose of caffeine required to raise the resting tension by 1.0 g (normal: ≥ 2.0 mM) or halothane (normal: >2.0 g) required to produced a threshold contracture. In Japan the MH trait is detected by means of measuring calcium–induced calcium release in single chemically skinned fibers. Microscopy should be preformed to rule out other myopathies, in particular **central core disease**. Some MH patients have internal nuclei, small angular or split or atrophic fibers, and/or fiber grouping.

Once diagnosed, MH patients should be encouraged to obtain a Medic Alert bracelet. They ought to be warned that obtaining life insurance may be difficult. Travel to remote, third world countries, where the expertise, drugs, and equipment to manage an elective anaesthetic or an emergency MH reaction are simply not available, may be inadvisable.

Known or suspected MH patients can be safely anesthetized with nitrous oxide, barbiturates, narcotics, ketamine, propofol, tranquillizers, or local anesthetics. The gas machine should be vapor free. Pretreatment with **dantrolene** is usually not necessary. Monitoring should include ETCO$_2$, SaO$_2$, temperature, EKG, blood pressure, heart rate, skin appearance, blood gases, electrolytes, and muscle enzymes.

When only isolated MMR is present triggering agents should be stopped and monitoring performed for signs of impending fulminant reaction. When a fulminant reaction occurs: triggering agents should be immediately discontinued; the patient must be hyperventilated with oxygen; sodium bicarbonate may be infused if the pH is low; dantrolene (60 cc of bacteriostatic free water in each vial of 20 mg of dantrolene, 2.0 g of mannitol and enough sodium hydroxide to raise the pH to 9.5) ought to be immediately started at 1.0 mg/kg/min until definite signs of improvement occur; procaine and propranolol may be administered to treat arrhythmias; furosemide and mannitol should be infused to prevent renal failure; and insulin plus 50% glucose may be necessary to return the high serum potassium to normal. Cooling is no longer considered to be necessary for treatment of most reactions since dantrolene alone will return the temperature to normal.

References

1. Maclennan DH, Phillips MS. The role of the RYR1 gene in malignant hyperthermia and central core disease. In: Dawson DC, Frizzell RA, eds. Ion channel and genetic diseases. New York: Rockefeller University Press, 1995;89–100.
2. Britt BA. Malignant hyperthermia. In: Lane RJM, ed. Handbook of muscle disease. New York: Marcel Dekker, 1994.
3. Britt BA. Malignant hyperthermia—a review. In: Milton AS. ed. Handbook of experimental pharmacology, pyretics and antipyretics. Heidelberg: Springer-Verlag, 1982;547–615.
4. Larach MG. Standardization of the caffeine halothane muscle contracture test. Anesth Analg 1989;69:511–5.
5. European MH Group. A protocol for the investigation of malignant hyperpyrexia (MH) susceptibility. Br J Anesth 1984;56:1267–9.
6. Endo M. Calcium induced calcium release test. Presented at the III International Symposium on Malignant Hyperthermia, Hiroshima, Japan, July 16, 1994.

PART VI

Cardiovascular and Cerebrovascular Disorders

27 Primary Hypertension and Sympathetic Nervous Activity

David A. Calhoun
Vascular Biology and Hypertension Program
University of Alabama at Birmingham
Birmingham, Alabama

Suzanne Oparil
Vascular Biology and Hypertension
Program of the Division of
Cardiovascular Disease
University of Alabama at Birmingham
Birmingham, Alabama

It is well established that elevations of **sympathetic nervous system activity** acutely raise blood pressure through stimulation of **the heart, kidney, and peripheral vasculature** causing, respectively, increases in **cardiac output, fluid retention, and vascular resistance.** Less certain is to what degree sustained or repeated elevations of sympathetic activity contribute to the development and/or maintenance of chronic hypertension. Using widely different methods of assessment, investigators have reported sympathetic nervous system activity to be elevated in both the early and chronic stages of primary hypertension. By inference, these data suggest that elevated sympathetic activity plays an important role in the development of hypertension. It is hypothesized that increased sympathetic nervous system activity induces **vascular smooth muscle cell hypertrophy** resulting in sustained increases in peripheral resistance and blood pressure.

Plasma Norepinephrine Levels

Norepinephrine is the predominant neurotransmitter released by postganglionic sympathetic nerve terminals. Most of the released norepinephrine is inactivated following reuptake into the nerve terminal. A portion of the released norepinephrine, however, diffuses out of the synaptic cleft prior to reuptake and enters the bloodstream. Because the majority of sympathetic nerves innervate blood vessels, particularly arterioles, circulating levels of norepinephrine are thought largely to reflect arteriolar stimulation.

Varied methods of assessment confirm that **plasma norepinephrine** levels correlate with the level of sympathetic nervous system activity: (1) **Regional sympathectomy** corresponds to reduced regional release of norepinephrine; (2) the level of **sympathetic nervous system activity recorded** directly from peripheral nerves correlates with norepinephrine levels; and (3) **circadian fluctuations** in blood pressure correlate with similar circadian fluctuations in plasma norepinephrine levels.

While elevations of circulating norepinephrine levels are generally specific for increases in sympathetic nervous system activity, they are not particularly sensitive. Only a small percentage of the norepinephrine released form the nerve terminal avoids reuptake, such that large changes in sympathetic nerve activity are necessary to significantly alter plasma levels. In addition, **large**

intra- and interlaboratory variations in the measurement of plasma norepinephrine limit sensitivity. Lastly, and potentially compromising both specificity and
sensitivity, variations in norepinephrine levels reflect differences not only in
release but also in clearance. Individual and group differences in clearance of
released norepinephrine have been demonstrated, particularly in relation to
age, which might confound interpretation of norepinephrine levels.

In spite of the limitations of interpreting plasm norepinephrine levels, most
studies have reported greater circulating levels of norepinephrine in hypertensive subjects than in normotensive controls. A review of 64 studies comparing
plasma norepinephrine levels found that 52 of the 64 studies (81%) reported
higher norepinephrine levels in hypertensive compared to normotensive subjects, but the higher norepinephrine levels were significant in only 25 of the
64 studies (39%). More compelling was the observation that in almost all
studies comparing younger subjects (<40 years of age), norepinephrine levels
were found to be significantly greater in the hypertensive versus the normotensive subjects. These results are consistent with the hypothesis that sustained
increases in sympathetic activity contribute significantly to the development
of hypertension. Once hypertension is established, however, measurement of
circulating norepinephrine levels suggests that sympathetic output subsides—
perhaps related to progressive blunting of the baroreflex—and does not contribute to the maintenance of chronic hypertension. Instead, vascular changes
induced by the previously elevated sympathetic output, such as smooth muscle
cell hypertrophy, likely serve to maintain the elevated blood pressure in spite
of decreases in sympathetic activity.

Autonomic Blockade

One of the earliest techniques suggesting that sympathetic nervous system
activity is elevated in subjects with primary hypertension was comparison of
the relative efficacy of sympatholytic agents or adrenoceptor antagonists in
subjects with and without evidence of heightened sympathetic activity. Hypertensive subjects have been shown to be more sensitive to β-blockade than
normotensive controls. In other studies, the degree of blood pressure reduction
following clonidine administration correlates with pretreatment plasma norepinephrine levels (Fig. 1). Similarly, reduction of forearm vascular resistance
during α_1-adrenergic receptor blockade correlates with plasma norepinephrine
levels, suggesting indirectly, that sympathetic overactivity contributes in large
part to chronic blood pressure elevation.

Regional Norepinephrine Spillover

To minimize the confounding influence of variations in norepinephrine clearance, techniques have been developed to measure norepinephrine spillover,
allowing for estimation of norepinephrine release. According to this technique,
tissue clearance of norepinephrine is determined by the degree of dilution of
a small amount of intravenously infused radiolabeled norepinephrine, allowing
for calculation of norepinephrine spillover. The norepinephrine spillover rate

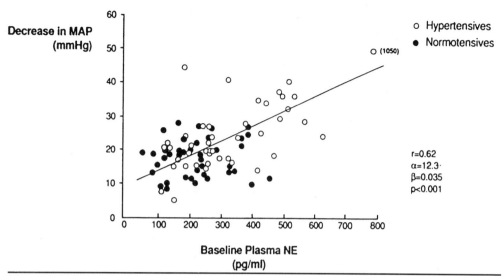

Figure 1. Plot showing decrease in mean arterial pressure (MAP) as a function of baseline plasma norepinephrine (NE) 3 hr after administration of 0.3 mg clonidine in patients with essential hypertension and in normotensive controls. Linear regression line is for the hypertensive group. Reprinted, with permission, from Goldstein *et al.* (4).

is thought to reflect norepinephrine release from the sympathoeffector terminal and, thereby, sympathetic activity.

Using this technique, investigators from Australia have reported that **whole body norepinephrine spillover is elevated in young hypertensive subjects** compared to normotensive controls, suggesting that heightened sympathetic activity contributes to the development of hypertension. Regional application of norepinephrine spillover techniques indicate that the greater sympathetic activation observed in young hypertensives is **primarily attributable to greater sympathetic outflow to the kidneys and heart.** Norepinephrine spillover has also been found to be greater in normotensive offspring of hypertensive parents compared to normotensive offspring of normotensive parents, suggesting that increases in sympathetic activity predisposing subjects to the development of hypertension, are, in large part, genetic in origin.

Evaluation of total body norepinephrine spillover suggests that the greater norepinephrine plasma concentrations observed in **older hypertensive subjects** compared to normotensive counterparts may be attributable to **differences in norepinephrine clearance** and not to persistent elevation of sympathetic activity. This and the above studies support the role of sympathetic overactivity in the development of hypertension in younger subjects, but do not support a persistent role of sympathetic activity in the maintenance of hypertension in older subjects.

Reliable interpretation of the norepinephrine spillover assumes that: (1) significant amounts of the radiolabeled norepinephrine is not rereleased after it is cleared from the circulation which would confound the dilution measurements of the infused isotope, and (2) both the infused and the naturally released norepinephrine are well-mixed in a central plasma pool. Recent studies seemed to have confirmed the validity of the former assumption, while use of arterial samples to determine isotope dilution minimize the potential consequences of the latter assumption.

Microneurography

In the 1960s, Swedish neurophysiologists developed a technique referred to as microneurography **to directly record sympathetic activity** from peripheral nerves in humans. Since then, microneurography has been widely used to record efferent muscle sympathetic nervous system activity (MSNA) both at rest and after various pharmacologic and nonpharmacologic interventions.

Several maneuvers suggest that microneurography records postganglionic sympathetic nerve activity: (1) the nerve activity is abolished by **anesthetic nerve blockade** proximal but not distal to the recording site, (2) the nerve activity is conducted along the nerve at a speed consistent with **conduction speeds** recorded from unmyelinated nerve fibers in experimental animals, (3) the nerve signal is reversibly abolished by infusion of a **ganglionic blocker,** and (4) MSNA is clearly under **baroreflex control** and increases during stimuli known to increase sympathetic nervous system activity, such as the Valsalva maneuver, and during the cold pressor test.

Several studies have used microneurography to compare MSNA in hypertensive and normotensive subjects. The largest study to date compared resting MSNA recorded from the tibial nerve in 63 Japanese hypertensive subjects (48 males and 15 females) and from 43 Japanese normotensive subjects (32 males and 11 females). When MSNA is compared between groups, the integrated MSNA signal is reported as bursts or spikes per minute. The Japanese investigators found that resting MSNA values were significantly greater in the hypertensive compared to the normotensive subjects (31 versus 21 bursts/min; $P < 0.01$). MSNA was found to increase with age, but even when corrected for this factor, MSNA values remain elevated in the hypertensive subjects. Preliminary data from investigators at the University of Milan confirm that MSNA is elevated in patients with established hypertension. In this study, resting **MSNA was found to be progressively higher in subjects with mild, moderate, and severe hypertension, respectively.**

Resting MSNA has also been found to be greater in the developing stages of hypertension. Investigators at the University of Iowa found that MSNA was significantly greater in 12 young males with "borderline" or intermittent hypertension compared to 15 age-matched normotensive controls, regardless of high or low dietary NaCl ingestion. In a similar comparison, Canadian investigators found resting MSNA to be significantly greater in young subjects with JNC V Stage 1 hypertension (systolic 140–149/diastolic 90–99 mm Hg) than normotensive controls. The greater MSNA in the hypertensive subjects correlated with greater peripheral vascular resistance of the lower extremities. Both the greater MSNA and the peripheral resistance were present during two separate recording sessions at least 1 month apart, suggesting that the greater values were not attributable to a greater arousal and alerting response in the hypertensive subjects during the initial recording session.

Because **microneurography** measures nerve activity directly, it can be **more sensitive and specific** than other indirect assessments of sympathetic activity. Resting MSNA has been shown to generally correlate with plasma norepinephrine in both hypertensive and normotensive subjects. During provocation, however, small but significant changes in MSNA may be observed without significant change in plasma norepinephrine levels, reflecting the greater sensitivity of microneurography.

Limitations of microneurography include: (1) it is minimally invasive and technically difficult, prohibiting broad application of its use; (2) there is a large interindividual variation in resting MSNA, decreasing its power to identify differences between groups; (3) it records only efferent sympathetic efferent activity to the musculature which may not reflect sympathetic activity to other regions of importance, such as the kidneys and heart; (4) microneurography can only be attempted in stationary, prone, or semiprone subjects. Comparisons outside of the laboratory or in ambulatory subjects are not possible.

Power Spectrum Analysis

Heart rate and blood pressure do not vary randomly but instead manifest periodicities of fairly constant frequency. Power spectrum analysis is a computer-based technique used to identify the relative preponderance of these different frequencies of variation. One such **high-frequency component** occurs **in synchrony with respiration.** A **lower frequency component** has been identified that is significantly reduced during sleep and is thought to represent **sympathetic activity.** The relative power of this frequency in heart rate variation has been reported to be elevated in hypertensive subjects versus normotensive controls, consistent with sympathetic overactivity.

While spectral analysis of heart rate variability is thought to be capable of reliably quantifying sympathetic versus parasympathetic tone, questions remain regarding the same type of analysis applied to blood pressure variation. In some situations, as during sleep, **blood pressure spectra** are consistent with known changes in sympathetic activity, while in other situations, such as in heart failure patients or during exercise, blood pressure spectra have not accurately reflected known changes in sympathetic activity. In addition, the low-frequency domain in blood pressure variation seems to contain a **large nonsympathetic component** that remains unidentified. Until these inconsistencies have been clarified, power spectral analysis of blood pressure must be interpreted cautiously.

Sympathetic and Vascular Reactivity

Hypertensive subjects have been repeatedly demonstrated to manifest greater vasoconstrictive responses to infused norepinephrine than normotensive controls. In normotensive subjects, greater levels of circulating norepinephrine generally induce down-regulation of norepinephrine receptors. In hypertensive subjects, however, such down-regulation appears not to occur, resulting in the greater sensitivity to norepinephrine. The **combination of enhanced sensitivity to and greater circulating levels of norepinephrine** likely contributes significantly to sympathetic nervous system activity-related hypertension. Greater sensitivity to norepinephrine also has been observed in normotensive offspring of hypertensive parents compared to control subjects without a family history of hypertension, suggesting that the phenomena may be genetic in origin and not simply a consequence of elevated blood pressure.

Exposure to **stress** is well known to increase sympathetic output. A vicious circle is hypothesized to link stress and increases in sympathetic activity to the development of hypertension. According to this hypothesis, repeated stress-induced vasoconstriction causes **vascular hypertrophy,** which promotes even more vigorous vasoconstrictive responses to stress, leading to progressive increases in peripheral vascular resistant and blood pressure. Stress-induced hypertension has been observed in certain laboratory animals. Such an occurrence may explain in part the greater incidence of hypertension in lower socioeconomic groups, since such persons must endure greater levels of stress associated with day-to-day living.

Numerous studies have evaluated the responses of normotensive or hypertensive groups to different laboratory stressors in an effort to determine if greater vascular reactivity is correlated with the development or presence of hypertension. The findings of these studies have not been consistent. Overall, the data seem most consistent in suggesting that young subjects, adolescents and young adults, with a genetic predisposition to develop hypertension, that is, a **positive family history of hypertension,** do manifest **greater vasoconstrictive responses to laboratory stressors,** such as mental stress, cold pressor testing, or physical exercise. In some studies, but not all, this greater vascular reactivity has been shown to correlate with a greater likelihood of developing hypertension.

The results of stress testing are perhaps most consistent in **young African Americans.** The majority of studies have reported young, normotensive or mildly hypertensive blacks, particularly in response to cold pressor testing, to manifest greater stress-induced vascular reactivity than age-matched whites. A recent study used microneurography to record muscle sympathetic nervous system activity responses in young normotensive black and white subjects and found that **the greater pressor response** to cold pressor testing observed in blacks was **attributable to greater increases in peripheral sympathetic nervous system activity** (Fig. 2). It is hypothesized that greater stress-induced increases

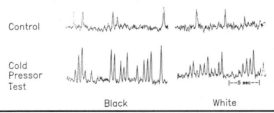

Figure 2.   Tracings show muscle sympathetic nerve activity as recorded by microneurography (each spike represents an efferent burst) in black normotensive subject and white normotensive subject at rest (control) and during cold pressor test. Sympathetic nerve activity increased in both subjects during cold stress, but the magnitude of the increase was greater in the black subject. Reproduced, with permission, from Calhoun *et al.* (1).

in sympathetic activity, in combination with the greater socioeconomic stress that blacks must endure, likely contributes to the significantly greater incidence of hypertension in African Americans compared to American whites.

References

1. Calhoun DA, Mutinga ML, Collins AS, Wyss S, Oparil S. Normotensive blacks have heightened sympathetic response to cold pressor test. Hypertension 1993;22;801–5.
2. Esler M, Jennings G, Biviano B, Lambert G, Hasking G. Mechanism of elevated plasma noradrenaline in the course of essential hypertension. J Cardiovasc Pharmacol, 1986; 8(suppl 5):S39–43.
3. Folkow BS. Physiological aspects of primary hypertension. Physiol Rev 1982;62:347–504.
4. Goldstein DS, Levinson PD, Zimlichman R, Pitterman A, Stull R, Keiser HR. Clonidine suppression testing in essential hypertension. Ann Intern Med 1985;102:42–48.
5. Guzzetti E, Piccaluga E, Casati R, Cerutti S, Lamardi F, Pagani M, Malliani A. Sympathetic predominance in essential hypertension: a study employing spectral analysis of heart rate variablility. J Hypertens 1988;6:711–7.
6. Mancia G, Grassi G, Parati F, Daffonchio A. Evaluating sympathetic activity in human hypertension. J Hypertens 1993;11(suppl 5):S13–8.

28   *Cardiac Arrhythmias and Sudden Death*

Katherine T. Murray
*Division of Clinical
Pharmacology
Vanderbilt University
Nashville, Tennessee*

Dan M. Roden
*Division of Clinical Pharmacology
Vanderbilt University
Nashville, Tennessee*

Sudden death, usually due to **ventricular fibrillation,** kills 500,000 Americans every year. There is no doubt that the autonomic nervous system modulates cardiac electrophysiology, and considerable evidence suggests that abnormalities of autonomic function can increase or decrease the risk of sudden death, particularly in patients with heart disease.

In Vitro Correlates

Both sympathetic and parasympathetic systems can affect cardiac electrophysiology. Adrenergic stimulation produces complex changes in cardiac electrical activity and ionic currents. For example, **norepinephrine** may exert a biphasic effect on cardiac **action potential duration** (APD), with either prolongation or shortening of APD depending on factors such as concentration or relative abundance of α and β receptors. *In vivo*, **selective β-adrenergic stimulation,** which increases intracellular cAMP, increases heart rate, AV nodal conduction, and contractile force, and shortens atrial and ventricular refractoriness. The plateau of the action potential and contractility are enhanced due to **an increase in current through L-type Ca^{2+} channels** (I_{Ca}), while repolarization is accelerated by an increase in both the slowly activating component of the **delayed cardiac rectifier current** (I_{Ks}) and **the chloride current** (I_{Cl}). Thus, β-stimulation may shorten or prolong APD, depending on whether effects on I_{Ca} or on I_{Ks}/I_{Cl} predominate. Beta-receptor stimulation also shifts activation of the pacemaker current (I_f) to more positive potentials causing more rapid pacemaker activity in the sinus node. All these modulatory effects on ion channel function are most likely due to **phosphorylation of channel proteins,** although direct interactions with GTP-binding proteins may also play a role, particularly with I_{Ca}.

Depending on receptor subtype, α-adrenergic receptors can either decrease intracellular cAMP concentrations or activate turnover of the membrane phospholipid phosphatidylinositol with activation of protein kinase C. Alpha receptor stimulation prolongs APD in Purkinje fibers and ventricular muscle with enhancement of contractility due to Ca^{2+} influx. One important arrhythmogenic effect of adrenergic stimulation *in vitro* is the **development of afterdepolarizations and triggered beats.** Multiple ionic mechanisms are involved, and elevated intracellular calcium is a common feature.

The electrophysiologic effects of **acetylcholine** and **muscarinic receptor** stimulation are likely related to the reduction in intracellular cAMP which occurs with antagonism of β-adrenergic-mediated effects. *In vivo,* this results in a slowing of heart rate and automaticity, due to a shift of I_f activation to more negative potentials, reduced contractility associated with suppression of I_{Ca}, and an increase in ventricular refractoriness. Another well-described effect of parasympathetic stimulation is activation of an atrial K^+ current (I_{KAch}), which **hyperpolarizes atrial cells** and shortens their APD. Some patients develop **atrial fibrillation at night** (during periods of **high vagal tone**), and APD shortening as a consequence of I_{KAch} activation may contribute to this effect. In such patients, **digitalis** should be avoided because of its **vago-mimetic actions.**

In Vivo Studies

In most cases, sudden cardiac death is due to development of sustained ventricular tachycardia or ventricular fibrillation which results in hemodynamic collapse. In some cases, acute myocardial ischemia triggers these arrhythmias. In other cases, acute ischemia is not evident, and fatal arrhythmias are thought to arise as a result of a combination of factors such as myocardial scarring or hypertrophy; in these cases, numerous studies indicate a role for the **sympathetic nervous system** in triggering **the development of these arrhythmias,** while increased **parasympathetic tone** appears to **inhibit** them. In patients with congestive heart failure, high circulating levels of norepinephrine predict an increased incidence of sudden cardiac death. The **protective effect** of **β-adrenergic receptor blockers** to reduce the incidence of sudden death following **acute myocardial infarction** has been well documented. Adrenergic activation using either stellate ganglion stimulation or catecholamine infusion results in a reduction of the electrical stimulus threshold to induce ventricular fibrillation, as well as an increase in the likelihood of spontaneous ventricular arrhythmias in animal models of ischemia. Beta-receptor blockade inhibits these effects. Recent data indicate that following coronary occlusion, sympathetic denervation occurs in normal tissue apical to the myocardial infarction. This can contribute to increased dispersion of refractoriness following β-adrenergic stimulation with enhanced shortening of refractoriness in denervated tissue compared to innervated areas, a potentially arrhythmogenic action. This effect can be prevented by β blockers. Evidence for denervation in patients can be obtained using **myocardial uptake of radiolabeled metaiodobenzylguanidine (MIBG),** an analog of norepinephrine which is concentrated in postganglionic presynaptic fibers. Defects in MIBG uptake are found more frequently in patients with spontaneous ventricular arrhythmias following acute myocardial infarction than those without such arrhythmias.

Enhanced **parasympathetic tone** has been shown to be **protective against sudden cardiac death** in certain circumstances. This effect is probably due to a reduction in both the threshold to induce ventricular fibrillation and the risk of ventricular arrhythmias in animal models of ischemia and myocardial infarction. The mechanism(s) of these effects are unknown but may relate to antagonism of sympathetic activation. Parasympathetic activity can be estimated by determining the relationship between changes in blood pressure and heart rate following administration of a vasoconstrictor such **phenylephrine.** The slope of this relationship is termed the **baroreflex slope,** and its **steepness** correlates with **parasympathetic tone.** Following **myocardial infarction,** the baroflex slope is **reduced** in patients with extensive coronary artery disease, ventricular tachyarrythmias, and poorest long-term survival. This reduction in slope is typically transient following an MI, and its occurrence correlates with the period of greatest risk from arrhythmias. Another index of parasympathetic activity is **heart rate variability.** Using multivariate analysis, a reduction in this parameter (indicative of lowered vagal tone) has been shown to be an independent risk factor for mortality following an MI. Spectral analysis of heart rate variability using fast Fourier transform demonstrated a reduction in a high-frequency component following myocardial infarction paralleling a reduction in baroreflex slope. However, enhanced parasympathetic activity may not always be protective. **Vasodepressor syncope** and sudden death can occur during periods of **severe psychological stress,** usually due to threat of injury associated with uncertainty as to outcome. Anecdotal data suggest that arrhythmias in this situation are precipitated by simultaneous activation of both the adrenergic and parasympathetic nervous systems.

A clinical abnormality which highlights the role of the autonomic nervous system in the modulating cardiac electrophysiology is the **congenital long QT syndrome.** These patients have markedly **abnormal repolarization,** manifest on the ECG as a prolonged QT interval with abnormal T and U waves, and the occurrence of a **polymorphic ventricular tachycardia** known as **Torsades**

de Pointes. Slow heart rates are also common. Torsades de Pointes can cause syncope or sudden death and in these patients is usually precipitated by physical or emotional stress; β blockers are thought to reduce episodes of syncope. An imbalance of sympathetic innervation has been postulated to contribute to abnormal repolarization in this syndrome, given historical data that **stimulation of the left stellate ganglion** or interruption of the right **causes QT prolongation.** However, experimental data, including a lack of evidence by MIBG for sympathetic imbalance in these patients, makes this hypothesis less tenable. In patients with the congenital long QT syndrome, **interruption of the left stellate ganglion** seems to **reduce syncope** in patients in whom this symptom persists despite treatment with β-adrenergic receptor blockers. This suggests a role for α-mediated effects in precipitating arrhythmias in this syndrome. The mechanism by which adrenergic activity causes arrhythmias in these patients is probably the development of triggered activity.

In summary, the **autonomic nervous system** plays an important role in modulating cardiac electrophysiology acting as **a trigger for the lethal arrhythmias** which cause sudden cardiac death. This risk seems greatest in patients who have advanced underlying heart disease; this may be regional (e.g., myocardial infarction) or global (e.g., the congenital long QT syndrome; dilated cardiomyopathy with, possibly, elevated intracellular calcium). Additional studies are necessary to determine the utility of interventions which either block adrenergic stimulation or enhance parasympathetic tone in reducing the incidence of sudden death in patients recovering from a myocardial infarction and other groups at risk for sudden death.

References

1. Schwartz PJ, Priori SG, Napolitano C. Role of the autonomic nervous system in sudden death. In Josephson ME, ed. Sudden cardiac death. Cambridge, MA: Blackwell Scientific Publications, 1993: pp 16–37.
2. Wharton JM, Coleman RE, Strauss, HC. The role of the autonomic nervous system in sudden cardiac death. Trends Cardiovasc Med 1992;2:65–71.
3. Engel GL. Psychologic stress, vasodepressor (vasovagal) syncope, and sudden death. Ann Intern Med 1978;89:403-412.
4. Zipes DP. The long QT interval syndrome: A rosetta stone for sympathetic related ventricular tachyarrhythmias. Circulation 1991;84:1414-19.

29

Cerebral Autonomic Regulation Underlying Cardiovascular Disease

James E. Skinner
Totts Gap Medical Research Institute
Bangor, Pennsylvania

Cerebral Defense and Homeostasis

Why the brain regulates the heart is itself a most interesting question. Walter B. Cannon had an early hypothesis that the focus for natural selection among the higher primates involved what he called a **cerebral defense system**. This was described as an integrated brain/autonomic system which enabled an animal to provide cardiovascular support for behaviors **before** as well as during an attack on prey or an escape from predators. He specifically hypothesized that an **orchestrator** of the sensory input channels and the autonomic output effectors would be found in the most highly encephalized cerebral tissues. Paul MacLean developed a similar theory, but it incorporated the independent development of **three** separate cognitive systems, each with its own separate mechanism for the autonomic support of attendant behaviors.

The **orchestration** seems to be the basis for autonomic outflow during at least one type of sensory "attention," that associated with a **higher cognitive evoked-potential** called the **expectancy wave** or the **contingent negative variation**. The cerebral mechanism underlying this higher cognitive process is, at least, a **noradrenergic** one. During an event-related slow potential evoked by presenting a novel stimulus, NE is released from presynaptic terminals in the frontal cortex thus stimulating the β **receptors** and in turn inducing intracellular cyclic AMP accumulation; this second-messenger effect then turns off a slow outward potassium current in the frontocortical neurons of the conscious subject and induces an extracellular negative potential.

At least for the frontal lobes, Cannon's concept regarding an "orchestrator" appears to be correct, as this bilateral structure not only has important bilateral projections to the brainstem autonomic centers, but also has bilateral projections into the **thalamus** that control the ascent of sensory information into the cerebral cortex during selective perception.

The Problem Is Patterned Autonomic Tone, Not Sympathetic Outflow Alone

In the anesthetized animal, complete **cardiac denervation** will prevent lethal **ventricular fibrillation** (VF) following coronary artery occlusion. Also in the anesthetized preparation high cervical transection will normalize blood pressure elevations. In the conscious animal (pig), **psychological "stress"** evoked by an abundance of novel stimuli (i.e., being in a new environment) must be present for coronary artery occlusion to result in VF. **Bilateral cryogenic blockade** of the output pathways to the brainstem autonomic centers, from either the frontal lobes or the amygdalae (i.e., two of MacLean's intracranial systems), also prevents VF after coronary occlusion, even in the stressed animal. These same two cerebral blockades also normalize blood pressure elevation in experimental hypertension. Thus the cardiovascular disorders have a neural component that is necessary for their manifestations.

This conclusion is underscored by recent findings. It has been found that the antimortality effect of the β-blocker cardiac drugs (which were developed initially as antihypertensives) is mediated by an **action in the brain** and not an action in the heart or peripheral autonomic nerves. The goal now is to explain how these cerebral effects on the cardiovascular disorders are mediated through the autonomic nervous system.

The cause of death in many **stroke** patients is **cardiac arrhythmogenesis.** **Epileptic discharges** induced in the cortex also result in sudden cardiac ectopy. Intense **psychological stress** in both animals and humans can quickly result in sudden cardiac death. In some, but not all, of the latter cases, a transient stress cardiomyopathy may be detected. It is apparent from these observations together that the brain perturbations alone can produce ectopic cardiac arrhythmias in the apparently normal heart. The descending autonomic perturbations must indeed be significant.

Electrical stimulation or stroke in the **frontal cortex of the pig,** or intense psychologic stress, produce malignant cardiac ectopies, including ventricular tachycardia. These all occur in a normal myocardium. In none of these experimental perturbations, however, is a simple excitatory or inhibitory autonomic disturbance produced; rather, a complex pattern in established in which the arrhythmias arise during concomitant sinus tachycardia, bradycardia, or with no change at all.

The study of how the autonomic nerves regulate each heartbeat may reveal important clues about the causes of VF. Some investigators believe that the deleterious neural regulation is reflected in the reduced variability of the heartbeats. Low parasympathetic tone is thought to be the culprit, as the patients that later manifest VF not only have a reduced variability, but also manifest smaller heart rate reductions in response to induced blood pressure elevations (i.e., reduced baroreflex sensitivity), and reduced peaks in the heartbeat power spectrum indicative of cholinergic activity.

But it is not **low cholinergic activity** *per se* that is the problem, for increased parasympathetic tone can be dangerous if sympathetic tone is also high. High **dual autonomic** tone occurs naturally during **slow wave (SW) sleep.** Pigs with a previous myocardial infarction manifest a markedly increased total number of ventricular arrhythmias during SW sleep compared to quiet wakefulness or to the rapid eye movement stage of sleep (REM), in which cases low autonomic-tones are present. In the **waking** pig, using a precise measure of sympathetic β-receptor activation of the myocardium (i.e., phosphorylase activation), it is observed that when the animal is placed in an unfamiliar environment, sympathetic tone is very high, but in the hemodynamically resting heart. In this case parasympathetic tone must also have been high, as the sympathetic tone alone would have increased heart rate and blood pressure.

Furthermore, when running on a treadmill, an animal with a myocardial infarction does not usually manifest VF, even though sympathetic tone is very high at this time. When the treadmill is turned off, however, and parasympathetic tone begins to increase while sympathetic tone is still high, arrhythmias quickly develop and VF often results.

A simple demonstration that it takes activation of **both** the sympathetic and parasympathetic nerves to evoke ventricular arrhythmias was provided in an early study in which it was found in the isolated heart that stimulation of either type of autonomic nerve separately did not evoke arrhythmias, whereas their joint stimulation produced premature ventricular complexes.

Together these experiments indicated that it is a heartbeat **pattern** resulting from dual autonomic tones that is likely to be the basis of cardiovascular risk, not just a simple failure of cholinergic tone and cardiac reflexes.

Heart Rate Variability and Risk of Sudden Cardiac Death

Identification of risk of sudden cardiac death has focused on the analysis of the variability of the heartbeat intervals. In a multicenter study of postinfarction patients, it was shown that when the standard deviation of 5-min means of heartbeat intervals is made over a 24-hr period, lower values are found, on average, for the group of patients who later manifest VF than for the survivors. Similarly it was found that when the power in a high-frequency band related to cholinergic activity was divided by total power related to both adrenergic and cholinergic activity that the resultant was another significant indicator of risk. But in neither of these studies do the sensitivity and specificity of the result of the analysis predict risk at the level of the individual; that is, the measure is good for distinguishing between large groups that either manifested VF or not, but it is not good for distinguishing among the individuals, because too many false-negative and false-positive predictions result.

The two sections above suggest that it is the integrated brain–autonomic outflow from specific cerebral systems that results in the descending **pattern** of sympathetic and parasympathetic control of the cardiovascular system that is responsible for increased risk. The type of measurement technique used to assess this variability may be very important in determining the sensitivity and specificity of the predictor. For example, the **stochastic measures,** such as the standard deviation or the power spectrum, regard the data as **intrinsically noisy about a mean** and therefore each beat-to-beat variation is random. In contrast, the **deterministic measures** regard each beat as **caused** and the variation as a nonrandom pattern.

Chaos theory suggests that some patterns might be revealed when the data are plotted in a time-delayed phase space, instead of the time or frequency domain that are the more common methods. The plot of the data in **phase space forms an object called an attractor.** The dimensions of these attractors represent a condensed measure of the "pattern" that exists in phase space. Thus dimensional measures might enable one to discriminate among data series with a greater sensitivity and specificity than can be achieved using a stochastic measure, such as the mean, standard deviation, or Fourier transform.

The methods of determining the dimensions of the **attractors** that had been developed for physics and chemistry (e.g., the correlation dimension, abbreviated D2) do not work well for biological data. This failure is because biological systems keep changing state following input from the nervous system and the data are thus quite nonstationary. The problem of **data nonstationarity,** however, seems to have been resolved by **an algorithm that does not require data nonstationarity.** This algorithm, called the point D2 or PD2i, has been used on heartbeat data with very encouraging results.

In heartbeat data from the pig model of experimental myocardial infraction, it is found that within 1 min after coronary occlusion the PD2i reduced from around 3 to less than 1.2 in those cases which later manifested VF, whereas PD2i was greater than 1.2 in all cases which did not later manifest VF. Neither the standard deviation nor the power spectrum (i.e., stochastic measures) were able to make such a discrimination when applied to the **same** data. Similarly, when analyses were made of samples of heartbeat intervals from 24-hr tape recordings of 43 high-risk ambulatory patients with nonsustained ventricular tachycardia and low left ventricular ejection fractions, it was found that PD2i (i.e., PD2i < 1.2) predicts VF within a span of 12 hr with very good sensitivity (100%) and specificity (86%). The stochastic measures were unable to make significant predictions in these same subjects.

In the conscious pig either **psychological stress** (touching) or transient **coronary artery occlusion** will evoke a **reduction in the PD2i** of the heartbeat intervals, whereas **stress-reduction** (adaptation to a novel environment) or intracerebral **β blocker** injection (levo propranolol) will evoke a dimensional increase. These data suggest that external and internal signals may operate together in a simple manner to determine whether or not the dimension of the heartbeats will approach the critical level of 1.2.

The conclusion is that the PD2i is able to detect a phase-space pattern in heartbeat intervals that is indicative of future risk of VF. This pattern appears to result from the sympathetic and parasympathetic outflow evoked by the cerebral integration of external and internal signals. It is not yet known what the significance is for the 1.2 dimensional character of the heartbeat intervals that precedes VF. This pattern in phase space, however, may be considered a dynamical pathology.

References

1. Skinner JE, Carpeggiani C, Landisman CE, Fulton KW. The correlation-dimension of heartbeat intervals is reduced in conscious pigs by myocardial ischemia. Circ Res 1991;68:966–76.
2. Skinner JE, Pratt CM, Vybiral T. A reduction in the correlation dimension of heart beat intervals proceeds imminent ventricular fibrillation in human subject. Am Heart J 1993;125:731–43.
3. Skinner JE. Neurocardiology: Brain mechanisms underlying fatal cardiac arrhythmias. Neurol Clin 1993;11:325–51.
4. Elbert T, Ray WJ, Kowalik ZJ, Skinner JE, Graf KE, Birbaumer N. Chaos in physiology. Physiol Rev 1993;74:1–48.
5. Skinner JE, Molnar M, Tomberg C. The point correlation dimension: performance with nonstationary surrogate data and noise. Integr Physiol Behav Sci 1994;29:217–34.

30 Transient Myocardial Ischemia and Infarction

Richard L. Verrier
Institute for Prevention of
Cardiovascular Disease
Deaconess Hospital
Harvard Medical School
Boston, Massachusetts

Peter Y. D. Taylor
Cardiovascular Division
Deaconess Hospital
Harvard Medical School
Boston, Massachusetts

James E. Muller
Institute for Prevention of
Cardiovascular Disease
Cardiovascular Division
Deaconess Hospital
Harvard Medical School
Boston, Massachusetts

Recent progress in our understanding of the role of the autonomic nervous system in transient myocardial ischemia and infarction has been the result of diversified research strategies. Clinical investigations of the timing of onset and the activities of patients prior to ischemic events have disclosed the importance of **sympathetic nervous system activation** and **coagulative factors** in precipitating **ischemia** and **infarction**. Experimental studies not only have provided detailed information concerning neural mechanisms involved in arrhythmogenesis but also have led to new noninvasive methodologies for exploration of autonomic function by heart rate variability analysis and for **tracking cardiac electrical instability** by quantification of **T-wave alternans,** a beat-to-beat fluctuation in waveform area.

Time of Onset and Triggering of Transient Myocardial Ischemia

Ambulatory monitoring of patients with transient myocardial ischemia disclosed a peak incidence of ST segment depression in the morning. This is associated with increases in several physiologic variables including systemic and arterial pressure and catecholamine levels. The morning peak in ischemia in patients with stable angina is dependent on the activity that occurs after awakening. If the patients were kept in bed, the time of the peak in transient levels of ischemia was shifted to the hours after beginning the activities of the day. Most ischemic episodes in the morning and afternoon were associated with increases in heart rate, suggesting increases in myocardial oxygen demand due to sympathetic nervous system activation. The important sympathetic contribution was confirmed by the finding that β-adrenergic blockade with **nadolol diminished the morning increase in ambulatory ischemia.**

Triggering of transient myocardial ischemia may also be attributed to either mental or physical activities at other times of the day. Recurrent episodes of ST segment depression during daily life in patients with stable angina often occurred during ordinary tasks such as conversing, driving a car, or holding a meeting at work, and were not correlated with fluctuations in heart rate. The investigators concluded that **transient impairment of coronary artery blood flow** was frequently the underlying basis for these ischemic events. A link between silent ischemia and mental stress was subsequently demonstrated. By measuring the uptake of rubidium-82 with positron tomography, they assessed regional myocardial perfusion and ischemia after mental arithmetic or physical exercise. During **mental arithmetic,** 12 of 16 (75%) patients exhibited **regional perfusion abnormalities** accompanied in 6 by ST segment depression and in 4 of these 6 by angina. The remaining 6 patients with perfusion abnormalities had neither pain nor electrocardiographic changes. Following exercise, all of the patients exhibited abnormal regional myocardial perfusion in the segments that had become ischemic with mental arithmetic. This was associated with ST segment depression in all and angina in 15 (94%) individuals. The investigators concluded that the interaction between mental activity and myocardial ischemia may operate continuously during everyday life and could be responsible for many transient and symptomless electrocardiographic changes in patients with coronary disease. Further evidence of a direct link between acute mental stress and myocardial ischemia has been provided by a battery of behavioral tests in patients with coronary artery disease. Especially significant is the demonstration that a personally relevant, emotionally arousing speaking task provoked more frequent and greater regional wall-motion abnormalities than did less specific cognitive tasks and the changes induced were of the magnitude of those induced by exercise.

Anger has been shown to decrease myocardial perfusion and to induce arrhythmias. In experimental animals, an angerlike state elicited by a confrontation paradigm involving food-access denial enhanced vulnerability in both the normal and ischemic heart, as evidenced by a reduction in the repetitive extrasystole threshold and by significant increases in T-wave alternans magnitude. The post-anger state is marked by a propensity to develop myocardial ischemia which is thought to be due to renormalization of blood pressure at a time when catecholamines may be persistently elevated.

Time of Onset and Triggering of Myocardial Infarction

While Obraztsov and Strazhesko proposed as early as 1910 that activities frequently trigger infarction, only recently has intensive research been directed to understanding the events immediately preceding infarction. In 1960, a study by Master, which was retrospective and not controlled, led to the view that activities were of little importance in the triggering of infarction. This concept prevailed for approximately 30 years but recently has been challenged by various authors. The primary impetus to a new interest in triggering onset of myocardial infarction was provided by data from the MILIS study, which showed that infarction is three times more likely to begin in the morning compared to the evening. A new case-crossover design was employed to identify activities of patients that serve as triggers of infarction at any time of day. Over 1700 patients were interviewed on an average of 4 days after myocardial infarction. Information was collected regarding the usual annual frequency of physical activity and the time, type, and intensity of physical activity in the 26 hr before the onset of myocardial infarction. With the use of appropriate control data, it was found that **heavy physical exertion increases the risk by 5-fold** that the onset of myocardial infarction would occur in the subsequent hour. The risk was increased by 100-fold in sedentary individuals. These investigators also demonstrated that there is a heightened risk of onset of myocardial infarction in the 2 hr **following anger.** It is now estimated that approximately **15% of myocardial infarctions have an identifiable trigger** such as exertion or anger.

It has been hypothesized that acute coronary ischemic events begin when a **vulnerable plaque disrupts** secondary to physical or psychological stress, associated with an increase in sympathetic input (Fig. 1). After plaque disruption, the final result can be altered by the amount of thrombosis that develops. If the thrombus is large and occludes the lumen, the final result may be an acute Q-wave myocardial infarction or sudden death. If the thrombus is smaller and nonocclusive, the result may be unstable angina, non Q-wave myocardial infarction, or asymptomatic plaque growth.

Aspirin and **β blockers** have been shown to prevent the onset of myocardial infarction. These agents may exert their protective effect by blocking important steps in the triggering process. Aspirin is thought to reduce occlusive coronary thrombosis by its antiplatelet effect. Observational data from the MILIS and the ISAM studies indicate that β blockers reduce the morning incidence of myocardial infarction. In the randomized BHAT trial, a morning peak in sudden death was found in the placebo group but not in the β-blocker group. These findings that β blockers prevent morning events suggest that the morning surge in sympathetic input is responsible for MI onset.

Autonomic Influences on Arrhythmias Following Ischemia and Infarction

In addition to contributing to the onset of myocardial ischemia and infarction, the autonomic nervous system also influences the type and severity of arrhythmias which are elicited by the disorders. This influence varies markedly with time after onset of ischemia or infarction. It is well established that within 2 to 3 min of coronary artery occlusion, there is a marked increase in cardiac electrical instability, as evidenced by the occurrence of ventricular premature beats, tachyarrhythmias, and ventricular fibrillation (Fig. 2). Reflex activation of the sympathetic nervous system is a critical element in the ischemia-induced electrical instability, as the arrhythmia can be significantly blunted by sympathectomy or β-adrenergic blockade. If the coronary obstruction is abruptly terminated, **a second period of heightened vulnerability** to fibrillation ensues within 15 to 30 sec and persists for less than 1 min. **Arrhythmias** occurring during this **reperfusion phase** are highly **lethal and refractory** to therapy. Most antifibrillartory agents including β blockers are ineffectual against reperfusion-induced arrhythmia. However, the nondihydropyridine calcium channel blockers, including **diltiazem** and **verapamil,** have been shown to exert significant protection. Whereas the exact mechanism for reperfusion-induced arrhythmias is uncertain, it is thought that washout of ischemic by-products is likely to be involved. Since reperfusion must occur rapidly to elicit these arrhythmias, an event such as abrupt disaggregation of platelets rather than cessation of vasospasm is a more probable clinical counterpart to reperfusion as modeled in experimental laboratories. If the occlusion persists for more than 30 min,

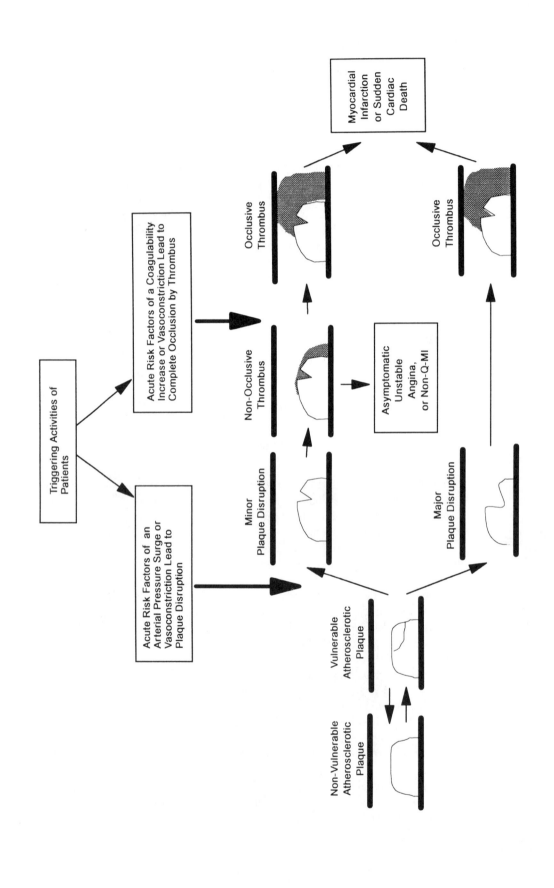

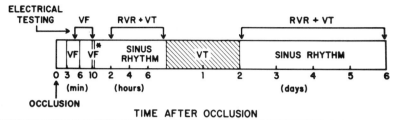

Figure 2. Time course of changes in ventricular electrical stability following left anterior descending coronary artery occlusion in the dog. Cardiac response to electrical testing is designated above the bar, while the spontaneous rhythm is denoted inside the bar. VF, ventricular fibrillation; RVR, repetitive ventricular response; VT, ventricular tachycardia. [Reprinted, with permission, from Verrier RL, Lown B. Influence of neural activity on ventricular electrical stability during acute myocardial ischemia and infarction. In: Sandøe E, Julian DC, Bell JW, eds. Management of ventricular tachycardia: role of mexiletine (International Congress Series No. 458). Amsterdam; Excerpta Medica 1978:133–150.)

reperfusion no longer elicits ventricular tachyarrhythmias because of a no-reflow effect which results from microvascular degeneration. This phenomenon and the prolonged reperfusion during thrombolysis probably account for the relatively low incidence of lethal arrhythmias during thrombolytic therapy.

In humans as well as in animals, late-phase ventricular arrhythmias ensue following hours of coronary occlusion. **Persistent susceptibility to arrhythmias** is present **when the myocardial infarction is of a mottled nature** with interpolated areas of viable and nonviable tissue, a substrate considered to be conducive to electrophysiologic inducibility. The electrophysiologic basis of late-phase arrhythmias appears to be electrical inhomogeneity and depressed conduction, which create conditions predisposing to reentry. Sympathetic nervous system stimulation by electrical excitation of nerves or exposure to behavioral stress is capable of eliciting ventricular tachyarrhythmias in animals recovering from myocardial infarction.

T-Wave Alternans and Ventricular Arrhythmias during Myocardial Ischemia and Infarction

There is growing experimental evidence that T-wave alternans, defined as a beat-to-beat alternation in T-wave area, constitutes a means for tracking

Figure 1. A hypothesis of the mechanisms through which daily activities may trigger occlusive coronary thrombosis. Three triggering mechanisms are presented: (1) physical or mental stress producing hemodynamic changes leading to plaque disruption; (2) activities causing an increase in coagulability; and (3) stimuli leading to vasoconstriction. The scheme depicting the role of coronary thrombosis in unstable angina, myocardial infarction, and sudden cardiac death has been well described by numerous investigators. The novel portion of this figure is the addition of triggers. See text and Muller *et al.* (1) for detailed discussion. Non-Q-MI, non-Q wave myocardial infarction. [Reprinted with permission from the American College of Cardiology (Journal of the American College of Cardiology, 1994, 23, 809–13).]

vulnerability to ventricular tachycardia and fibrillation. Using spectral analysis techniques to quantify T-wave alternans magnitude, it is possible to delineate the time course of vulnerability to fibrillation under diverse conditions in the experimental laboratory, most particularly during acute myocardial ischemia and reperfusion (Fig. 3). The enhanced vulnerability associated with sympathetic nervous system stimulation during coronary occlusion can be accurately evaluated and the profibrillatory influence predicted. The **antifibrillatory action** of **vagus nerve stimulation** has also been demonstrated. The technique is also sensitive to the impact of behavioral stress in conscious animals. Utilizing the anger paradigm, it was demonstrated that intense arousal can elicit a significant degree of T-wave alternans even in the normal state and that this effect is markedly enhanced during the superimposition of a coronary artery occlusion. Cardioselective β-adrenergic blockade with metoprolol reduced the degree of alternans, an observation which is consistent with the agent's cardioprotective effect against stress-induced vulnerability.

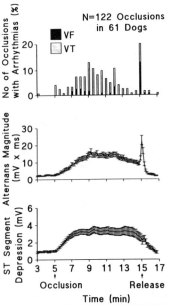

Figure 3.   Simultaneous time course of spontaneous ventricular fibrillation (VF) and tachycardia (VT), T-wave alternans, and ST segment depression during 10 min of left anterior descending (LAD) coronary artery occlusion and reperfusion in 61 chloralose-anesthetized dogs monitored with a left ventricular ECG catheter. Two occlusion/release sequences were performed in each dog. Incidence of spontaneous VT and VF was summed for each 30-sec period. T-wave alternans and ST segment changes were summed for each 10-msec interval. The waxing and waning of T-wave alternans magnitude closely parallels the spontaneous occurrence of malignant ventricular arrhythmias during both occlusion and reperfusion ($r^2 = 0.98, P < 0.01$). By contrast, ST segment changes were dissociated from arrhythmogenesis during the initial and latter minutes of the occlusion ($r^2 = 0.07$,NS) and upon reperfusion. The alternans and ST segment values are means, error bars represent SEM. VT was defined as four or more successive ventricular ectopic beats. (Reprinted, with permission, from Nearing BD, Oesterle SN, Verrier RL. Quantification of ischaemia-induced vulnerability by precordial T-wave alternans analysis in dog and human. Cardiovasc Res 1994; 28:1440–1449.)

Repolarization alternans has been observed in humans under diverse conditions conducive to myocardial ischemia, including **Prinzmetal's angina, angioplasty, bypass graft occlusion,** and **the postexercise period.** A detailed study during angioplasty in patients with mid-LAD coronary occlusion demonstrated that T-wave alternans magnitude delineates the time course of vulnerability associated with both myocardial ischemia and release–reperfusion. Adgey, Pantridge, and co-workers found a significant degree of alternans associated with ventricular premature beats in a patient in the early phase of anterior myocardial infarction. Following administration of **atropine** (0.6 mg, iv), which would be expected to diminish potentially protective vagal influences, the alternans level was significantly increased and ventricular fibrillation ensued (Fig. 4). Drug-induced acceleration in heart rate, which is known to exacerbate ischemia and cardiac vulnerability, may also have contributed to the arrhythmia. Repolarization alternans was shown to be a significant and independent predictor of inducible arrhythmias in 83 patients with and without organic heart disease referred for **electrophysiologic (EP) testing.** The presence of T-wave alternans in the microvolt range was found to be as significant a predictor of arrhythmia-free survival ($P < 0.001$) as the results of EP testing.

These studies thus point to the **pivotal role of autonomic nervous system activity** in causing **myocardial ischemia and infarction.** In addition, autonomic influences can alter the responses to ischemia and infarction, thereby determining the occurrence of life-threatening **arrhythmias.** It has become apparent that the sympathetic component of the autonomic nervous system is the main culprit, while enhanced vagal activity may exert a salutary influence as a result of

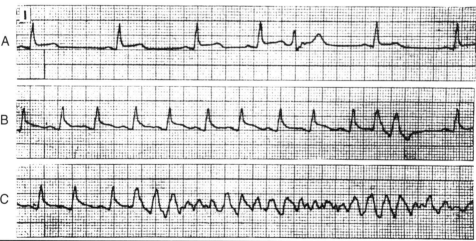

Figure 4. Sinus tachycardia after atropine leading to ventricular fibrillation. Patient with anterior infarction, lead I. (A) Sinus bradycardia (rate, 55 beats/min) with ventricular ectopics. (B) Record 2 min after atropine 0.6 mg, iv. Sinus tachycardia (rate, 110 beats/min) with consecutive ventricular ectopics. (C) Record 3 min after atropine showing development of ventricular fibrillation. (Reprinted, with permission, from Pantridge JF. Autonomic disturbance at the onset of myocardial infarction.In: Schwartz PJ, Brown AM, Malliani A, Zanchetti A, eds. Neural mechanisms in cardiac arrhythmias. New York: Raven, 1978:7.)

presynaptic inhibition of catecholamine release and antagonism of adrenergic influences at the receptor level. Exciting new methods permit noninvasive assessment of the interaction between nervous system activity and cardiac vulnerability by spectral analysis of heart rate variability and T-wave alternans. These powerful techniques may improve our understanding of the impact of neural activity on coronary hemodynamic and cardiac electrical function and thereby result in improved methods of prevention, diagnosis, and therapy.

Acknowledgment

This work was supported by grants HL41016 and HL50078 from the National Institutes of Health.

References

1. Muller JE, Abela GS, Nesto RW, Tofler GH. Triggers, acute risk factors and vulnerable plaques: The lexicon of a new frontier. J Am Coll Cardiol 1994;23:809–13.
2. Verrier RL, Dickerson LW. Autonomic nervous system and coronary blood flow changes related to emotional activation and sleep. Circulation 1991;83:II-81—9.
3. Verrier RL, Nearing BD. Electrophysiologic basis for T-wave alternans as an index of vulnerability to ventricular fibrillation. J Cardiovasc Electrophysiol 1994;5:445–61.
4. Parker JD, Testa MA, Jimenez AH, Tofler GH, Muller JE, Parker JO, Stone PH. Morning increase in ambulatory ischemia in patients with stable coronary artery disease. Importance of physical activity and increased cardiac demand. Circulation 1994;89:604–14.
5. Rozanski A, Bairey CN, Krantz DS, Friedman J, Resser KJ, Morell M, Hilton-Chalfen S, Hestrin L, Bietendorf J, Berman DS. Mental stress and the induction of silent myocardial ischemia in patients with coronary artery disease. N Engl J Med 1988;318:1005–12.
6. Rosenbaum DS, Jackson LE, Smith JM, Garan H, Ruskin JN, Cohen RJ. Electrical alternans and vulnerability to ventricular arrhythmia. N Engl J Med 1994;330:235–41.

31 *Congestive Heart Failure*

Murray Esler
Monash University
Baker Medical
Research Institute
Prahran
Melbourne, Australia

David Kaye
Cardiovascular
Division
Brigham and
Women's Hospital
Boston,
Massachusetts

Gavin Lambert
Human Autonomic
Function Laboratory
Baker Medical
Research Institute
Prahran
Victoria, Australia

Garry Jennings
Alfred Baker
Medical Unit
Prahran
Melbourne, Australia

Activation of the sympathetic nervous system is commonly observed in **heart failure,** reflected by **increased sympathetic nerve firing rates** in sympathetic fibers passing to skeletal muscle, **high rates of overflow of the sympathetic**

nervous transmitter, norepinephrine, to plasma, and **high plasma norepinephrine concentrations.** This sympathetic nervous stimulation has been ascribed
a pivotal role in the pathophysiology of the condition.

Although increased sympathetic outflow to the peripheral circulation and kidneys in cardiac failure may have adverse effects, through vasoconstriction, sodium retention, and ventricular overfilling, it is the sympathetic overactivity in the
heart which is potentially most damaging. Stimulation of the cardiac sympathetic
outflow may for a time provide inotropic support for the failing myocardium,
but at a cost. A **strong link** has been demonstrated between **cardiac sympathetic
nervous stimulation** and the development of **ventricular arrhythmias,** both under
experimental conditions and clinically. Further, norepinephrine in high concentrations, similar to those thought to exist in the myocardium in heart failure,
exerts a direct **toxic effect on cardiac myocytes** grown in cell culture, suggesting
that chronic cardiac sympathetic nervous activation in heart failure patients may
cause progressive damage to the myocardium.

Sympathetic Nervous Function in the Failing Human Heart

The concentration of norepinephrine in peripheral venous plasma, although
useful as a guide to overall sympathetic nervous activity, for several reasons does
not provide information specific to the heart. First, the plasma concentration is
dependent not only on the rate of release of norepinephrine from sympathetic
nerves but also on its clearance from plasma; **norepinephrine clearance is reduced
in cardiac failure** due to the lowered cardiac output and reduced regional blood
flows in organs, such as the liver and kidneys, which remove norepinephrine
from the circulation. Second, the anatomical and functional organization of the
sympathetic nervous system is into regional outflows, with each outflow being
capable of differentiated responses to a variety of physiological and pathophysiological stimuli. Global measures of sympathetic activity, such as plasma norepinephrine measurements, fail to identify sites of norepinephrine release and cannot identify sympathetic nervous activation in the heart. Only a small fraction
of the norepinephrine in plasma is derived from the heart.

The application of **tracer kinetic techniques** using radiolabeled norepinephrine avoids these deficiencies, and has allowed demonstration that the sympathetic nervous outflow to the heart is preferentially stimulated in congestive
cardiac failure, with rates of norepinephrine spillover from the heart to plasma
being **up to 100 times normal.** This increased spillover of the neurotransmitter
from the heart seems to be largely attributable to increased rates of sympathetic
nerve firing, as it is accompanied by increased overflow from the heart of
the noradrenaline precursor, **dopa** (indicating that norepinephrine synthesis is
increased), and of the sympathetic cotransmitter, **neuropeptide Y** (Fig. 1).
Neuronal reuptake of norepinephrine seems to be essentially unimpaired, as
the extraction of tritiated norepinephrine from plasma by the heart and its
conversion to the radiolabeled intraneuronal metabolite DHPG is normal or
very little reduced in cardiac failure. These observations of normally retained
capacity for neuronal reuptake of norepinephrine in the failing human heart
studied *in situ* contrast with those obtained from studies with myocardial

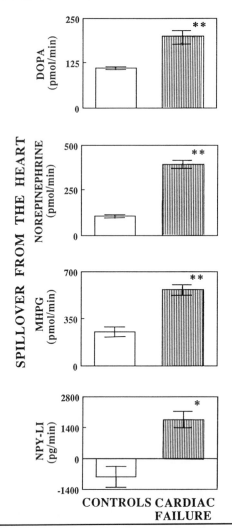

Figure 1. In cardiac failure, there is increased spillover from the heart to plasma of norepinephrine, of its precursor, dihydroxyphenylalanine (DOPA), and its extraneuronal metabolite, 3-methoxy-4-hydroxyphenylglycol (MHPG), and of the sympathetic cotransmitter, neuropeptide Y (NPY-LI). *$P < 0.05$, **$P < 0.01$.

tissue slices. The latter may be misleading, partly because of problems with diffusibility of the tracer *in vitro,* in the absence of hemoperfusion.

Responsiveness of the failing myocardium to sympathetic neural stimulation is **subnormal,** attributable in part to a **reduction in myocardial β adrenoceptor numbers,** preferentially involving β_1 adrenoceptors, and to **diminished postreceptor signal transduction.** The marked diminution in heart rate spectral power in congestive heart failure, studied using spectral analysis techniques, is presumably an expression of these changes.

The Basis for Sympathetic Nervous System Activation in Heart Failure

The afferent circulatory stimulus responsible for sympathoexcitation in congestive heart failure and the central nervous system neuronal circuitry involved remains to be elucidated. Recently, a strong relationship was demonstrated

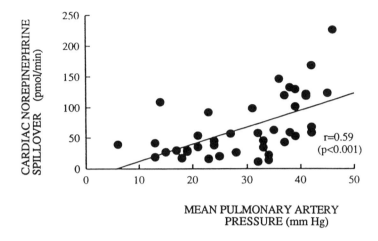

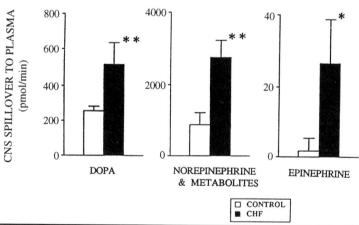

Figure 2. Consideration of possible mechanisms of sympathetic nervous stimulation in cardiac failure. (*Top*) A positive relation exists between pulmonary artery pressure and sympathetic nervous activity in the failing human heart, suggesting that intracardiac and pulmonary pressures act as a signal for reflex sympathoexcitation. (*Bottom*) The overflow into the internal jugular veins of norepinephrine, and its precursor, DOPA and major lipophilic CNS metabolites, MHPG and 3,4-dihydroxyphenylglycol (DHPG), is increased in congestive heart failure, indicative of elevated brain turnover of norepinephrine. Internal jugular venous overflow of epinephrine is present in heart failure patients, but not healthy subjects, suggesting that there is also activation of CNS epinephrine containing neurons. $^*P < 0.05$, $^{**}P < 0.01$.

between biochemical measures of cardiac sympathetic activity and pulmonary artery and pulmonary wedge pressures in heart failure patients, raising the possibility of reflex linkage of **cardiopulmonary baroreceptors** with efferent cardiac sympathetic activity (Fig. 2). This finding of intracardiac pressures being a probable direct determinant of the degree of sympathetic activation in patients with cardiac failure is contrary to an alternative explanation of the sympathetic nervous stimulation present, which emphasizes a desensitization of low-pressure baroreflexes as a basis for withdrawal of tonic inhibition of peripheral sympathetic activity. Whether elevated pulmonary pressures, in fact, provide the hemodynamic signal for increased sympathetic outflow to the myocardium does remain an open question.

There have been recent attempts to investigate **central nervous system monoamine neuronal mechanisms** which may underlie sympathetic nervous stimulation in human heart failure. **Norepinephrine, epinephrine,** and **serotonin** releasing neurons in the brainstem and forebrain have an important regulatory influence over sympathetic nervous outflows to the cardiovascular system. Cardiopulmonary volume receptor afferents do project to the noradrenergic nuclei of the locus coeruleus, and the firing rate of locus coeruleus neurons is changed by alterations in cardiopulmonary pressures. By combining direct sampling of internal jugular venous blood with isotope dilution methods, it is possible to study the **turnover of brain monoamine and indoleamine neurotransmitters** and investigate their association with efferent sympathetic outflow. Although a diffusional barrier limits the passage of catecholamines from the circulation to the brain, movement in the reverse direction, from the brain to plasma, is less restricted. **Raised internal jugular venous spillover** of **epinephrine,** and of **norepinephrine** and its lipophilic metabolites, occurs in cardiac failure (Fig. 2). An association between activation of central monoaminergic neurons, in particular, epinephrine neurons, and sympathetic nervous tone in the heart is suggested by these results. Epinephrine neurons in the brain (possibly **sympathoexcitatory adrenergic neurons of the C1 region** of the medulla) may play the dominant role, with activation of sympathoexcitatory noradrenergic neurons, most likely those of the forebrain, also being involved.

Adverse Consequences of High Sympathetic Nervous Activity

Despite recent important therapeutic advances involving in particular the clinical use of **angiotensin-converting enzyme inhibitors,** the mortality rate in patients with advanced cardiac failure remains high. In an attempt to modify the natural history of heart failure by the application of more specific therapeutic interventions, investigators have endeavored to identify pathogenic mechanisms in heart failure additional to those involving the renin angiotensin system. In this regard, the probable importance of the sympathetic nervous system in the pathogenesis of heart failure has been underlined by clinical investigations in which the concentration of norepinephrine in peripheral venous plasma, used as a simple semiquantitative measure of overall sympathetic nervous system activity, has been identified as a prognostic marker in patients with chronic heart failure. Indirect support also comes from several additional clinical sources, such as from studies of **β-blockade therapy in heart failure** which have reported beneficial effects on myocardial function and survival, and from neurochemical evidence that there is overactivity of the cardiac sympathetic nerves in those patients with mild cardiac failure most likely to suffer out of hospital ventricular tachycardia or fibrillation.

Although the rate of release of norepinephrine from the heart is, on average, higher in heart failure patients than in healthy subjects, **cardiac norepinephrine spillover rates differ widely.** Among patients with heart failure encompassing a broad spectrum, from mild to very severe, the extent of sympathetic stimulation is related to heart failure severity, but even in patients with profoundly impaired left ventricular function, sympathetic nervous activity in the heart can differ markedly. The basis of this differing degree of sympathetic nervous activation is not clear. It appears not to be due to the etiology of the heart failure, as cardiac norepinephrine spillover is identical in patients with idiopathic and ischemic cardiomyopathy. When the prognostic value of cardiac norepinephrine spillover measurements was recently prospectively compared with other hemodynamic, biochemical, and electrocardiographic predictors of outcome in heart failure, the cardiac norepinephrine spillover rate was the only variable which was significantly associated with outcome in a multivariate model. In these patients, all of whom had severe heart failure, plasma norepinephrine concentrations in peripheral venous and arterial plasma were unrelated to clinical outcome, in contrast to an earlier report, in which patients with all severity grades of heart failure were included. A confounding effect of heart failure severity on the plasma concentration of norepinephrine in the earlier studies may be partly responsible for this different finding. These results suggest that **activation of the sympathetic nervous system,** specifically of the cardiac sympathetic nerves, **contributes to the progression of heart failure and sudden death.** In this recent study, deaths were sudden, or attributable to progressive heart failure, in equal numbers, so it was not possible to implicate a specific effect of overactivity of the cardiac sympathetic nerves, in having either a toxic action on the myocardium underlying progressive cardiac decompensation, or in triggering ventricular arrhythmias. Both effects may possibly be operating.

These recent findings suggest that measurement of the cardiac norepinephrine spillover rate in patients with severe heart failure may provide **novel prognostic information.** General clinical applicability of the methodology to the determining of prognosis in patients on heart transplant waiting lists is unlikely, however, as it involves right heart catheterization and specialized neuroanalytical radiotracer chemistry. These results, however, do not provide the most direct clinical evidence to date of a deleterious effect of sympathetic nervous overactivity on the heart in patients with severe cardiac failure, and emphasize that the potential value of protecting against this with agents such as β-adrenergic blockers and **centrally acting sympathetic nervous system suppressants** needs to be tested.

References

1. Cohn J, Levine T, Olivari M, Garberg V, Tura D, Francis G, Simon A, Rector, T. Plasma norepinephrine as a guide to prognosis in patients with chronic congestive heart failure. N Engl J Med 1984;311:819–23.

2. Packer M. The neurohormonal hypothesis: a theory to explain the mechanism of disease progression in heart failure. J Am Coll Cardiol 1992;20:248–54.
3. Kaye DM, Lambert GW, Lefkovits J, Morris M, Jennings G, Esler MD. Neurochemical evidence of cardiac sympathetic activation and increased central nervous system norepinephrine turnover in severe congestive heart failure. J Am Coll Cardiol 1994;23:570–78.
4. Meredith IT, Eisenhofer G, Lambert GW, Dewar EM, Jennings GL, Esler MD. Cardiac sympathetic activity in congestive heart failure: evidence for increased neuronal norepinephrine release and preserved neuronal uptake. Circulation 1993;88:136–45.
5. Bristow MR, Anderson FL, Port DJ, Skerl L, Hershberger RE, Larrebee P, O'Connell JB, Renlund DG, Volkman K, Murray J, Feldman AM. Differences in β-adrenergic neuroeffector mechanisms in ischemic versus idiopathic dilated cardiomyopathy. Circulation 1991;84:1024–39.
6. Kaye DM, Lefkovits J, Jennings GL, Bergin P, Broughton A, Esler MD. Adverse consequences of high sympathetic nervous activity in the failing human heart. J Am Coll Cardiol 1995;26:1257–1263.

PART VII

Paroxymal Autonomic Syncopes

32

Evaluation of a Patient with Syncope

Horacio Kaufmann
Autonomic Nervous System Laboratory
Mount Sinai School of Medicine
New York, New York

Syncope (Greek *synkope,* cessation, pause) is a transient loss of consciousness and postural tone with spontaneous recovery and no neurological sequelae. Syncope is caused by a global reversible reduction of blood flow to the **reticular activating system,** the neuronal network in the brainstem responsible for supporting consciousness. Temporary loss of consciousness caused by noncardiovascular mechanisms such as seizure and metabolic and psychiatric disorders may simulate syncope but can be distinguished from true syncope by clinical features.

Syncope is a very common clinical problem. In the 26 years of surveillance of the Framingham study, syncope occurred in **3% of men** and in **3.5% of women.** Moreover, syncope accounts for **6% of hospital admissions.**

Mechanisms of Syncope

Three hemodynamic abnormalities may produce syncope (Table 1): (a) a fall in blood pressure, usually in the standing position (i.e., orthostatic hypotension); (b) an acute decrease in cardiac output; and (c) an acute increase in cerebrovascular resistance.

Orthostatic Hypotension

In the standing position, arterial pressure at brain level is 15 to 20 mm Hg lower than arterial pressure at the level of the aortic arch. Local autoregulatory mechanisms keep cerebral blood flow fairly constant despite changes in cerebral arterial pressure. However, if cerebral arterial pressure falls below 40 mm Hg, cerebral autoregulation does not prevent decreases in cerebral blood flow. Thus, if a person is standing and mean aortic **pressure falls below 70 mm Hg,** cerebral blood flow is likely to decrease sufficiently for **syncope or presyncope** to occur.

Orthostatic hypotension can be secondary to **drugs,** to **chronic baroreflex failure** (covered elsewhere in this book), and **to neurally mediated syncope** (i.e., vasovagal syncope).

Orthostatic hypotension due to **drugs** is a common but often overlooked cause of syncope, particularly in the elderly in whom baroreflexes may be impaired. Another frequent reason for syncope in the elderly is **postprandial hypotension.** This is believed to be caused by impaired baroreflex-mediated vasoconstriction which fails to compensate for the splanchnic vasodilation induced by food.

Table 1.   Causes of Syncope

Orthostatic hypotension (reduction in vascular
   resistance or intravascular volume or both)
   Drugs
   Chronic baroreflex failure
   Neurally mediated syncope
Fall in cardiac output
   Cardiac arrhythmia
   Obstructions to flow
   Myocardial infarction
Increased cerebrovascular resistance
   Hyperventilation
   Increase intracranial pressure

The most frequent cause of syncope in apparently normal subjects is **neurally mediated syncope.** Neurally mediated syncope (also referred to as **vasovagal, vasodepressor,** or **reflex syncope**) is an acute hemodynamic reaction produced by a sudden change in autonomic nervous system activity. In neurally mediated syncope, the normal pattern of autonomic outflow that maintains blood pressure in the standing position (increased sympathetic and decreased parasympathetic activity) is acutely reversed. Parasympathetic outflow to the sinus node increases, producing bradycardia, while sympathetic outflow to blood vessels is reduced and there is profound vasodilation. Bradycardia is not the cause of hypotension as ventricular pacemakers prevent it but do not prevent syncope. Whether the reduction in sympathetic activity is the sole mechanism responsible for vasodilation is unknown. An increase in **nitric oxide-mediated vasodilation** may also be involved.

Neurally mediated syncope can be triggered centrally by stimuli such as **pain or fear;** presumably, by descending signals from cortical, limbic, or hypothalamic structures to autonomic control centers in the medulla. Neurally mediated syncope can also be triggered peripherally by stimulation of sensory receptors located in the arterial tree or viscera. These receptors respond to pressure or mechanical deformation and have afferent fibers in the **vagus** and **glossopharyngeal nerves** and when discharged excessively may inhibit vasomotor centers in the medulla (Fig. 1).

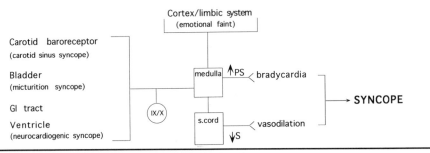

Figure 1.   Afferent and efferent pathways in neurally mediated syncope.

For example, neurally mediated syncopal syndromes occur after **compression of carotid baroreceptors** in the neck, following rapid **emptying of a distended bladder** or **distention of the gastrointestinal tract** and during glossopharyngeal or **trigeminal neuralgia.**

In addition, in susceptible individuals, neurally mediated syncope may occur with no obvious trigger while the subject is standing or walking. Several lines of evidence suggest that, in these cases, the source of abnormal afferent signals may be sensory receptors in the heart (i.e., **neurocardiogenic or "ventricular" syncope**). However, neurally mediated syncope has recently been induced in patients with heart transplants, in whom the ventricle is likely to be denervated. Perhaps, sensory receptors in the heart transplant patients are in the arterial tree rather than the ventricle.

Neurally mediated syncope needs to be distinguished from syncope in autonomic failure. In **autonomic failure**, orthostatic syncope is **persistent** and caused by chronic inability to appropriately activate efferent sympathetic fibers. In contrast, hypotension in neurally mediated syncope is an acute, self-limited event caused by a paroxysmal transient disruption of baroreflex function (Fig. 2). Between syncopal episodes, patients with neurally mediated syncope have normal or even increased autonomic cardiovascular responses.

Acute Decrease in Cardiac Output

A decrease in cardiac output resulting in syncope may be caused by cardiac **arrhythmias,** by obstruction to flow in **aortic stenosis** or **pulmonary embolism,** as a result of acute **myocardial infarction.** Episodes of profound sinus bradycardia or sinus arrest in patients with **sinoatrial disease** may present as recurrent syncope. Similarly, **supraventricular tachyarrhythmias** and the sinus pauses that follow, as well as rapid **ventricular tachycardia** that progress to ventricular fibrillation before reverting spontaneously to normal, may be responsible for recurrent episodes of syncope or near syncope.

Acute Increase in Cerebrovascular Resistance

Rarely, syncope may occur when blood flow to the reticular activating system is compromised by acute increases in cerebrovascular resistance or intracranial pressure. A **reduction in carbon dioxide** in blood induced by alveolar hyperventilation, as it occurs in **panic attacks,** may produce **diffuse cerebral vasoconstriction** severe enough to induce syncope, particularly if the person is standing. A rise in intracranial pressure induced by **coughing** or straining against a closed glottis may precipitate syncope particularly in patients with **craniocervical malformations or chronic obstructive pulmonary disease.**

Atherosclerotic disease involving the **posterior cerebral circulation** is an infrequent cause of syncope and is usually accompanied by other neurological abnormalities.

A very rare cause of syncope is the **subclavian steal syndrome.** It is caused by occlusive disease of the subclavian artery, proximal to the origin of the vertebral artery, usually **on the left side.** Syncope occurs during upper arm

A) 36 y.o. male with autonomic failure

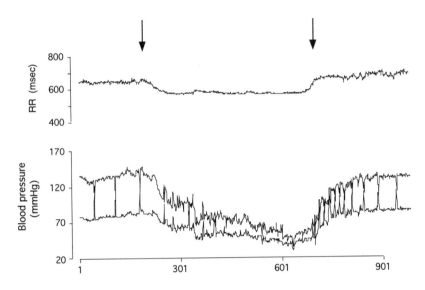

B) 28 y.o. male with neurally mediated syncope

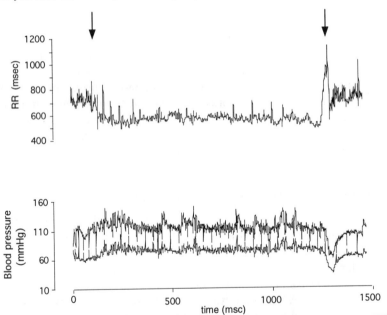

Figure 2.   Continuous RR intervals and blood pressure (Finapress) recordings during passive head up tilt in (A) subject with primary autonomic failure and (B) subject with neurally mediated syncope. First arrow indicates tilt up and second arrow tilt down after syncope occurred.

exercise because blood is shunted via the circle of Willis retrogradely through the vertebral artery to the distal subclavian artery to the arm.

Diagnosis

A thorough history may reveal the cause of syncope in a substantial number of cases. Accounts of witnesses must be sought to rule out a seizure disorder. A few **myoclonic jerks, tonic contractions of the limbs,** or "**rolling of the eyes**" can occur in syncope, but frank tonic clonic convulsions suggest seizure. **Urinary incontinence** is rare in syncope but frequent with seizures, and **post-ictal confusion is almost diagnostic of seizure activity.**

A complete **drug history** is essential. The use of antihypertensives, neuroleptics, tricyclic antidepressants and dopaminergic agonists is a frequent cause of orthostatic hypotension and syncope, particularly in the elderly.

When syncope is preceded **by emotionally stressful or painful situations** or by nausea, abdominal discomfort, pallor, diaphoresis, and blurred vision (all symptoms of autonomic activation) neurally mediated syncope should be suspected. When the victim falls, the horizontal position improves cerebral blood flow and consciousness is quickly regained, but hypotension and bradycardia may persist for several minutes, so that, on attempting to stand, consciousness is frequently lost again. A characteristic setting is typical in several well known neurally mediated syncopal syndromes. For example, syncope after **standing immobile,** particularly in **hot weather** or **after a period of bedrest** as well as syncope occurring **during micturition** or coughing or while playing a wind instrument such as the trumpet, and syncope with trigeminal or glossopharyngeal neuralgia are likely to be neurally mediated.

In marked contrast to the prodromal symptoms characteristic of neurally mediated syncope, syncope in patients with autonomic failure is **never preceded by signs of autonomic activation.**

Syncope during or **after exercise** suggests fixed or dynamic **aortic stenosis.** Syncope in aortic stenosis can be caused by obstruction to flow, arrhythmias, or reflex vasodilation. The latter results from increased ventricular mechanoreceptor discharge (Bezold–Jarisch reflex), a mechanism similar to that of neurally mediated syncope.

On physical examination, blood pressure and heart rate should be taken in the supine and upright position, checking for orthostatic hypotension with or without a compensatory increase in heart rate. Special attention should be given to signs of cardiac valvular disease, autonomic failure, or other neurological abnormalities commonly associated with autonomic failure, such as **parkinsonism, cerebellar ataxia,** or the presence of **deafness** as in **Romano Ward syndrome (congenital long QT syndrome).** A **bruit** over the **supraclavicular** area and induction of symptoms by **exercise of the arm** are suggestive of **subclavian steal syndrome.**

Because of its potential severity, the possibility of a cardiac arrhythmia causing syncope should always be considered first. A severe or potentially severe conduction defect such as third degree atrioventricular block or the long QT syndrome are easily identified by 12-lead electrocardiography. In most cases, however, an arrhythmic cause of syncope is difficult to prove.

Ambulatory electrocardiographic monitoring for 24 hr may be diagnostic but the test is frequently inconclusive because arrhythmias which do not correlate with clinical symptoms are common. **Portable loop electrocardiographic recorders** that a patient can wear for weeks or months and that can be activated after a syncopal episode are now available and may prove useful in identifying arrhythmias. Invasive electrophysiologic studies, by introducing extra electrical stimuli into the heart, identify susceptibility to ventricular arrhythmias that can cause syncope. The procedure has shown some predictive value only in patients with structural heart disease. The use of **signal-averaged EKG to identify late potentials in the terminal portion of the QRS complex** (indicative of heterogeneous myocardial activation and a possible substrate of sustained ventricular tachycarrhythmias) has been reported to be useful.

Tilt Testing

In patients with syncope in whom a cardiac arrhythmia cannot be documented by electrocardiography, hemodynamic monitoring during passive tilt (i.e., tilt table test) is the best available diagnostic procedure. Passive head-up tilt by preventing the pumping effect of skeletal muscle contraction exaggerates the reduction in venous return of the upright posture and triggers neurally mediated syncope in susceptible individuals.

During prolonged tilt, between 30 and 80% of patients with recurrent unexplained syncope suffer neurally mediated syncope with symptoms similar to those they experience spontaneously. Their initial response to tilt is normal. However, following a variable period of time with well maintained blood pressure and tachycardia, hypotension and sudden bradycardia develops. As shown in Fig. 2, this picture clearly differentiates between these patients and those with classic autonomic failure because in patients with autonomic failure blood pressure falls progressively immediately following tilt and there is no bradycardia.

Although tilt-induced neurally mediated syncope appears to be identical to spontaneous syncope, the mechanism responsible for triggering this abnormal reflex response and the reason for individual susceptibility are still unknown. Increased discharge from ventricular mechanoreceptors is the currently postulated but disputed mechanism.

The tilt table test is also useful to assess the effect of drugs in orthostatic intolerance. Orthostatic hypotension due to drugs may not be evident following a few minutes in the standing position but may become apparent during prolonged tilt. False positive studies sometimes limit the usefulness of tilt.

Prognosis

The prognosis of syncope depends on the underlying cause. The 1-year mortality risk for patients with syncope associated with cardiac disease varies from 19 to 33%, while for patients with syncope unassociated with cardiac disease it varies from 0 to 12%.

References

1. Savage DD, Corwin L, McGee DL, Kannel WB, Wolf PA. Epidemiologic features of isolated syncope: the Framingham study. Stroke 1985;16(4):626–29.

2. Lipsitz LA, Nyqvist RP, Wei JY, Rowe JW. Postprandial reduction in blood pressure in the elderly. N Engl J Med 1983;309:81–3.
3. Kaufmann H. Neurally mediated syncope. Pathogenesis, diagnosis, and treatment. Neurology 1995; 45:S12–8.
4. Kapoor WN. Evaluation and management of the patient with syncope. JAMA 1992;268(18):2553–60.

33   *Neurocardiogenic Syncope*

Blair P. Grubb
Department of Medicine
Division of Cardiology
Medical College of Ohio
Toledo, Ohio

Daniel J. Kosinski
Department of Medicine
Division of Cardiology
Medical College of Ohio
Toledo, Ohio

Pathophysiology

The precise pathophysiologic mechanisms responsible for **neurocardiogenic syncope** are not completely understood; however, a basic outline can be constructed (Figs. 1 and 2). In normal subjects spontaneous or induced volume changes are compensated. As preload decreases there is a decrease in activation of **ventricular mechanoreceptor C-fibers**. In addition, aortic arch and carotid sinus **baroreceptors** react in a similar fashion. As these receptors decrease afferent neural traffic to the brainstem, a reflex increase in sympathetic stimulation occurs. Thus, the normal subject has an increase in heart rate, an increase in diastolic blood pressure, and an unchanged or slightly decreased systolic blood pressure.

In patients with **neurocardiogenic syncope**, the above described compensatory reflex is at some point replaced by a **paradoxical decrease in blood pressure and/or heart rate.** It is believed that when ventricular preload rapidly decreases and sympathetic stimulation occurs, patients with neurocardiogenic syncope develop an exaggerated myocardial inotropic response. This **hypercontractive state** produces a decrease in end systolic area and volume, an increase in fractional shortening, and an increase in intracavitary pressure. These changes then presumably activate cardiac mechanoreceptor C-fibers and produce an abrupt increase in neural traffic to the **nucleus tractus solitarii** of the brainstem. However, this hypothesis has been challenged and it is conceivable that other mechanisms, both cardiac and extracardiac, may be in part responsible.

The efferent reflex arc is also incompletely understood. It is possible that at the brainstem level, alterations in **serotonin** levels are in some fashion involved in the initiation of the efferent reflex. However, whether serotonin is a

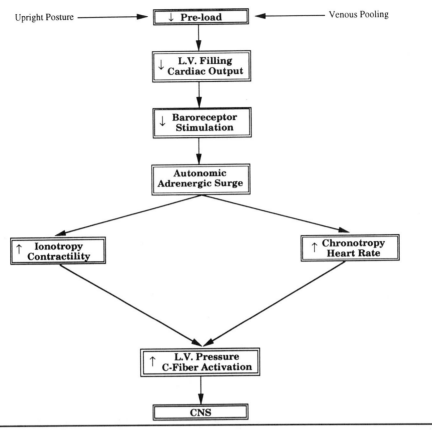

Figure 1.   Afferent reflex arc.

primary or secondary mediator is not known. Other mediators such as **nitric oxide** and **adenosine** may also have a role.

Recent data are now also sufficient to support that sympathetic withdrawal is responsible for the bradycardia and hypotension that are observed clinically. Vagal mechanisms have a comparatively minor role.

Role of the Cerebral Vasculature

Several authors have demonstrated that in neurocardiogenic syncope, there exists an abnormality of cerebral blood flow during symptomatic episodes. In symptomatic patients with hypotension, in whom one would expect to see cerebral arteriolar vasodilation, a **paradoxic profound cerebral vasoconstriction** occurs. These changes may augment cerebral hypoperfusion and enhance the probability of clinical syncope. It has been demonstrated that in patients with neurocardiogenic syncope who are successfully treated, these changes are improved or eliminated.

Diagnosis

Head-upright tilt table testing was first described as a diagnostic modality for neurocardiogenic syncope in 1986. Since that point, this test has come to be

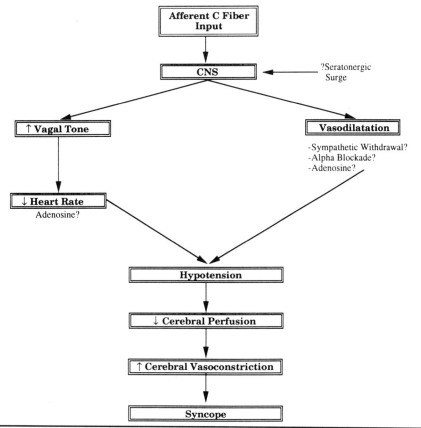

Figure 2. Efferent reflex arc.

recognized as the standard for diagnosis. However, considerable disagreement exists as to the optimal angle of tilt and duration of testing that should be utilized. It is generally agreed that an angle of tilt of at least 60° be utilized. Steeper tilt angles have not been demonstrated to improve test sensitivity, but may shorten the time to syncope. The optimal test duration is still an area of controversy.

Isoproterenol is also commonly utilized as an adjunct to testing in patients who do not respond to passive tilt alone. Controversy also exists regarding this practice. Isoproterenol improves the overall sensitivity of tilt table testing; however, concern exists over whether specificity is significantly adversely affected. Many investigators believe that reasonable doses of isoproterenol (0.5– 3 μg/min) administered for a 10- to 15-min tilt test duration improve sensitivity without a significant decrease in test specificity.

Tilt Test Response

Three basic response patterns may be observed in patients who are tilt table positive. (i) A primary **cardioinhibitory** response predominated by bradycardia or asystole; (ii) a primary **vasodepressor** response predominated by hypotension without bradycardia; (iii) a "classic" or **mixed response** whereby both elements are present.

Debate also continues over what is a satisfactory clinical end-point of a positive tilt table response. Certainly, **syncope** is an agreed end-point. However, most experts would also agree that **presyncope** accompanied by hypotension with or without bradycardia is also an acceptable end-point.

Indications for Head-Upright Tilt Testing

Clearly, patients with syncopal episodes accompanied by a characteristic "vagal" prodrome should be considered for testing. These patients have presyncopal symptoms such as dizziness, nausea, headache, and "hot" feelings. Often patients will be able to abort episodes by sitting or lying down.

Sufficient data also exist to suggest the indication for tilt table testing in a variety of patients with various clinical presentations.

There are also certain populations of **patients in whom a positive tilt test may be a nonspecific finding** and must be interpreted carefully. Among these groups are patients who are **trained athletes** and patients with **hypertrophic cardiomyopathy.**

Therapy

If symptomatic events are accompanied by a sufficient prodromal warning, pharmacologic therapy may be unnecessary. The patient is simply instructed to lie down at the fist sign of an episode.

For patients without a sufficient prodromal warning, multiple pharmacologic agents, either alone or in combination, are effective, These agents include **β blockers, calcium channel blockers, theophylline, serotonin re-uptake inhibitors, scopolamine, disopyramide,** and **fludrocortisone.** The therapeutic mechanism of action of most of these agents for this disorder is unknown.

For patients with **severe bradycardia or asystole, cardiac pacing** may be helpful. This is an area of controversy as some data have been generated to suggest medical therapy as equivalent to pacing in this subgroup of patients. However, many of this subgroup of patients are refractory to pharmacologic therapy and although pacing usually does not entirely abort episodes, pacing may provide a prodrome sufficient to prevent injury. For this subgroup of patients, cardiac pacing in conjunction with pharmacotherapy is often effective.

References

1. Kosinski D, Grubb BP. Neurally mediated syncope with an update on indications of usefulness of head-upright tilt table testing and pharmacologic therapy. Curr Opin Cardiol 1994;9:53–64.
2. Samoil D, Grubb BP, Kip K, Kosinksi D. Head up tilt table testing in children with unexplained syncope. Pediatrics 1993;92:426–30.
3. Rubin A, Rials S, Marinchak R, Kowey P. The head up tilt table test and cardiovascular neurogenic syncope. Am Heart J 1993;125:476–82.
4. Samoil D, Grubb BP, Brewster P, Moore J, Temesy-Armos P. Comparison of single and dual chamber pacing techniques in prevention of upright tilt induced vasovagal syncope. Eur J Cardiac Pacing Electrophysiol 1993;1:36–41.

5. Sra J, Jazayeri M, Avitall B, Dhala A, Deshpande S, Blanck Z, Akhtar M. Comparison of cardiac pacing with drug therapy in the treatment of neurocardiogenic syncope with bradycardia and asystole. N Eng J Med 1993;328:1085–90.

34

Syncope in the Athlete

Victor A. Convertino
Physiology Research Branch
Armstrong Laboratory/AOCY
Brooks Air Force Base, Texas

Over the past half century, anecdotal reports have described common experiences of dizziness, nausea, and symptoms of syncope in endurance-trained athletes. From these observations emerged the hypothesis that aerobically fit athletes were predisposed to **orthostatic hypotension and intolerance.** Although numerous investigations reported in the literature have failed to support a relationship between aerobic fitness and orthostatic intolerance, a few studies have demonstrated that individuals who habitually participate in endurance exercise training demonstrate some degree of symptomatic othostatism.

The **mechanisms** underlying syncope in athletes are unclear. An early cross-sectional investigation demonstrated that lower orthostatic tolerance was associated with greater venous compliance in the legs of athletes compared to unfit subjects. However, more recent cross-sectional and longitudinal studies have failed to demonstrate differences in leg compliance between trained and untrained states. **High cardiac vagal tone** and depressed carotid and aortic baroreceptor reflex responsiveness have been implicated as possible mechanisms that may limit the ability of athletes to increase heart rate during orthostatism. However, cross-sectional and longitudinal data have demonstrated little difference in carotid-cardiac baroreflex responsiveness associated with exercise training. Further, **expanded blood volume,** which is associated with endurance exercise training, is known to reduce heart rate and vasoconstrictive baroreflex responses to baroreceptor stimulation. Since endurance athletes are hypervolemic, their reduced heart rate and vasoconstrictive responses may therefore represent a greater reserve for tachycardia and vascular resistance compared to untrained individuals. It is important to emphasize that **blood pressure** is the product of **heart rate × stroke volume × peripheral resistance.** Athletes who have large stroke volumes secondary to **eccentric hypertrophy** and a large end-diastolic volume may require smaller baroreflex-mediated tachycardia and vasoconstriction in response to arterial hypotension to affect an appropriate corrective increase in cardiac output than a nonathlete with a smaller stroke volume. This concept is supported by the observation that the lower orthostatic tachycardia observed in athletes during an orthostatic challenge is compensated for by higher stroke volume, thus maintaining cardiac output at or above levels of unfit subjects. Therefore, it is difficult to contend that syncope in athletes can be attributed to increased compliance of the lower extremities or attenuated arterial or cardiopulmonary baroreflex control of cardiac and vascular responses.

With the lack of evidence to support the role of attenuated baroreflex function in athletes to explain their predisposition to syncope, a new hypothesis has emerged which describes evidence that athletes have structural changes in the cardiovascular system that, although beneficial during exercise, can lead to an excessively large decrease in stroke volume during orthostatism. This hypothesis is based on the evidence that endurance-trained athletes demonstrate a **greater effective left ventricular compliance and distensibility** than nonathletes and a **steeper slope of the Frank–Starling relationship** between left ventricular filling pressure and stroke volume. Thus, this greater reduction in stroke volume for the same reduction in filling pressure may represent the most likely mechanism predisposing the athlete to syncope.

It should be emphasized that syncope in athletes occurs in very few highly endurance-trained individuals. Since there is an important genetic component to being an elite athlete, it is not unreasonable to speculate that a steeper Frank–Starling curve may be an innate characteristic of some athletes, thus predisposing them to syncope. It is important that the predisposition to syncope in a few elite athletes not detract from the health benefits to be gained by sedentary individuals who undertake aerobic exercise programs. The phenomenon of syncope in the elite athlete most likely represents a **mechanical change in the cardiovascular system** that benefits the athlete during exercise and should not be interpreted as a clinical abnormality.

References

1. Convertino VA. Aerobic fitness, endurance training and orthostatic intolerance. Exer Sports Sci Rev 1987;15:223–59.
2. Convertino VA. Endurance exercise training: conditions of enhanced hemodynamic responses and tolerance to LBNP. Med Sci Sports Exer 1993;25:705–12.
3. Levine BD. Regulation of central blood volume and cardiac filling in enduranace athletes: the Frank Starling Mechanism as a determinant of orthostatic tolerance. Med Sci Sports Exer 1993;25-727–32.
4. Mack GW, Convertino VA, Nadel E R, Effect of exercise training on cardiopulmonary baroreflex control of forearm vascular resistance in humans. Med Sci Sports Exer 1993;25:722–6.
5. Raven PB, Pawelczyk JA. Chronic endurance exercise training: a condition of inadequate blood pressure regulation and reduced tolerance to LBNP. Med Sci Sports Exer 1993;25:713–21.

PART VIII

Catecholamine Disorders

35

Pheochromocytoma and Neuroblastoma

William M. Manger
New York University Medical Center
Columbia Medical Center
National Hypertension Association
New York, New York

Ray W. Gifford, Jr.
Department of Nephrology and
Hypertension
Cleveland Clinic Foundation
Ohio State University College
of Medicine
Cleveland, Ohio

Pheochromocytoma, a rare neuroendocrine tumor, secretes catecholamines, and 50% cause sustained hypertension in at least 0.01% of patients with diastolic hypertension; 45% cause only paroxysmal hypertension. Rarely, patients remain normotensive or have orthostatic hypotension. Pheochromocytomas arise from neuroectodermal **chromaffin** cells in the **adrenal medulla** (90%) and from **paraganglia** chromaffin cells of the sympathetic nervous system elsewhere in the abdomen, pelvis, chest (<2%), and neck (<1%). Tumors occur at any age, especially in the 4th and 5th decades. There is no sex predilection except, before puberty, it is more common in boys. Multiple and extraadrenal tumors are more frequent in children than in adults. Ten percent are familial (autosomal dominant inheritance) and nearly always in the adrenal, frequently bilateral and multicentric. Mutations of the RET proto-oncogene on chromosome 10 and multiple gene abnormalities are probably involved in tumor pathogenesis.

About **10% of pheochromocytomas are malignant,** but this cannot be determined from histopathology; metastases or invasion of tissues establish malignancy. Nondiploid DNA patterns and paucity of sustentacular cells appear characteristic of malignancy.

Most tumors weigh less than 70 g, but can vary from microscopic to 3600 g. Cells contain secretory granules which release catecholamines by diffusion and/or exocytosis (along with dopamine beta hydroxylase, neuropeptide Y, and chromogranins), which exert cardiovascular and metabolic effects by stimulating adrenergic α and β receptors. Prolonged exposure to excess catecholamines can decrease receptor responsiveness (desensitization). Other peptides may be secreted and contribute to clinical manifestations.

Pathologic complications (**stroke, myocardial infarction, arrhythmias, catecholamine cardiomyopathy, ischemic enterocolitis,** shock, multisystem organ failure) result from hypertension and/or increased circulating catecholamines. Compression of adjacent structures and metastases can cause additional complications.

Hemodynamic and metabolic effects of hypercatecholaminemia may suggest many diseases, some with increased excretion of catecholamines and metabolites (Table 1). About 95% of patients periodically have **severe headache** and/or **generalized sweating** and/or **palpitations** with tachy- or bradycardia. Anxiety,

Table 1.   Differential Diagnosis

All hypertensives (sustained and paroxysmal)
Anxiety, panic attacks, psychoneurosis, tension states
Hyperthyroidism
Paroxysmal tachycardia
Hyperdynamic β-adrenergic circulatory state
Menopause
Vasodilating headache (migraine and cluster headaches)
Coronary insufficiency syndrome
Acute hypertensive encephalopathy
Diabetes mellitus
Renal parenchymal or renal arterial disease with hypertension
Focal arterial insufficiency of the brain; cerebral vasculitis
Intracranial lesions (with or without ↑ intracranial pressure)
Autonomic hyperreflexia
Diencephalic seizure; Page's syndrome; dopamine surges
Toxemia of pregnancy (**or eclampsia with convulsions**)
Hypertensive crises associated with monoamine oxidase inhibitors
Carcinoid
Hypoglycemia
Mastocytosis
Familial dysautonomia
Acrodynia
Neuroblastoma; ganglioneuroblastoma; ganglioneuroma
Acute infectious disease; **acute abdomen** (cardiovascular catastrophe)
Unexplained shock
Neurofibromatosis (with or without renal arterial disease)
Rare causes of paroxysmal hypertension: **adrenal medullary hyperplasia; acute porphyria; lead poisoning;** tabetic crisis; encephalitis; **clonidine withdrawal;** hypovolemia with inappropriate vasoconstriction; pulmonary artery fibrosarcoma; pork hypersensitivity; dysregulation of hypothalamus; **baroreflex failure; tetanus; Guillain–Barré syndrome; pseudopheochromocytoma;** factitious (induced by **certain illegal,** prescription, and nonprescription drugs); **fatal familial insomnia;** sickle cell crisis

Modified from Manger WM, Gifford RW Jr. Pheochromocytoma. New York: Springer-Verlag, 1977.

pallor (rarely flushing), tremor, weight loss, chest and abdominal pain, constipation, nausea, vomiting, and orthostatic hypotension are not uncommon.

Symptomatic attacks may occur every few months or many times daily; they usually last less than 5 min and may be caused by physical maneuvers, psychic stimulation, and certain drugs. Attacks caused by micturition or bladder distention suggest a bladder tumor.

Familial pheochromocytoma is designated **multiple endocrine neoplasia (MEN) type-2** when associated with **medullary thyroid carcinoma** (MTC) and/or **hyperparathyroidism; MEN type-3** is characterized by **MTC, mucosal neuromas, thickened corneal nerves,** and **alimentary-tract ganglioneuromatosis.** Hypercalcitonemia is almost diagnostic of MTC or premalignant thyroid cells. Patients with familial pheochromocytoma are often normotensive and/or asymptomatic.

Symptomatic patients with sustained or paroxysmal hypertension should be screened for pheochromocytoma; asymptomatic patients with hypertension of unknown etiology should be screened, especially if they have diseases known sometimes to coexist (e.g., cholelithiasis, neurofibromatosis, Cushing's syndrome, von Hippel–Lindau disease, acromegaly) with pheochromocytoma or if laboratory abnormalities caused by hypercatecholaminemia are present. Also first-degree relatives of patients with MEN type-2 or type-3 should be screened. Measurement of 24-hr urinary metanephrines or plasma catecholamines will detect 95% of patients with pheochromocytomas. For a preoperative diagnosis of pheochromocytoma, it is essential to demonstrate increased plasma or urinary catecholamines and/or their metabolites. Some patients with neurogenic or essential hypertension have elevated plasma catecholamines and manifestations suggesting pheochromocytoma. The **clonidine suppression test** permits differentiation of these conditions by suppressing plasma norepinephrine concentrations in patients without tumors but not in those with tumors.

Rarely, detecting pheochromocytomas in normotensive patients with normal plasma and urinary catecholamines and metabolites requires determining plasma catecholamines during attacks occurring spontaneously or induced by **glucagon**. Normal urinary catecholamine and metabolite excretion and substances interfering with their quantitation are indicated in Table 2. Physical stress and that occurring with various diseases, hypotension, acidosis, and hypoglycemia can cause hypercatecholaminemia.

Localization of pheochromocytomas preoperatively is essential. **Imaging with CT** identifies 95% of pheochromocytomas. **Scintigraphy with** ^{131}I-MIBG identifies 85% of tumors and is highly specific and more reliable than CT if tumors are small and metastatic (uptake may occur in neuroblastomas, MTC, carcinoids, and small cell lung cancers; some drugs prevent ^{131}I-MIBG uptake). MRI is superior to CT in locating extraadrenal, recurrent, and metastatic pheochromocytomas; T_2-weighted images are usually characteristic of pheochromocytomas, although similar images may be seen in certain tumors, including neuroblastoma. **MRI is more sensitive than** ^{131}I-MIBG and is valuable in identifying intrapericardial pheochromocytomas; also, it involves no radiation and can be used during pregnancy. Central venous blood sampling for catecholamine assay may rarely help localize pheochromocytomas.

Diagnosis of pheochromocytoma is crucial, since 90% are successfully removed by surgery; if unrecognized, they are almost always fatal. Preoperative α and β blockade may be needed to control hypertension and arrhythmias, respectively. Because of the danger of causing hypertensive crises, β **blockers should never be given before inducing α blockade.** Morphine and phenothiazines are avoided, since they may precipitate hyper- or hypotension.

Surgical and anesthetic expertise are essential and a transperitoneal approach is mandatory for abdominal tumors, since they may be multiple and extraadrenal. Hypertension during operation is controlled with **nitroprusside** or **nitroglycerin;** arrhythmias are managed with β **blockers** and/or **lidocaine.** Operative mortality should be <3%. Chemotherapy and radiotherapy may be helpful in managing some malignant pheochromocytomas, whereas adrenergic blockers and metyrosine may successfully control manifestations of hypercatecholaminemia.

Neuroblastoma, the most common extracranial solid tumor of childhood (85% occurring before 6 years old), arises from immature, undifferentiated

Table 2.   Effects of Drugs and Interfering Substances on Excretion of Catecholamines and Their Metabolites[a]

	Upper limit of normal (adults) (mg/24 hr)	Effects	
		Increase apparent value	Decrease apparent value
Catecholamines		Catecholamines	Fenfluramine (large doses)
Epinephrine	0.02	Drugs containing catecholamines	α-Methyltyrosine
Norepinephrine	0.08	Isoproterenol	
Total	0.10	Levodopa	
Dopamine	0.40	Methyldopa	
		Labetalol[b]	
		Tetracyclines[b]	
		Erythromycin[b]	
		Chlorpromazine[b]	
		Other fluorescent substances (e.g., quinine, quinidine, bile in urine)[b]	
		Rapid withdrawal from clonidine	
		Ethanol	
Metanephrines		Catecholamines	Methylglucamine (in radiopaque agents)
Metanephrine	0.4	Drugs containing catecholamines	
Normetanephrine	0.9	Monoamine oxidase inhibitors	Fenfluramine (large doses)
Total	1.3	Benzodiazepines	α-Methyltyrosine
		Labetalol[b]	
		Rapid withdrawal from clonidine	
		Ethanol	
Vanilmandelic acid (VMA)	6.5	Catecholamines (minimal increase)	Clofibrate
		Drugs containing catecholamines (minimal increase)	Disulfiram
		Levodopa	Monoamine oxidase inhibitors
		Labetalol[b]	Fenfluramine (large doses)
		Nalidixic acid[b]	α-Methyltyrosine
		Rapid withdrawal from clonidine	
Homovanillic acid (HVA)	8.0	Catecholamines	α-Methyltyrosine
		Drugs containing dopamine	Monoamine oxidase inhibitors
		Levodopa	
		Methyldopa	

Note. Modified from Manger WM, Gifford RW Jr. Cardiovasc Med 1978;3:289–303. Reproduced with permission.

[a] As determined by most reliable assays.

[b] Probably spurious interference with fluorescence and high-pressure liquid chromatography assays.

neuroblasts of neural crest origin. They may vary in size from several centimeters to massive retroperitoneal tumors. In the United States, 1 per 7000 children develop neuroblastomas, with no sex predilection. Two-thirds of neuroblastomas occur in an adrenal gland (rarely bilaterally) but also wherever sympathetic nerves occur elsewhere in the abdomen, pelvis, chest, and neck. Clinical presentation may include anorexia, fever, weight loss, anemia, weakness, abdominal discomfort and a mass, bone pain, pallor, proptosis, periorbital ecchymoses, easy bruising, neurological manifestations (motor weakness, Horner's syndrome, myoclonus, ataxia), and metastatic subcutaneous nodules. Tumors may elaborate **dopa, dopamine,** and **norepinephrine** and cause hypertension. Rarely, they produce paroxysmal hypertension with tachycardia, palpitations, diaphoresis, pallor, flushing, irritability, polyuria, and polydipsia. Neuroblastoma may even occur in the **fetus** and cause manifestations of excess catecholamines in the mother.

Diagnostic evaluation should include CT or MRI of the abdomen, pelvis, and chest, a bone scan with ^{99m}Tc, and bone marrow aspiration or tumor biopsy. CT will detect almost 100% of abdominal neuroblastomas, whereas MRI may define extent of tumors and spinal canal involvement. Total body scan with ^{131}I-MIBG is especially valuable in detecting metastases. Increased urinary excretion of dopa, dopamine, norepinephrine, vanilmandelic acid (VMA), and homovanillic acid (HVA) usually occurs (VMA and HVA are elevated in >90%). Epinephrine excretion is almost invariably normal; therefore, increased excretion of epinephrine is valuable in differentiating neuroblastoma from pheochromocytoma. Several peptides have also been identified in neuroblastomas; **vasoactive intestinal peptide** (VIP) may cause **diarrhea.**

Neuroblastomas cured by **surgical removal** appear to have differentiated cells which lack multiple copies (**amplification**) of the N-myc proto-oncogene and which fail to grow *in vitro.* N-myc amplification, a diploid DNA pattern, chromosome 1_p deletion, and undifferentiated cells which proliferate in tissue culture portend a poor prognosis. Approach to treatment and prognosis also depend on tumor staging, defined by CT, bone scan, bone marrow aspiration, and tumor biopsies. About 60% of neuroblastomas are fatal, but they are **radiosensitive** and may respond to a variety of chemotherapeutic agents. **Marrow-ablative chemotherapy** or chemoradiotherapy may be effective, but recurrences are frequent. Survival rates are best when tumors are detected under 1 year of age and before metastatic disease. Screening for urinary dopamine, VMA, and HVA has been utilized for early detection of neuroblastomas. Rarely, antenatal ultrasound can detect neuroblastomas.

References

1. Manger WM, Gifford RW, Jr. Pheochromocytoma. New York: Springer-Verlag, 1977.
2. Manger WM, Gifford RW, Jr., Hoffman BB. Pheochromocytoma: a clinical and experimental overview. Curr Probl Cancer 1985;9:5–89.
3. Manger WM, Gifford RW, Jr. Pheochromocytoma: current diagnosis and management. Clev Clin J Med 1993.
4. Smith EI, Castleberry, RP. Neuroblastoma. Curr Probl Surg 1990;27:573–620.
5. Seeger MC, Reynolds CP. Neuroblastoma. Cancer medicine, Vol. 2, 3rd edition. Philadelphia/London: Lea and Febiger, 1993: 2172–84.

36

Chemodectoma and the Familial Paraganglioma Syndrome

James L. Netterville
Head and Neck Surgical Oncology
Department of Otolaryngology
Vanderbilt University
Nashville, Tennessee

Robert Sinard
University of Texas
Dallas, Texas

Introduction

The **carotid body** is one of the paraganglia located along the course of the vagus nerve in the head, neck and chest. It functions as a **chemoreceptor** to stimulate respiration. Located on the medial surface of the carotid bifurcation, it is about 2×5 mm in size. (Fig. 1) The carotid body is composed of clusters of epithelium-like cells in a richly vascular connective tissue stroma. Two cell types make up the cell nests. **Chief cells** (type I, epithelioid cells) are the larger polygonal cells. They have an epithelioid appearance and, ultrastructurally, contain neurosecretory granules. **Sustentacular cells** (type II cells, supporting cells) are smaller, irregularly shaped cells situated between the sinusoids and the type I cells. They are devoid of neurosecretory granules. These cell clusters are encased in a network of myelinated nerve fibers mixed with a rich vascular plexus.

Although there are no known tumors which arise from the carotid sinus, neoplastic growth of the carotid body can occur either as an isolated tumor or as part of the **familial paraganglioma syndrome.** Due to the chemoreceptor function of the carotid body these tumors were first called **chemodectomas** or **carotid body tumors (CBT)**, but **carotid body paraganglioma** is the most accurate histologic terminology for these lesions. Paragangliomas that develop from the paraganglia adjacent to the vagus nerve and the jugular bulb are usually described in the literature as **glomus vagale** and **glomus jugulare**, respectively.

Fewer than 1000 CBT cases had been reported prior to 1980, indicating the rarity of these tumors. About 5% of these patients presented with bilateral carotid body tumors. Multiple paragangliomas, including those arising from the carotid, jugular, vagal, and tympanic regions, are commonly seen in patients with familial paraganglioma syndrome. At Vanderbilt over the last 10 years, 34 patients presented with CBT. Of these, 19 were part of various kindreds with familial paraganglioma syndrome, and 17 presented with or subsequently developed other paragangliomas. Only 6 of the nonfamilial cases presented with other paragangliomas.

The inheritance pattern of familial occurrence appears to be **autosomal dominant** modified by **genomic imprinting.** In genomic imprinting the imprintable gene is transmitted in a Mendelian manner but the expression of the gene is determined by the sex of the transmitting parent. In the case of paragangliomas, the gene does not result in the development of tumors when maternally inherited. Thus male and female children of a male positive for the genetic

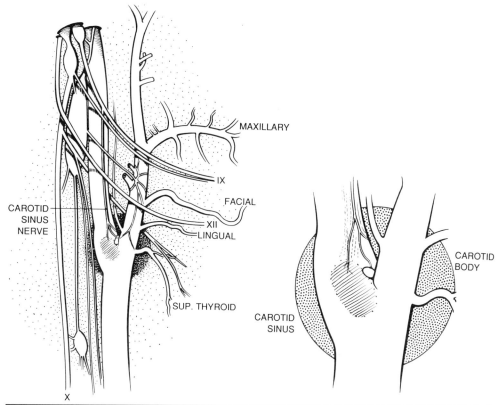

Figure 1.   The carotid body lies on the medial surface of the carotid bifurcation adjacent to the carotid sinus in the lateral wall of the carotid bifurcation. The afferent signals travel up the carotid sinus nerve (nerve of Hering) to join with the glossopharyngeal nerve.

defect have a 50% chance of manifesting paragangliomas. Children of a female positive for the abnormal trait will not develop paragangliomas, but may pass the abnormal gene on to their children. Thus, the abnormal gene can be passed silently down through several generations, making it difficult to determine accurately the incidence of familial inheritance of these tumors.

Symptoms of cervical paragangliomas include dysphagia, dysphonia, aspiration, tinnitus, hearing loss, pain, chronic cough, and shoulder weakness, all of which occur because of tumor encroachment on cranial nerves. However, most patients with an isolated CBT present with an asymptomatic mass either in the high cervical region or in the lateral pharyngeal wall. On physical exam, if the tumor is larger than 2 cm, a mass is palpable just inferior to the angle of the mandible. The mass has moderate side to side mobility with a limitation in up and down mobility due to its attachment to the carotid artery.

There are multiple imaging modalities used in the **diagnosis** of cervical paragangliomas. Initial evaluation with duplex doppler scanning is often recommended. The MRI is more helpful in differentiating the soft tissue interfaces of the tumors. It has the ability to identify CBT down to 8 mm in size. Thus for the evaluation of suspected CBT we initially evaluate the patient with MRI with and without contrast (Fig. 2). The CT scan is only performed if bony details are needed to evaluate skull base extension of the tumor.

Unlike pheochromocytomas, less than 5% of paragangliomas secrete **catecholamines.** Other paragangliomas such as jugular and vagal tumors have a higher rate of catecholamine secretion than CBT. In spite of this low rate of secretion, it is still prudent to evaluate each patient with a 24-hr urinalysis to determine if catecholamine excretion is elevated. If elevated levels of catecholamines are detected on the 24-hr screening, the tumor may be secreting these catecholamines, but such elevations may also occur as part of tumor-induced **baroreflex failure.**

Most carotid body tumors grow from 1–2 mm per year. Some tumors, however, appear to advance at an even slower rate with minimal change over a several year period. Rarely, paragangliomas progress at a much faster rate. Due to this slow rate of enlargement it is reasonable initially to observe some tumors to establish their rate of progression prior to deciding on a treatment course.

Surgical excision has been the mainstay of treatment for CBT. Surgical resection is indicated for unilateral isolated CBT. This decision becomes more

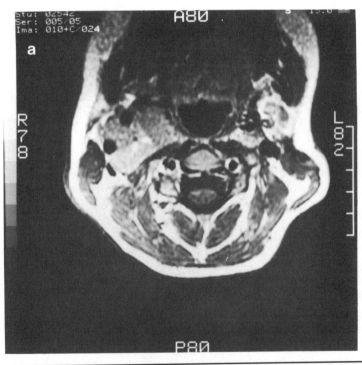

Figure 2.   Carotid body tumors have a very characteristic appearance on most imaging studies. (a). An axial MRI slice at the midcervical level demonstrates a 5-cm carotid body tumor splaying the right internal and external carotid arteries. On the contralateral side a 1.5-cm tumor is seen in the same location with minimal separation of the carotid bifurcation. (b). The classic splaying of the carotid bifurcation, and the hypervascular blush of a CBT is seen after injection of the common carotid artery during an arteriogram.

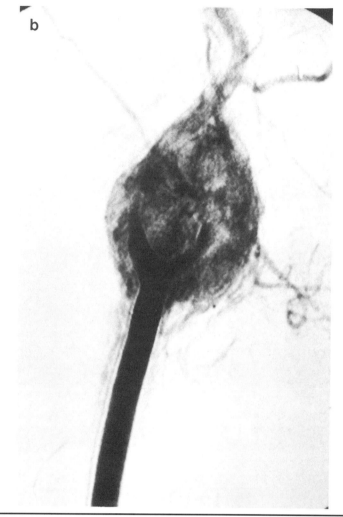

Figure 2. *(continued)*

complicated in patients with bilateral CBT or patients with multiple bilateral paragangliomas. Tumors less than 4.0 cm in size have minimal neural involvement and can usually be separated away from the carotid with minimal damage to the artery. The complication rate, which is very low for these smaller tumors, increases as the tumors enlarge over 5 cm.

Cranial nerve loss is the most common complication with surgical excision. In various series the rate of loss ranges from 10 to 50%. The most commonly injured nerve is the **superior laryngeal nerve** which provides sensory feedback from the superior half of the larynx and motor function to the cricothyroid muscle. Due to its location deep to the carotid bifurcation, it is usually enveloped within the vascular capsule on the medial surface of the tumor. Loss of the superior laryngeal nerve results in moderate **dysphagia** with mild aspiration due to loss of sensory function and a decrease in the vocal pitch range with the loss of motor function. Although the vocal pitch range rarely returns to normal, compensation for the dysphagia occurs within several weeks to months after injury. Infrequently the **vagus** and or the **hypoglossal** nerves must be resected with the tumor secondary to tumor involvement. More commonly these nerves are injured due to retraction as they are separated away from the tumor. The hemilaryngeal and hemiglossal paralysis which develops with retraction injury to these nerves causes voice weakness, dysarthria, and significant aspiration. Other nerves that are occasionally injured during surgical resection include the **glossopharyngeal, spinal accessory,** and the **sympathetic trunk.**

First bite syndrome can occur after resection of carotid body tumors. This is manifested by pain in the region of the parotid gland which occurs with the first few bites of each meal. This pain results from the loss of the postganglionic sympathetic innervation to the parotid gland. These postganlionic fibers lie within the periadventitial tissue of the external carotid artery. This loss results in a denervation supersensitivity of the sympathetic receptors on the myoepithelial muscle cells within the parotid. It is hypothesized that crossover stimulation occurs during parasympathetic stimulation of the gland resulting in spasm of the myoepithelial cells. The pain decreases over time, but most patients alter their diets to stay away from strong sialogogues.

Baroreceptor dysfunction is very mild and transient after unilateral CBT resection if there is normal innervation to the contralateral carotid sinus. With bilateral carotid body tumor resection most patients manifest baroreflex failure to some degree. With **baroreflex failure** the regulation of acute changes in blood pressure is impaired. This results in wide swings in systolic pressure to any stimulus which results in a release in catecholamines. An in-depth discussion of baroreflex failure is presented in the following chapter.

Radiation therapy has had a limited role in the treatment of CBT. Although the series are small, it appears that radiation therapy can control tumor growth in a significant percentage of patients treated. Averaging several series, 25% of the tumors completely regressed, 25% of the tumors underwent a partial regression, and the final 50% either stayed the same size with no further growth or continued to advance in size. Stereotatic radiation therapy holds promise as a very selective treatment of these tumors when the hardware is developed to deliver the irradiation to the mid to lower neck.

Observation is a reasonable form of treatment in selected individuals. Due to the slow growth rate, these tumors can be observed to establish their rate of progression prior to final treatment planning. A few patients have been observed in some series for over a decade with minimal or no progression in the size of their tumors. We routinely observe tumors in patients over 65 years of age, or individuals whose life expectancy is decreased due to some other disease process. During this period of observation the size of the tumor is monitored to be sure that rapid growth does not unexpectedly occur.

References

1. Hallett JW, Nora JD, Hollier LH, Cherry KJ, Pairolero PC, Trends in neurovascular complications of surgical management for carotid body and cervical paragangliomas: A fifty year experience with 153 tumors. J Vasc Surg, 1988;7:284–9.

2. Grufferman S, Gillman MW, *et al.* Familial carotid body tumors: case report and epidemiologic review. Cancer, 1980;46:2116–22.

3. Netterville JL, Reilly KM, Robertson D, Reiber ME, Armstrong WB, Childs P, Carotid body tumors: a review of 46 tumors in 30 patients. Laryngoscope 1995;105:115–26.

4. McCaffrey TV, Meyer FB, Michels VV, Piepgras DG, Marion MS, Familial paragangliomas of the head and neck. Arch Otolaryngol Head Neck Surg 1994;120:1211–16.

5. Valdagni R, Amichetti M. Radiation therapy of carotid body tumors. Am J Clin Oncol 1990;13,45–8.

37

Baroreflex Failure

Rose Marie Robertson
Division of Cardiology
Vanderbilt University
Nashville, Tennessee

Introduction

Efferent autonomic activity controlling blood pressure in man is determined at the level of medullary brainstem nuclei, which receive multiple inputs as diverse as visual and auditory stimuli routed from the cortex, and visceral stimuli from abdominal, retroperitoneal, thoracic, and neck structures. The input information is integrated in these brainstem nuclei, where it serves to determine the balance of efferent parasympathetic and sympathetic activity.

An essential portion of the input information comes from the **baroreflexes,** whose function is to maintain arterial pressure within a narrow range. This serves both to protect blood flow to critical organs, especially the brain, and to protect the vasculature from large, potentially deleterious fluctuations in pressure. Vascular baroreceptors are found in the **carotid sinus,** where they transduce changes in stretch of the arterial wall and transmit that information via the **glossopharyngeal nerve** to the nucleus tractus solitarii (NTS), the site of the first synapse of the baroreflex. They are also found in the **aortic arch** and great vessels of the thorax, sending similar information to the NTS via vagal fibers. There are in addition **low-pressure receptors** in vascular structures in the thorax that transmit information regarding central intravascular volume via the **vagus.**

The **baroreflex** as a system can potentially be damaged at any site, i.e., at the baroreceptor in the vasculature, in the course of the glossopharyngeal or vagal nerves, or at the nuclei in the brainstem. Failure of the baroreflex at any point produces a characteristic clinical syndrome of volatility of blood pressure and heart rate, which will be described below. However, the terminology describing autonomic syndromes has not always been sufficiently precise, and **baroreflex failure** has often been confused with efferent **autonomic failure.** Diminished efferent parasympathetic and/or sympathetic activity produces an entirely different syndrome of autonomic failure, which is described in the section on **pure autonomic failure,** in which orthostatic hypotension is a prominent feature.

Clinical Presentation

Descriptions of case studies in the previous literature and data from patients with baroreflex failure seen at the Vanderbilt University Autonomic Dysfunction Center (11 patients out of 500 referred with severe disorders of autonomic function) allow us to begin to define the presentation of this syndrome, a number of varying etiologies, and approaches to effective therapy.

Patients ultimately determined to have **baroreflex failure** are sent to tertiary care centers for a number of reasons, including, in the cases we have seen, evaluation for **essential hypertension, uncontrolled severe hypertension, pheochromocytoma,** or, less commonly, recognition that there had been **damage to the glossopharyngeal or vagal nerves.** "Labile hypertension" is a frequent descriptor.

Patients with baroreflex failure may present with **severe hypertension,** either **sustained** or **episodic.** Hypertensive crises are often seen, and pressures during these episodes may be extremely high, in the range of 170–280/110–135. Concomitant tachycardia often suggests the diagnosis of pheochromocytoma, and this is further supported by subjective sensations of warmth or **flushing, palpitations, headache,** and **diaphoresis.** This diagnosis is almost always given serious consideration at some point in the course of evaluation of these patients, but is excluded by computed tomography (CT) or MIBG scanning, by venous sampling for norepinephrine, or by arteriography. In addition, there is either **stability or improvement of hypertensive episodes over time** in baroreflex failure, and this is not the case in pheochromocytoma. An historical feature helping to differentiate these two syndromes is the presence of emotional lability or nervousness in the great majority of patients with baroreflex failure, especially prominent at the times of blood pressure elevations. The cause for this is not known.

The degree of **blood pressure lability** is shown in Fig. 1, which depicts the mean extremes of blood pressure during monitoring as inpatients during both the acute and chronic phases of this disorder. Note that the peak blood pressures seen in these patients are much greater than those seen in normal control subjects; in addition, the lowest blood pressures, which usually occur at night, are lower than those in the control group. **Excessively high heart rates** paralleled the elevated blood pressures. However, while many patients had minimal heart rates lower than normal, in two subjects the minimal heart rate exceeded 90 bpm. This may have been due to partial loss of parasympathetic influence on the heart from damage of the right vagus nerve.

As would be expected with a loss of the buffering capacity of the baroreflex, other inputs to the vasomotor centers have a more pronounced and sustained effect in these patients. Cortical influences that normally elevate blood pressure,

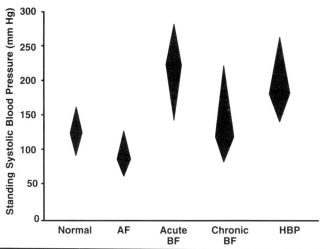

Figure 1. Representative standing systolic blood pressures recorded in inpatients and normal subjects. The widest point of each diamond depicts the most common standing systolic pressure seen in typical patients, while the height depicts the range of pressures seen throughout the day. Patients with autonomic failure (AF) have the lowest standing pressure. In the acute phase (Acute BF), e.g., as in the days to weeks immediately following acute bilateral damage to cranial nerves IX and X, extremely high pressures are seen, in some cases exceeding those seen even in severe hypertension (HBP). After several months (Chronic BF), the standing systolic pressure is usually near normal, but great variability is still seen.

such as **pain, emotion,** visual attention, or engaging in tasks such as mental arithmetic, may have a profound effect. For example, the response of systolic blood pressure to the **cold pressor test** (placing the patient's hand in a combination of ice and water for 1 min) in normal subjects is an increase of 24 ± 7 mm Hg; in patients with baroreflex failure, we have reported responses of 56 ± 14 mm Hg. While the increased blood pressure produced by this stimulus in normal subjects abates over a few minutes once the hand is rewarmed, in patients with baroreflex failure a significant increase may persist for more than 30 minutes (see Figure 2 below). The high blood pressures seen during the day, and, conversely, the low pressures seen at night, likely reflect the differences in arousal and cortical input in these two situations.

Etiologies for baroreflex failure have included **surgery** and **irradiation for cancer of the throat,** surgical section of the glossopharyngeal nerve for glossopharyngeal neuralgia in a patient who had previously sustained injury to the contralateral glossopharyngeal and vagus nerves, the **familial paraganglioma syndrome** (discussed elsewhere in this book), and cell loss bilaterally in the nuclei of the solitary tract (NTS, found at subsequent autopsy) in the setting of a degenerative neurologic disease of medullary and higher structures. In several patients, no etiology could be documented. In a number of the patients who had had radiation therapy, the hypertensive syndrome did not appear until several months to years later, obscuring the etiologic connection. Patients with tumor involvement who sustained damage to glossopharyngeal and vagal nerves with **resection** exhibited **especially severe and sustained hypertension,**

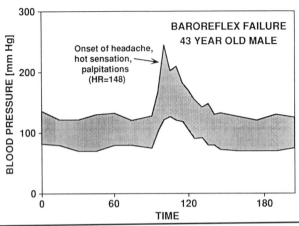

Figure 2.   Blood pressure monitoring over a 200-minute period in a 43-year-old man approximately two weeks following surgical removal of a second carotid body tumor, 5 years after removal of the initial (contralateral) carotid body tumor. While blood pressure was being monitored at normal baseline levels, a cold pressor test with immersion of the hand in ice water for 60 seconds was performed. The blood pressure immediately rose, and continued to rise for several minutes following discontinuation of the cold stimulus. The symptoms appeared during this time and resolved as blood pressure and heart rate returned to normal over the succeeding half hour.

particularly in the days to weeks following surgery. It appears that the most severe symptoms occur when the interruption of the baroreflex is sudden. In this circumstance, the hypertension may be so severe as to require continuous **nitroprusside** or **phentolamine** infusion for the first 24–72 hr. Apneic spells can be seen during the first 24 hr when carotid body input to the CNS is lost. Over time, the hypertension tends to become more episodic, although it may remain problematically high episodically for years. Orthostatic hypotension was not seen early unless the patients were volume depleted or were receiving phenoxybenzamine, but over a period of years, some patients who initially had only hypertension began to experience it.

The **diagnostic abnormality** in these patients is their ability to increase their heart rate with stress and decrease it with sedation or rest in the absence of a bradycardic response to pressor agents or a tachycardic response to vasodilators. Normal subjects will decrease the heart rate 7–21 bpm in response to a pressor dose of phenylephrine that raises the blood pressure by 20 mm Hg and will raise the heart rate 9–28 bpm in response to a dose of nitroprusside that lowers blood pressure by 20 mm Hg. In contrast, these patients did not alter their heart rate by more than 4 bpm with either maneuver. Patients with autonomic failure, of course, exhibit denervation hypersensitivity to these agents and show no overlap with patients who have baroreflex failure.

Biochemical assessment of patients with baroreflex failure demonstrates surges of sympathetic activity associated with hypertensive-tachycardic episodes, and plasma norepinephrine levels as high as 2660 pg/ml have been seen. Conversely, levels drawn during quiescent periods may be normal (111–360 pg/ml). **Clonidine** (0.1 mg po) has a dramatic depressor effect in these patients, generally twice the effect seen in normal subjects, although its effect is greatest when blood pressure is highest. It reliably reduces plasma norepinephrine levels to essentially normal levels. Clonidine is quite effective in decreasing the number and the severity of hypertensive crises, although tailoring of the dose to the individual patient is important, with doses from 0.3 to 2.4 mg/day required in our patients. It is more effective than **phenoxybenzamine,** which can reduce blood pressure, but does not limit the associated tachycardia or diminish the frequency of attacks. In follow-up, we are able to gradually reduce the clonidine dosage in many patients, and some have been able to be tapered off entirely. These patients still require modest doses of **diazepam** (5 mg po tid) to control blood pressure and still have episodic hypertension during times of stress.

References

1. Aksamit TR, Floras JS, Victor RG, Aylward PE. Paroxysmal hypertension due to sinoaortic baroreceptor denervation in humans. Hypertension 1987;9:309–14.
2. Robertson D, Goldberg MR, Hollister AS, Wade D, Robertson RM. Baroreceptor dysfunction in man. (Letter). Am J Med 1984;76:A49–58.
3. Robertson D, Hollister AS, Biaggioni I, Netterville JL, Mosqueda-Garcia R, Robertson RM. The diagnosis and treatment of baroreflex failure. N Engl J Med 1993;329:1449–55.
4. Kochar MS, Ebert TJ, Kotrly KJ. Primary dysfunction of the afferent limb of the arterial baroreflex system in a patient with severe supine hypertension and orthostatic hypotension. J Am Coll Cardiol 1984;4:802–5.
5. Kuchel O, Cusson JR, Larochelle P, Buu NT, Genest J. Posture- and emotion-induced severe hypertensive paroxysms with baroreceptor dysfunction. J Hypertens 1987;5:227–83.

38

Tetrahydrobiopterin Deficiency and Aromatic L-Amino Acid Decarboxylase Deficiency

Keith Hyland
Institute of Metabolic Disease
Baylor University Medical Center
and Department of Neurology
University of Texas Southwestern Medical Center
Dallas, Texas

Biochemistry

Tetrahydrobiopterin (BH_4) is the cofactor for **tyrosine hydroxylase** (TH) and **tryptophan hydroxylase** (TRYPH), the rate-limiting enzymes required for

the synthesis of the catecholamines (dopamine, norepinephrine, and epinephrine) and serotonin (5HT). BH_4 is formed from **guanosine triphosphate** (GTP)
in a multistep pathway and defects in its biosynthesis have been described at
the level of GTP cyclohydrolase and 6-pyruvoyltetrahydropterin synthetase
(6PTPS). In addition, **deficiency of dihydropteridine reductase** (DHPR) leads
to the inability to regenerate BH_4 following its oxidation in the hydroxylase
reactions (Fig. 1). The various defects of BH_4 metabolism that occur within
the CNS lead to a deficiency of serotonin and the catecholamines. There are,
however, peripheral forms of 6PTPS deficiency in which central neurotransmitter metabolism is normal. BH_4 is also the cofactor for phenylalanine hydroxylase (PH); hence, defects in BH4 metabolism lead to hyperphenylalaninemia.
Another enzyme, pterin-4a-carbinolamine dehydratase, is involved in the hydroxylation of phenylalanine; deficiency again leads to hyperphenylalaninemia
but effects on central 5HT and catecholamine metabolism are minimal, if
present at all.

   Dopa and **5-hydroxytryptophan** (5HTP), the products of the TH and
TRYPH reactions, are decarboxylated by vitamin B6 requiring **aromatic L-
amino acid decarboxylase** (AADC) to form the respective neurotransmitters
(Fig. 1). A defect in this enzyme also leads to deficiencies of both 5HT and
the catecholamines.

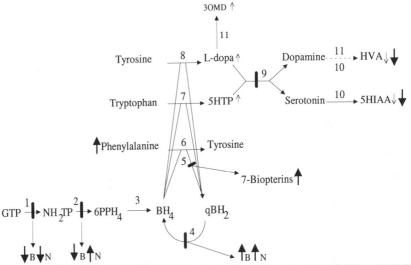

Figure 1.   Biosynthesis of serotonin and dopamine, showing sites of metabolic block and abnormal metabolite
profiles. GTP, guanosine triphosphate, NH_2TP, dihydroneopterin triphosphate, $6PPH_4$, 6-pyruvoyl-
tetrahydropterin; BH_4, tetrahydrobiopterin; qBH_2, quinonoid dihydrobiopterin; 5HTP, 5-hydroxy-
tryptophan; HVA, homovanillic acid; 5HIAA, 5-hydroxyindoleacetic acid; 3OMD, 3-O-methyl-
dopa; 1, GTP cyclohydrolase; 2, 6-pyruvoyltetrahydropterin synthetase; 3, sepiapterin reductase;
4, dihydropteridine reductase; 5, pterin-4a-carbinolamine dehydratase; 6, phenylalanine hydroxylase; 7, tryptophan hydroxylase; 8, tyrosine hydroxylase; 9, aromatic L-amino acid decarboxylase;
10, monoamine oxidase; 11, catechol-O-methyltransferase; B, biopterin; N, neopterin. ↑ and ↓
represent changes seen in aromatic L-amino acid decarboxylase deficiency. ⬆ and ⬇ represent
changes seen in the central forms of tetrahydrobiopterin deficiency. | shows the position of a
metabolic block.

Presentation and Neurological Symptoms

The neurological symptoms of **central BH₄ deficiency** and **AADC deficiency** are very similar and reflect the neurotransmitter deficiency. Patients present between 2 and 8 months of age with a fairly well characterized syndrome. Symptoms include hypersalivation, temperature instability, pinpoint pupils, ptosis of the eyelids, oculogyric crises, hypokinesis, distal chorea, truncal hypotonia, swallowing difficulties, drowsiness, and irritability. Some patients with DHPR deficiency develop **long tract signs** associated with multifocal perivascular calcification located mainly in the **basal ganglia** and to a lesser degree in areas of white and gray matter. These changes are thought to occur as a result of an **insidious folate deficiency** which has been postulated to arise as a result of inhibition of folate metabolism by the unusual forms of biopterin that accumulate in this disease. The neurological signs associated with peripheral forms of 6PTPS deficiency and pterin-4a-carbinolamine dehydratase deficiency are minimal and disappear following correction of the hyperphenylalaninemia. A peripheral form of 6PTPS deficiency progressing to give a central phenotype has been reported, thus all patients should be reevaluated in terms of their central neurotransmitter status at a later age.

Diagnosis of Tetrahydrobiopterin Deficiencies

Defective BH₄ metabolism should be considered in all cases of **hyperphenylalaninemia** and in any child who presents with the above neurological syndrome. Methods for diagnosis rely initially on the appearance of **characteristic HPLC profiles of neopterins and biopterins in urine**. The changes expected in each condition are shown in Fig. 1.

A **BH₄ loading test** can also distinguish between BH₄ defects and primary PH deficiency. Administering 2–20 mg/kg orally leads to a drop in plasma phenylalanine in deficiencies of GTP cyclohydrolase, pterin-4a-carbinolamine dehydratase, and 6PTPS; however, some cases of DHPR deficiency fail to respond.

Further tests are required in suspected cases of **6PTPS and DHPR deficiency**. The biopterin/neopterin profiles are similar in DHPR deficiency and PH deficiency. Therefore, it is necessary to measure DHPR activity in blood spots or erythrocytes. Pterin analysis also cannot distinguish between the peripheral and central forms of 6PTPS deficiency; here it is necessary to measure CSF levels of 5-hydroxyindole acetic acid (5HIAA) and homovanillic acid (HVA), the major catabolites of serotonin and dopamine. These are normal in the peripheral condition but reduced in the central forms of the disease.

Diagnosis of Aromatic L-Amino Acid Decarboxylase Deficiency

AADC deficiency does not lead to abnormal profiles using traditional screening methods (blood spot screening, organic acid or amino acid analyses, etc.). Recognition requires the clinician to consider an abnormality in biogenic amine metabolism in a child with clinical signs similar to those described above. The pattern of biogenic amine metabolites is very characteristic. There is **marked** elevation of L-dopa, 5HTP, and 3-O-methyldopa in CSF, plasma, and urine. HVA and 5HIAA concentrations are greatly reduced in CSF, as are the levels of 5HT, catecholamines, and their catabolites in blood and urine. Positive diagnosis is accomplished by analysis of AADC activity in plasma.

Treatment of BH$_4$ Deficiencies

Hyperphenylalaninemia may be corrected using a low-phenylalanine diet, or in deficiencies of GTP cyclohydrolase, 6PTPS, and pterin 4a-carbinolamine, by administration of oral BH$_4$ (0.5–40 mg/day). BH$_4$ is usually ineffective in DHPR deficiency. Central neurotransmitter deficiency is corrected by oral administration of the precursors L-dopa (2–20 mg/kg/day) and 5HTP (0.8–12 mg/kg/day), in conjunction with carbidopa (0.3–4.0 mg/kg/day). Initial doses should be low with clinical monitoring of therapeutic effect. Adverse symptoms due to overtreatment are sometimes similar to the disease symptoms; therefore, monitoring by measuring CSF levels of HVA and 5HIAA is crucial. Folinic acid (3 mg/day) should be administered in DHPR deficiency with CSF 5-methyltetrahydrofolate levels measured at the same time as the neurotransmitter metabolites to ensure the adequacy of the dose.

Treatment of AADC Deficiency

Treatment in the index cases of the disease consisted of the dopamine agonist bromocriptine (2.5 mg bid), tranylcypromine (nonselective monoamine oxidase inhibitor, 4 mg bid), and pyridoxine (100 mg bid) in combination. Therapy led to a marked clinical and biochemical improvement. As AADC is a B6 requiring enzyme, high dose pyridoxine monotherapy should be tried in all future cases.

References

1. Dhondt JL. In: Milupa, ed. Register of tetrahydrobiopterin deficiencies. Les Mercurials, Bagnolet, 1991.
2. Hyland K, Surtees RAH, Rodeck C, Clayton PT. Aromatic L-amino acid decarboxylase deficiency: clinical features, diagnosis and treatment of a new inborn error of neurotransmitter amine synthesis. Neurology 1992;42:1980–88.
3. Hyland K. Abnormalities of biogenic amine metabolism. J Inherit Metab Dis 1993;16:676–90.
4. Smith I, Hyland K, Kendall B, Leeming R. Clinical role of pteridine therapy in tetrahydrobiopterin deficiency. J Inherit Metab Dis 1985;8(Suppl. 1):39–45.
5. Hyland K, Howells DW. Analysis and clinical significance of pterins. J Chromatogr 1988;429:95–121.

39 Dopamine-β-Hydroxylase Deficiency

Anton H. van den Meiracker
*Department of Internal
Medicine I
University Hospital Dijkzigt
Rotterdam, The Netherlands*

Frans Boomsma
*Department of Internal
Medicine I
University Hospital Dijkzigt
Rotterdam, The Netherlands*

Arie J. Man in't Veld
*Department of Internal
Medicine I
University Hospital Dijkzigt
Rotterdam, The Netherlands*

Introduction

The syndrome of **dopamine β-hydroxylase (DβH) deficiency** is characterized by sympathetic noradrenergic denervation and adrenomedullary failure, but **intact vagal and sympathetic cholinergic function.** It is a rare, congenital, nonhereditary form of severe orthostatic hypotension, caused by complete absence of DβH, the enzyme involved in the conversion of dopamine to norepinephrine. The genetic defect in DβH deficiency has yet to be clarified.

After the description of the first two patients with DβH deficiency in 1986 and 1987 by Robertson *et al.* and Man in't Veld *et al.,* four cases, of which two are siblings, have been reported. This chapter is based on the reports of these six patients.

Clinical Presentation

Despite congenital sympathetic noradrenergic failure, presence of **orthostatic hypotension,** curiously enough, has not been documented before the age of 20 years in any of the reported patients with DβH deficiency. During childhood **impaired exercise tolerance, fatigue,** and episodes of **fainting** and **syncope,** usually worsening after exercise, are frequently present. Two of six patients have been treated with antiepileptic medications during childhood, although their EEGs showed no evidence of epileptiform activity. One of the reported patients with DβH deficiency was repeatedly admitted to the hospital in her first year of life, because of vomiting, dehydration, hypotension, hypothermia, and profound hypoglycemia, whereas one of the other patients did not open his eyes until 2 weeks of age. Gestation and delivery were uneventful in all patients.

Symptoms due to orthostatic hypotension become worse in late adolescence and early adulthood. As is typical of autonomic failure, symptoms are more severe in the morning hours, during hot weather, and after alcohol, but, interestingly, not after food ingestion. Physical and mental development and sexual maturation are normal in DβH deficiency. Sexual function is normal in female patients. In male patients **ejaculation is retrograde or unachievable.**

Physical examination in DβH deficiency reveals a low normal supine blood pressure and a low supine heart rate due to unopposed cardiac vagal innervation. In the upright position, systolic blood pressure always falls below 80 mm Hg, but, contrary to most other types of autonomic failure, the **compensatory rise in heart rate** is completely preserved. Pupils may be somewhat small, but respond to light and accommodation. **Sweating is normal.** Of the six patients with DβH deficiency reported, **blepharoptosis** is present in four, **hyperextensible/hyperflexible joints** and **sluggish deep tendon reflexes** in three, and **mild weakness of facial muscles** and **hypotonic skeletal musculature** in two patients.

Diagnosis

A 5- to 10-fold **elevated plasma dopamine** concentration (i.e., values as high as plasma norepinephrine concentration in normal subjects) together with **undetectable** concentrations of plasms **norepinephrine and epinephrine** is pathognomonic for DβH deficiency. As a reflection of these findings in plasma, urinary norepinephrine, and epinephrine and their metabolites are low or absent, whereas dopamine and its degradation products homovanillic acid and 3-methoxytyramine are increased. In cerebrospinal fluid (CSF) norepinephrine and epinephrine are also undetectable and dopamine is markedly increased. Although DβH, measured either as enzymatic activity or immunologically, is absent, its measurement is not suitable as a key diagnostic criterion in DβH deficiency, because extremely low DβH values, genetically determined, are present in 3–4% of the population.

The markedly elevated plasma dopamine concentration in DβH deficiency is explained by **induction of tyrosine hydroxylase** (see Fig. 1), the first and rate-limiting enzyme in the formation of norepinephrine. Most likely, loss of the inhibitory feedback of norepinephrine in sympathetic nerves accounts for this induction and explains why the concentration of L-dopa, the precursor of dopamine, is elevated as well.

Interestingly, the elevated plasma dopamine concentration of DβH deficiency responds to various physiological and pharmacological stimuli as does norepinephrine in normal subjects. Thus, in response to **upright posture** a two- to three-fold increase in dopamine occurs. Likewise, in response to **insulin-**

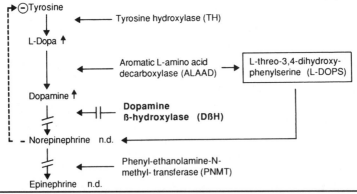

Figure 1.   Biochemical consequences of DβH deficiency and conversion of L-DOPS to norepinephrine. Due to deficiency of DβH, norepinephrine and epinephrine are not formed. Loss of negative feedback of norepinephrine leads to induction of tyrosine hydroxylase, so that L-dopa and dopamine are elevated. L-DOPS is converted to norepinephrine by ALAAD, thereby bypassing DβH. nd, Not detected; ↑, elevated.

induced hypoglycemia, infusion of **tyramine,** which liberates neurotransmitters from sympathetic nerve terminals, and ganglionic stimulation with **edrophonium,** plasma dopamine increases several times, whereas plasma norepinephrine and epinephrine remain undetectable. Conversely, a decrease in dopamine occurs in response to **clonidine,** a centrally acting sympatholytic agent. Microneurography preformed in one patient with DβH deficiency has shown the **existence of muscle sympathetic nerve activity,** modulated in a normal way by physiological and pharmacological interventions. All these observations imply that in DβH deficiency sympathetic nerves and reflex arcs are intact, but that in sympathetic nerves dopamine instead of norepinephrine is stored and released.

Analogous to other forms of autonomic failure, there is increased sensitivity to the hemodynamic effects of α- and β-adrenoceptor agonists in DβH deficiency, but because of complete (nor)adrenergic failure **denervation supersensitivity** is more extreme. Conversely, because of absent noradrenergic and adrenomedullary function, heart rate does not fall in response to β blockers and blood pressure does not fall in response to α blockers. As expected, heart rate rises normally in response to atropine, since parasympathetic innervation is intact.

Differential Diagnosis

On clinical grounds (**congenital orthostatic hypotension, intact cholinergic innervation**) and biochemical grounds (**markedly increased plasma dopamine and undetectable plasma norepinephrine and epinephrine levels**) DβH deficiency is easily differentiated from other types of autonomic insufficiency. **Familial dysautonomia** (Riley–Day syndrome) is another form of congenital orthostatic hypotension. In this autosomal recessive syndrome, however, there is **combined sympathetic–parasympathetic insufficiency** as well as other neurological abnormalities.

Therapy

The treatment of choice in DβH deficiency is DL, or L-**threo-3,4-dihydroxyphenylserine** (DOPS). L-threo-DOPS, an unnatural amino acid devoid of direct pressor activity, is in one step **converted into norepinephrine** by aromatic L-amino acid decarboxylase (AAAD), thereby bypassing DβH. AAAD is present in most tissues as well as in sympathetic nerves. Administration of **DOPS** in a dose of 250 to 500 mg, twice daily, produces a moderate rise in blood pressure and a **sustained dramatic relief of orthostatic symptoms,** although postural hypotension is not completely cured. Plasma norepinephrine becomes detectable and plasma dopamine moderately decreases during administration of DOPS. In response to standing and tyramine infusion plasma norepinephrine concentration increases further, indicating storage of norepinephrine in sympathetic nerves. Since in response to tyramine and standing **a rise in the plasma level of DOPS occurs as well,** it may be that *de novo* formation of norepinephrine from DOPS takes place in the sympathetic nerves. Alternatively norepinephrine may be formed extraneuronally and taken up by the sympathetic nerves.

Although norepinephrine becomes detectable, plasma epinephrine remains undetectable after DOPS, which raises the possibility of an associated deficiency of the enzyme phenylethanolamine N-methyl transferase (PNMT) in the adrenal medulla if DOPS is taken up there.

In conclusion, DβH deficiency is one of the more recently recognized causes of autonomic failure. With the more widespread availability of the simultaneous measurement of the concentrations of norepinephrine, epinephrine, and dopamine in plasma, it is to be expected that more cases will be detected in the future. Diagnosing DβH deficiency and differentiating it from other causes of autonomic failure is important, since with DOPS treatment almost complete relief of orthostatic symptoms is easily achievable.

References

1. Robertson D, Goldberg MR, Ornot J, Hollister AS, Wiley R, Thompson JG, Robertson RM. Isolated failure of autonomic noradrenergic neurotransmission. N Eng J Med 1986;314:1494–7.
2. Man in't Veld AJ, Boomsma F, Moleman P, Schalekamp MADH. Congenital dopamine-beta-hydroxylase deficiency. Lancet 1987; i:183–8.
3. Mathias CJ, Bannister RB, Cortelli P, Heslop K, Polack JM, Raimbach S, Springall R, Watson L. Clinical, autonomic and therapeutic observations in two siblings with postural hypotension and sympathetic failure due to the inability to synthesize noradrenaline form dopamine because of a deficiency of dopamine beta hydroxylase. Q J Med 1990;278:617–33.
4. Biaggioni I, Goldstein DS, Adkinson T, Robertson D. Dopamine β-hydroxylase deficiency in humans. Neurology 1990;40:370–3.
5. Robertson D, Haile V, Perry SE, Robertson RM, Phillips JA III, Biaggioni I. Dopamine β-hydroxylase deficiency. Hypertension 1991;18:1–8.

40

Menkes Disease

Robert Hoeldtke
Department of Medicine
Division of Endocrinology
West Virginia University Medical School
Morgantown, West Virginia

Menkes disease (trichopoliodystrophy, kinky hair disease) is a hereditary sex-linked degenerative disease of gray matter associated with widespread abnormalities in the central nervous system that typically become manifest during the first year of life and leads to death during early childhood. Danks noted a similarity between the peculiar "kinky" hair of affected patients and the wool of sheep grazing in copper deficient soil in Australia and suggested a deficiency in this cation played a role in the pathogenesis of the disease.

Biochemical Features and Pathology

A generalized abnormality in copper transport is the hallmark of Menkes disease. A basic **defect in copper efflux from cells** causes it to be trapped in the gut and connective tissue and unavailable for distribution elsewhere. The genetic defect has been localized to the long arm of the X chromosome (the Xq 13.3 region) **where a copper transporting ATPase is coded.** The resulting defect in intestinal copper absorption makes copper relatively unavailable for the synthesis of most copper-containing proteins including **ceruloplasmin, superoxide dismutase, cytochrome oxidase, lysyl oxidase, ascorbic acid oxidase,** and **dopamine β-hydroxylase. Norepinephrine production is decreased by about 50%** in affected patients and deficits in plasma norepinephrine as well as cerebrospinal fluid 3-methoxy-4-hydroxy-phenylglycol (the major metabolite of brain norepinephrine) have been documented.

Dysfunction of lysyl oxidase results in failure in **elastin** and **collagen cross-linking.** This is believed to be responsible for enhanced tortuosity of the vasculature and splitting of the intimal lining. The physiological significance of the reduced activity of cytochrome oxidase is poorly understood but may be linked to mitochondrial swelling and the presence of intramitochondrial electron dense bodies. A wide variety of vascular and neuronal changes in the brain have been described; their relationship, if any, to copper metabolism is poorly understood. Neuronal loss and degeneration is evident in the gray matter and cerebellum, where Purkinje cell loss is the predominant feature. Axonal degeneration is seen in the white matter, frequently associated with **cerebral atrophy** and **encephalomalacia.** Nearly all patients develop **subdural hematomas.**

Clinical Features

Inadequate feeding and impaired growth are frequently recognized during the neonatal period. **Mental retardation, seizures,** and **hypotonia** then dominate the clinical course. The most distinctive feature, **colorless friable scalp hair,** is the clue to the diagnosis. Microscopic examination of the hair reveals twisting and characteristic fractures of the hair shaft. Little is known about autonomic function, although it is recognized that patients are susceptible to hypothermia perhaps as a consequence of decreased norepinephrine biosynthesis.

Urological abnormalities, including **hydronephrosis** and **bladder diverticula,** are common and a variety of abnormalities of long bones, such as metaphyseal spurring, have been described. Although a few patients with mild disease have been described, more commonly a progressive downhill course ensues and patients rarely survive beyond 10 years of age.

Diagnosis and Treatment

The diagnosis is confirmed by **measuring copper and ceruloplasmin serially** during the first year of life. Typically these parameters fail to rise into the normal range for adults after 1 month of age. The diagnosis can be confirmed by documenting enhanced accumulation of radioactive copper into cultured fibroblasts. Intrauterine diagnosis can be made if the copper content of fibroblasts or chorionic villi is excessive.

Parenteral copper therapy (cupric acetate 550–850 μg/kg/day) should begin as soon as possible after the diagnosis is established. After serum copper and ceruloplasmin have normalized, lower doses of cupric acetate (200 μg/kg) once or twice weekly or oral copper (8–10 mg elemental copper administered as cupric trisodium nitrilotriacetate) should be given to maintain serum copper within the normal range. Although there is no evidence that copper therapy alters the natural history of the neurological dysfunction, or prolongs survival, it appears to help control seizures and pain in some patients. Copper therapy should be continued until the cerebral dysfunction is clearly irreversible.

References

1. Danks DM. Disorders of copper transport. In: The metabolic basis of inherited disease (Scriver CR, Beaudet AL, Sly WS, Valle D. eds). 6th ed., McGraw–Hill, New York: 1989: 1251–68.
2. Menkes JH. Metabolic diseases of the nervous system. In: Menkes JH, ed. Textbook of Child Neurology 4th ed. Philadelphia: Lea and Febiger, 1990: 121–2.
3. Vulpe C, Levinson B, Whitney S, Packman S, Gitschier J. Isolation of a candidate gene for Menkes disease and evidence that it encodes a copper transporting ATPase. Nature Genet 1993;3:7–9.
4. Hoeldtke RD, Cavanaugh ST, Hughes JD, Mattis-Graves K, Hobnell E, Grover WD, Catecholamine metabolism in kinky hair disease. Ped Neurol 1988;4:23–26.

41

Monoamine Oxidase Deficiency States

Xandra Breakefield
Massachusetts General Hospital
Charlestown, Massachusetts

The genes for monoamine oxidase A (MAOA) and monoamine oxidase B (MAOB) are located next to each other on human **chromosome Xp11.** This X chromosomal location means that **essentially only males are affected with MAO deficiency syndromes.** The first MAO-deficient individuals described had a contiguous gene syndrome caused by chromosomal deletions including both MAO genes and the adjacent gene for **Norrie disease** (NDP). The NDP gene is responsible for an X-linked **congenital blindness,** sometimes accompanied by mild mental retardation and progressive hearing loss. The rare, atypical Norrie patients with chromosomal deletions have **severe mental retardation, seizures, hypotonic crises,** and **poor growth.** These individuals, with no MAO activity, can live into their twenties, but are noncommunicative and have **hypertensive crises** in response to **dietary amine** intake.

Their levels of amines and their metabolites in urine, CSF, and plasma are markedly abnormal, including very low levels of **methoxyhydroxyphenol glycol** (MHPG), the deaminated norepinephrine metabolite, elevated levels of **nor-metanephrine,** and very high levels of **phenylethylamine** and other trace amines. In a few individuals chromosomal deletions remove the NDP and MAOB genes, sparing the MAOA gene. These individuals show a phenotype typical of NDP deficiency alone, indicating that **loss of MAOB,** with MAOA intact, is **not associated with any obvious symptoms.**

Levels of MAOA and MAOB activity **vary 50- to 100-fold in control humans** as assessed in cultured skin fibroblasts and platelets, respectively [for review see (4)]. These wide variations have not been associated with any marked differences in physiology, although they have been suggested to have a contributory role in some neurologic and psychiatric conditions. In 1993 a group led by Dr. Han Brunner carried out linkage analysis in one family which placed a gene responsible for an X-linked recessive condition of **borderline mental retardation and abnormal behavior** to the same chromosomal region as the MAO genes. Affected males were found to have **complete loss of MAOA activity,** with no decrease in MAOB activity, resulting from a single base pair substitution in the MAOA gene which changes a glutamine codon to a stop codon. Abnormal behavior, as described by family members included **aggressive acts under stress,** suggesting a possible decrease in impulse control. Affected males have **a shortened lifespan attributed to cardiovascular failure,** which may reflect sensitivity to dietary amines. These individuals also manifest abnormally low levels of MHPG and elevated levels of normetanephrine in body fluids. Carrier females in this syndrome appear normal. This condition of MAOA deficiency is likely to be rare, and further work is needed to characterize the associated traits. No individuals with singular MAOB deficiency have yet been described, but this would be predicted to have a mild phenotype.

References

1. Berger W, van de Pol D, Warburg M, Gal A, Bleeker-Wagemakers L, de Silva H, Meindl A, Meitinger T, Cremers F, Ropers H. Mutations in the candidate gene for Norrie disease. Human Mol Genet 1994;7:461–5.

2. Brunner HG, Nelen M, Breakefield XO, Ropers HH, van Oost BA. Abnormal behavior associated with a point mutation in the structural gene for monoamine oxidase A. Science 1993;262:578–80.

3. Brunner HG, Nelen MR, van Zandvoort NGGM, Abeling AH, van Gennip AH, Wolters EC, Kulper MA, Ropers HH, and van Oost BA. X-linked borderline mental retardation with prominent behavioral disturbance: phenotype, genetic localization, and evidence for disturbed monoamine metabolism. Am J Hum Gene 1993;52:1032–9.

4. Hsu Y-PP, Powell JF, Sims KB, Breakefield XO. Molecular genetics of the monoamine oxidases. J Neurochem 1989;53:12–8.

5. Murphy DL, Sims KB, Karoum F, de la Chapelle A, Norio R, Sankila EM, Breakefield XO. Marked amine and amine metabolite changes in Norrie disease patients with an X chromosomal deletion affecting monoamine oxidase. J Neurochem 1990;54:242–7.
6. Sims KB, de la Chapelle A, Norio R, Sankila EM, Hsu Y-PP, Rinehart WB, Corey TJ, Ozelius L, Powell JF, Bruns G, Gusella JF, Murphy DL, Breakefield XO. Monoamine oxidase deficiency in males with and X chromosome deletion. Neuron 1989;2: 1069–76.
7. Warburg M. Retinal malformations. Trans Ophthalmol Soc UK 1979;99:272–83.

42 *Disorders of Dopamine Metabolism*

Otto Kuchel
Clinical Research Institute of Montreal
Montreal, Quebec, Canada

Besides the main mode of catecholamine clearance from extracellular fluid by neuronal uptake, deamination by monoamine oxidase, and methylation by catechol-O-methyltransferase, **sulfoconjugation** represents **the only degradative pathway which is bidirectional** (Fig. 1). Catecholamines are mainly sulfoconjugated in man by **phenolsulfotransferase** (PST). Sulfation is particularly important in **dopamine inactivation** with a ratio of approximately 50 : 1 of sulfated to free dopamine in plasma and of approximately 1 : 1 in urine. Epinephrine and norepinephrine are sulfated less extensively with a 3 : 1 ratio of sulfated to free catecholamines in plasma and approximately equal amounts of sulfated and free compounds in urine. The **desulfation** of catecholamine sulfates, which are mostly biologically inactive, to active forms of free catecholamines is **catalyzed by arylsulfatase A.** The highest sulfatase concentration is in the **kidney**, and, in descending order, in the liver, intestine, and heart.

PST, **sulfatases,** and the **dopamine reuptake transporter** (DAT) have been identified by molecular biology techniques (Table 1). They mediate genetic influences, modulating not only sulfoconjugation of catecholamines but also regeneration of biologically active catecholamines from a reserve form of catecholamine conjugates. Such an additional source of free catecholamines is suggested by the reciprocity of changes of free and sulfated plasma catecholamines during their physiologic variation under stress, physical exercise, and nycthemeral cycles. Physiological stimulation may thus activate a reverse process in which conjugated catecholamines may become a source of free catecholamines additive to their neuronal or autocrine–paracrine release. **Glucocorticoids** have been experimentally demonstrated to stimulate arylsulfatases; since plasma cortisol during the above-mentioned physiological changes moves in the same direction as free catecholamines, but opposite to catecholamine sulfates,

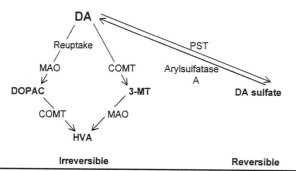

Figure 1. Schematic outline of dopamine (DA) metabolism via monoamine oxidase (MAO), catechol-O-methyltransferase (COMT), phenolsulfotransferase (PST), dopacetic acid (DOPAC), 3-methoxytyramine (3-MT), and homovanillic acid (HVA). Note the difference between irreversible (left) and reversible (right) pathways.

glucocorticoids may initiate the recovery of catecholamines from this reserve source under stress.

Genetically determined clinical **PST deficiency syndromes** are probably related to platelet PST distribution in normal populations suggestive of two alleles coding for low or high PST in homozygotes. This genetic polymorphism probably explains the considerable individual variability in sulfoconjugation of phenolic substances. In randomly selected healthy subjects receiving a borderline hypertensive infusion of dopamine, the catecholamine conjugated to the highest degree, reproducible patterns of **slow and fast conjugators** could be identified. **Slow conjugators showed a moderate increase of plasma norepineph-**

Table 1.

Enzyme	Identification of gene	Chromosome mapping	Clinical deficiency syndromes
Two phenolsulfotransferase (PST) isoenzymes (PST-P or TS, PST-M or TL)	cDNA codes for 291 AA	Chromosome 16p-11.2 (PST-TL)	Genetic polymorphism affecting sulfoconjugation of phenolic substances; slow conjugators; tyramine-sensitive migraine; pseudoheochromocytoma with low conjugated catecholamines
Family of sulfates	cDNA codes for 425 AA (arylsulfatase B)	Chromosome 22 Arylsulfatase A Chromosome 5 Arylsulfatase B	Subgroups of hypertension with increased DA sulfate and its decreased renal clearance? Chronic renal failure?
Dopamine transporter (DAT)	cDNA encoding human DAT cloned (620 AA)	Chromosome 5 p15-3	Limited role in the peripheral DA system; hyperdopaminergic states with partial dopamine reuptake defects?

rine and blood pressure while fast conjugators did not. This suggests that high conjugation drains dopamine away from alternative pathways, i.e., neuronal reuptake and conversion to norepinephrine. The action of some highly conjugated drugs (such as **minoxidil**) may also depend on sulfoconjugation velocity. Low conjugation of **tyramine,** a substance releasing catecholamines, has also been suggested to operate in patients with **tyramine-sensitive migraine.** Patients with severe therapy-resistant depressive illness also show a decreased ability to conjugate an oral tyramine load. **Sudden death** in asthmatic patients using **isoproterenol,** another phenolic substance, or its derivatives as bronchodilators, may be precipitated by an inborn conjugation defect resulting in undue drug toxicity. **Hyperadrenergic hypertensive patients,** occasionally found in families with **increased free catecholamines,** present a decrease in conjugated catecholamines. This again suggests a possible genetic defect in the conjugation component of the catecholamine metabolic pathway contributing to an overflow of free catecholamines.

Arylsulfatase A deficiency has to be viewed as a defect of a member of the sulfatase family responsible for the degradation of sulfated macromolecules in lysosomes. There are regions of homology between all cloned sulfatases. **Metachromatic leukodystrophy, mucopolysacharidosis, X-linked ichtyosis,** and **Hunter's syndrome** are clearly defined genetic defects of sulfatases. Arylsulfatase A deficiency, however, is based only on circumstantial evidence. The considerable increase of total (free + sulfates) circulating catecholamines in hypertension due essentially to elevated dopamine sulfate, associated with augmented levels of another sulfate (dehydroepiandrosterone), remains unexplained by platelet PST activity. Since arylsulfatase A and steroid sulfatase have the same 22-chromosome locus, in addition to considerable homology, the possibility of a partial defect within the sulfatase family may have to be considered. With catecholamines being trapped in tubules as sulfates, the mainly renally located arylsulfatase A may be responsible, if deficient, for **decreased renal clearance of dopamine sulfates in patients with essential hypertension.** Decreased clearance of catecholamine sulfates is further accentuated in patients with chronic renal failure. Thus, an additional acquired sulfatase deficiency (inhibition by uremic toxins?) may come into play in renal failure with increased plasma catecholamine sulfates partially remediable by hemodialysis.

Hyperdopaminergic states are rarely recognized because routine catecholamine determinations are usually limited to norepinephrine and epinephrine. Increased circulating and excreted free dopamine can be found in the rare genetic **dopamine β-hydroxylation deficiency** syndrome or **dopamine-secreting pheochromocytoma.** A hyperdopaminergic state based on increased urinary dopamine excretion was reported in a patient receiving chronic corticosteroid therapy. This increase was due to heightened renal dopamine synthesis since its blockade by carbidopa markedly reduced urinary dopamine output and sodium excretion. Since one of the sources of urinary free dopamine is dopamine sulfate, and corticosteroids are known to stimulate sulfatase, the possibility of steroid-induced dopamine sulfate deconjugation leading to free hyperdopaminuria has to be considered. Alternatively, it may represent a compensatory natriuretic adjustment to the sodium retention by steroids rather than primary hyperdopaminuria.

Recognition of hyperdopaminergic states can be improved by measurements of **free and sulfated dopamine** in plasma and urine. Dopamine has the highest affinity to the sulfoconjugating enzyme PST. Consequently, dopamine circulates to the highest degree (97–99%) in the form of dopamine sulfate which has a **half-life at least 60 times longer than that of free dopamine** (2–3 min). Therefore, **dopamine sulfate** in plasma is a better marker of free dopamine release than free dopamine. A hyperdopaminergic state unrecognizable by free dopamine was demonstrated by a **posture-induced excessive rise of total plasma dopamine** (almost exclusively dopamine sulfate) in patients with orthostatic hypotension. Another hyperdopaminergic state was characterized by plasma dopamine sulfate surges during hypertensive periods in patients with a **pseudo-pheochromocytoma** paradigm similar to that described by Page (Fig. 2). These patients had hypertensive episodes distinct from pheochromocytoma by the presence of **flushing, nausea, epigastric discomfort**, and **polyuria**, all extremely rare in pheochromocytoma. Comparison between baseline and crisis plasma concentrations showed that free dopamine levels overlapped considerably and were approximately twice as high while there were no differences in plasma NE and E. However, measurements of dopamine sulfate revealed an approximately 15-fold increase from baseline to values, even if widely dispersed, during hypertensive episodes. Increases of NE and E sulfates were minimal, suggesting that the moderate elevations of free NE and E were reflected by the longer half-life of NE and E sulfates. Similar changes were found in urine collected after the hypertensive episodes. Since dopamine sulfate appears to be a marker of the release of free dopamine which is rapidly sulfoconjugated, this indicates

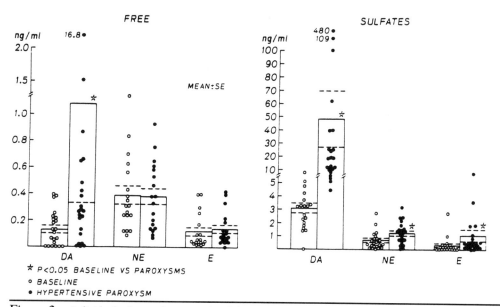

Figure 2. Individual values and means ± SE of plasma-free and sulfoconjugated dopamine (DA), norepinephrine (NE), and epinephrine (E) at baseline (open circles) and following hypertensive paroxysms (closed circles). *$P < 0.05$, baseline vs following paroxysms. Reprinted with permission from Arch Int Med 1986;146:1315–1320 © 1986 American Medical Association.

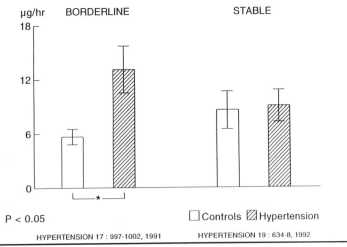

Figure 3. Urinary 3-methoxytyramine excretion in borderline and stable essential hypertensive patients compared to age-matched control subjects.

that these episodes are associated with dopamine release exceeding that of NE and E. Symptoms of flushing, epigastric discomfort, nausea, and polyuria after attacks are typical of the cutaneous, brain, and renal actions of dopamine and can be reproduced by an infusion of exogenous dopamine.

The causes of this **atypical sympathetic discharge** in which **dopamine release exceeds that of NE and E** are not clear. It apparently exists not only in extreme form in **paroxysmal hypertension** but also in a more subtle form in borderline essential hypertensive patients. In some of those patients, the hyperadrenergic features are reflected by higher baseline urinary excretion of the dopamine metabolite 3-O-methoxytyramine, indicating augmented exocytotic dopamine release or defective reuptake, while such a difference is not seen in stable hypertension (Fig. 3). This atypical sympathetic discharge in patients with borderline hypertension may be due to **a partial dopamine-β-hydroxylase deficiency,** as suggested by their decreased DβH release into plasma following various stimuli, or a **subtle defect in the dopamine transporter regulating dopamine reuptake.**

References

1. Kuchel O, Buu NT, Racz K, De Lean A, Serri O, Kyncl J. Role of sulfate conjugation of catecholamines in blood pressure regulation. Fed Proc 1986;45:2254–9.
2. Weinshilboum R. Biochemical genetic of catecholamines in humans. Mayo Clin Proc 1983; 58:319–30.
3. Kuchel O. Clinical implications of genetic and acquired defects in catecholamine synthesis and metabolism. Clin Invest Med 1994;17:369–88.
4. Schoors DF, Velkeniers B, Dupont AG. A case of hyperdopaminuria due to increased renal dopamine production. Nephron 1990;56:329–31.
5. Kuchel O, Buu NT, Larochelle P, Hamet P, Genest J Jr. Episodic dopamine discharge in paroxysmal hypertension: Page's syndrome revisited. Arch Intern Med 1986;146;1315–21.

PART IX

Central Autonomic Disorders

43

Parkinson's Disease

Thomas L. Davis
Department of Neurology
Division of Movement Disorders
Vanderbilt University
Nashville, Tennessee

Parkinson's disease (PD) is a common idiopathic neurodegenerative disorder that affects an estimated 1% of the population over the age of 65. The cardinal features of PD are resting tremor, **bradykinesia, rigidity,** and **loss of postural reflexes.** Signs and symptoms of altered autonomic dysfunction are also frequently present (Table 1).

PD results from a loss of pigmented, dopaminergic nerve cells within the **substantia nigra** that project to the **striatum (putamen and caudate).** The diagnosis is made clinically and confirmed only at autopsy when the substantia nigra shows a visible **loss of pigment on gross inspection** and a markedly reduced population of neurons containing intracytoplasmic inclusions (**Lewy bodies**) on histologic examination. Lewy bodies, sometimes associated with neuronal loss, may also be found in the preganglionic structures of the sympathetic and parasympathetic nervous system. **Shy–Drager syndrome or multiple system atrophy** (Chapter 44), characterized by autonomic failure plus parkinsonism or cerebellar ataxia, may mimic PD especially early in disease. This difficulty in making a correct early diagnosis complicates any study of the incidence of autonomic failure in PD.

Tests of Sympathetic Function

Sympathetic skin responses (SSR) represent a function of sympathetic sudomotor fibers. Studies have found abnormal SSR in 14% of PD patients while all age-matched controls were normal. Abnormal SSR correlated with duration of disease and with impotence. The abnormality of SSR seen in PD may be due to **intermediolateral column dysfunction.** Abnormalities in blood pressure responses to handgrip and standing have also been found in PD patients as compared to controls.

Tests of Parasympathetic Function

R–R interval variation (RRIV) is primarily indicative of the parasympathetic function of the vagus nerve. In one study approximately one-third of PD patients had abnormal RRIV during rest and deep breathing. Abnormal RRIV was not related to staging or duration of illness and was not affected by acute or chronic L-dopa treatment. Other studies have also shown mild abnormalities in parasympathetic testing in PD compared to controls.

Table 1.   **Autonomic Symptoms in
Parkinson's Disease**

Bladder dysfunction
Constipation
Dysphagia/drooling
Heat/cold intolerance
Syncope/near syncope
Seborrhea
Sexual dysfunction
Weight loss

Orthostatic Hypotension (OH)

Symptomatic OH may be present as a primary part of PD or as a complication of medications or inactivity. All dopaminergic drugs used to treat PD may exacerbate OH and should be initiated slowly to minimize this effect. Supine hypertension is uncommon in PD and its presence combined with a lack of response to L-dopa suggests the diagnosis of Shy–Drager syndrome. In addition to the general symptomatic measures used to treat OH (Chapters 65–68), the peripheral decarboxylase inhibitor carbidopa (Lodosyn) or the peripheral dopamine antagonist **domperidone** (Motilium) may be added to a patient's regimen to decrease the peripheral effects of dopamine.

Constipation

Constipation is eventually seen in almost all PD patients and is the chief complaint in some cases. The exact mechanism of the constipation remains unknown but increased transit time probably plays a major role. Initially symptoms may respond to increased dietary fiber and stool softeners, but many patients eventually require a daily bowel regimen that includes an osmotic laxative such as lactulose. The antimuscarinic effects of the anticholinergic medications used to treat parkinsonian tremor may also exacerbate constipation.

Dysphagia

Dysphagia is seen as a prominent symptom in some patients with PD, usually as part of end-stage disease. It typically occurs earlier in the course of other parkinsonian syndromes such as **multiple systems atrophy** (Chapter 44) and progressive supranuclear palsy. Although swallowing may improve with dopaminergic therapy, dysphagia is a relatively medication resistant symptom. **Anticholinergics** lead to drying of the oral mucosa and may make it more difficult to swallow. When anticholinergics are necessary for control of parkinsonism, artificial saliva may be used. Some patients may also benefit from a change in diet or speech therapy consultation for swallowing training.

Drooling

Drooling is a common late manifestation of the disease. Since saliva production is normal, drooling probably arises from the poverty of automatic swallowing. It would therefore be regarded as due to **hypokinesia, a cardinal motor feature,** rather than a strictly autonomic manifestation. It may respond somewhat to L-dopa. Some investigators have recommend treatment with a peripheral acting anticholinergic such as **propantheline** (15–45 mg/day in divided doses). Others have suggested that administration of antimuscarinics may further impair swallowing by increasing the viscosity of the saliva. Use of sugarless gum or hard candy may stimulate swallowing and decrease drooling.

Sexual Function

Little information exists concerning sexual function in PD. Recently 50 patients (36 men and 14 women) and their spouses were surveyed regarding sexual function since their diagnosis. Participants had a mean age of 67.3 years and an average duration of PD of 7 years. The majority of patients reported a sexual frequency that was less than before they had PD. A decrease in sexual interest was seen in 44% of men and 71% of women. Almost 50% of men were unable to ejaculate while 75% of women stated that the frequency of orgasm was less since the parkinsonism (38% anorgasmic). These changes were not felt to be solely due to depression. Although dopaminergic medications have been reported to lead to hypersexuality, this is rarely seen. On the other hand, these medications are one of the few families of medication not reported to impair sexual function. Erectile dysfunction in men may respond to the use of a **vacuum device, papaverine injections,** or **penile prosthesis.**

Bladder Dysfunction

It has been estimated that 50% of PD patients have some degree of bladder dysfunction. This is usually irritative symptomatology caused by involuntary bladder contraction, but obstructive symptoms may also be present. Because the pontine micturition center is spared, these patients have coordinated voiding. Formal urodynamics may be necessary to exclude a coexisting obstructive disorder such as prostatism. **Anticholinergics** may be used to help control symptoms if obstruction is not documented.

References

1. Awerbuch GI, Sandyk R. Autonomic functions in the early stages of Parkinson's disease. Int J Neurosci 1992;64:7–14.
2. Koller WC, Vetere-Overfield B, Williamson A, Busenbark K, Nash J, Parrish D. Sexual dysfunction in Parkinson's disease. Clin Neuropharm 1990;13:461–3.
3. Takahasi A. Autonomic nervous system disorders in Parkinson's disease. Eur Neurol 1991; 31(suppl 1):41–7.
4. van Dijk JG, Haan J, Zwinderman K, Kremer B, van Hilten BJ, Roos RAC. Autonomic nervous system dysfunction in Parkinson's disease: relationship with age, medication, duration and severity. J Neurol Neurosurg Psychiatry 1993;56:1090–5.
5. Wang SJ, Fuh JL, Shan DE, Liao KK, Lin KP, Tsai CP, Wu ZA. Sympathetic skin response and R-R interval variation in Parkinson's disease. Mov Dis 1993;8:151–7.

44 Multiple System Atrophy and Shy–Drager Syndrome

Ronald J. Polinsky
Clinical Pharmacology
Sandoz Research Institute
East Hanover, New Jersey

Multiple system atrophy (MSA) encompasses several overlapping degenerative neurological disorders that may be attended by autonomic failure. The relationship between MSA and Shy–Drager syndrome has been needlessly complicated by the multitude of terms utilized imprecisely in the medical literature. The pathological hallmark of MSA is neuronal loss and gliosis within several central nervous system regions including autonomic centers.

Clinical Manifestations

The average age of onset is in the sixth decade. Men are affected about twice as frequently as women. Autonomic symptoms compose the initial presentation in approximately 75% of patients with MSA. Genitourinary dysfunction is the most frequent initial complaint; impotence may precede other signs of autonomic failure by more than 10 years. Although syncope is uncommon as a presenting feature, headache, neck pain, dimming of vision, and frequent yawning may reflect impaired control of blood pressure. It is important to keep in mind that orthostatic hypotension is only one consequence of the abnormal cardiovascular control in MSA. Blood pressure responds in an exaggerated fashion to any physiologic or pharmacologic stimulus capable of raising or lowering blood pressure (e.g., postprandial or insulin-induced hypotension).

Imbalance, the most common presenting complaint when the illness begins with neurologic symptoms, causes a gait disorder related to cerebellar or parkinsonian features. Some patients also experience stiffness, clumsiness, or a change in handwriting as manifestations of parkinsonism at the onset of MSA.

The natural history in MSA is one of relentless progression. Most patients eventually manifest signs of sympathetic and parasympathetic dysfunction. Involvement of cerebellar, extrapyramidal, and pyramidal systems produces neurologic disability characterized primarily by the movement disorder. Dementia is fairly uncommon until the late stage of disease. Hoarseness and stridor may develop due to vocal cord paralysis. A mixed form of sleep apnea with obstructive and neurogenic components also occurs in MSA. Progression of autonomic and neurologic dysfunction is quite independent. Neurologic symptoms generally develop about 5 years after onset when autonomic symptoms herald the disease. In contrast, autonomic insufficiency appears about 2 years into the illness in patients who initially experience neurologic symptoms. These patterns facilitate clinical distinction among patients with MSA, PAF, and Parkinson's disease. As a general rule, it is wise to document at least 5 years of autonomic symptoms before a diagnosis of PAF can be made with certainty.

Primer on the Autonomic Nervous System

Three general patterns form the basis for a clinical subclassification of patients with MSA based on neurological signs. Imbalance, incoordination, and dysarthria are the predominant clinical features observed in the **olivopontocerebellar atrophy (OPCA)** variant. In those patients with the **striatonigral degeneration (SND)** form of MSA, rigidity and bradykinesia out of proportion to tremor contrast with the usual balance of these signs in Parkinson's disease. The OPCA and SND variants each comprise about 25% of patients with MSA. The others have features common to OPCA and SND, similar to the patients reported by Shy and Drager in 1960.

Diagnostic Evaluation

Routine cerebrospinal fluid examination is generally unrevealing. Similarly, the EEG shows only nonspecific changes. Electrophysiologic studies generally reveal normal latency and conduction times of sensory and motor nerves unless there are objective clinical signs of neuropathy. Denervation in laryngeal muscles and the rectal sphincter has been reported.

Voluntary and involuntary aspects of bladder control are affected in MSA. Patients cannot initiate a micturition reflex; filling of the bladder elicits **involuntary detrusor contractions.** Urethral tone may be compromised in severe cases. Some patients with MSA have detrusor areflexia while others are hyperreflexic.

Brain stem auditory evoked potentials are useful in differentiating MSA from PAF and Parkinson's disease. Abnormal latency and amplitude in most patients with MSA is not present in PAF patients and occurs uncommonly in Parkinson's disease.

Although CT scanning is most revealing in those cases with obvious cerebellar involvement, cerebellar and brainstem atrophy can be seen even in the absence of clinical signs. An abnormal decrease in putaminal signal intensity can be visualized using MRI with a strong (1.5 Tesla) magnetic source in combination with a T2-weighted spin–echo pulse sequence. Involvement of the posterior and lateral portions of the putamina distinguishes the findings in MSA from the changes seen in older normal subjects. Rigidity and putaminal signal dropout correlate in patients with MSA.

PET scanning reveals regional reductions in cerebral glucose metabolism in areas involved by the degenerative process. The changes in striatal dopa uptake and dopamine receptor binding also parallel neuropathological involvement in the extrapyramidal system.

The approaches for physiological and biochemical assessment of patients with autonomic failure have been discussed in several chapters of this book. More detailed reviews have also been recently published. Suffice it to say that the results of many investigative strategies support the suggestion of primary CNS involvement as the basis for autonomic and neurologic symptoms/signs in MSA. From the cardiovascular perspective, resting levels, neuronal stores, and uptake of NE are generally normal, indicative of the functional integrity of postganglionic sympathetic neurons. The exaggerated nonspecific pressor responses reflect **defective baroreflex modulation** of blood pressure. Parasympathetic and adrenal medullary function are also affected. Low levels of monoamine metabolites in CSF are consistent with the neurochemical findings observed by PET scanning and postmortem analysis of brain tissue in MSA.

Prognosis

Patients with MSA die on the average 8.5 years after the onset of their illness. Rare patients have survived for more than 20 years. **Aspiration, apnea,** and presumably arrhythmias contribute to the premature demise of MSA patients. Although swallowing may be impaired it is rarely necessary to employ a feeding tube or gastrostomy. Restriction of the airway can result from a combination of abductor paralysis and rigidity. The ability to handle secretions is clearly compromised in many patients. The changes in blood pressure and arrhythmias during sleep may well be secondary to apneic episodes. Abnormal respiratory control and laryngeal obstruction promote episodes of **sleep apnea** and **respiratory stridor.** The value of tracheostomy except in critical situations remains a matter of debate.

Pathological and Neurochemical Correlates

The degenerative process is characterized by neuronal loss and gliosis in many central nervous system areas. The nonspecific nature of these morphologic changes highlights the importance of documenting their geographic distribution to establish the diagnosis. More recently, **argyrophilic cytoplasmic inclusions** (Fig. 1) have been observed in **oligodendroglial cells** in the brains from all variants of MSA. These **glial cytoplasmic inclusions** react with antibodies to a variety of brain proteins (e.g., ubiquitin, MAP5). Although the pathologic findings in SND resemble Parkinson's disease, **Lewy bodies are notably absent.** The Lewy body has been used to classify patients with autonomic failure. However, the significance of Lewy bodies is unclear because they occur in normals and less frequently in MSA and other neurologic disorders.

Autonomic insufficiency results from loss of preganglionic neurons in the **intermediolateral columns (ILC)** of the spinal cord. Quantitative studies demonstrate a dramatic reduction in the number of ILC neurons. Comparable quantitative investigations of parasympathetic neurons are lacking though cell loss in the dorsal vagal nuclei has been reported. **Sacral parasympathetic outflow (Onuf's nucleus)** also appears to be affected by the degenerative process in MSA. The question of whether sympathetic ganglia are primarily involved has not been adequately answered.

A variety of neurochemical abnormalities have been found in the brains of MSA patients. The levels of **norepinephrine** and **dopamine** are reduced in several brain regions including the striatum, nucleus accumbens, substantia nigra, septal nuclei, hypothalamus, and locus ceruleus. Binding sites for dopamine are also decreased in the **substantia nigra. Low choline acetyltransferase** activity in hypothalamus, dentate, red nucleus, pons, and olive parallels some of the sites exhibiting morphologic signs of degeneration. Benzodiazepine receptors are normal in cerebellar cortex, but increased in the dentate nucleus from OPCA brains. Muscimol binding is diminished in the granule layer. Muscarinic cholinergic receptor density is also lower than normal in the molecular and

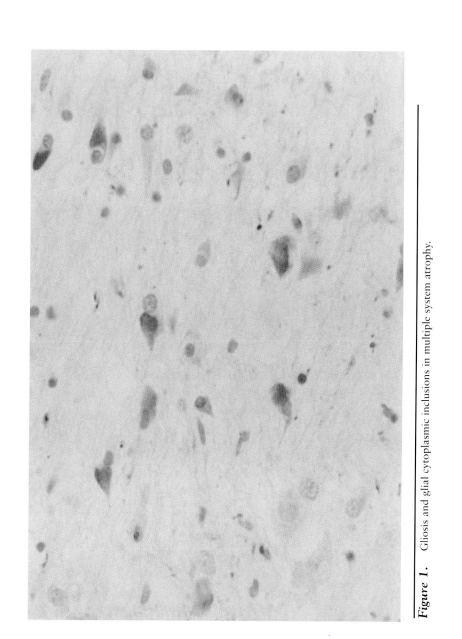

Figure 1. Gliosis and glial cytoplasmic inclusions in multiple system atrophy.

granule cell layers, but increased in the dentate. The marked depletion of **tyrosine hydroxylase** immunoreactive neurons in the A1 and A2 medullary regions of brainstem in SND patients may be particularly important in relation to blood pressure control.

Peptides have also been measured in the brain and spinal cord. The levels of substance P are dramatically reduced in the basal ganglia. Reduced neuropeptide concentrations are most apparent in the dorsal aspect of the cord. This includes substance P, substance K, calcitonin gene-related peptide (CGRP), somatostatin, and galanin.

Potential Etiologies

Although no definite etiology has been identified, preliminary evidence suggests a possible role for genetic, immune, and toxic mechanisms. Occasional familial cases have been reported; however, the association between HLA-Aw32 and autonomic failure was not confirmed in a larger study. Deficient DNA repair is another potential mechanism for neuronal degeneration. Cultured lymphoblasts from MSA patients show reduced survival after exposure to mutagenic agents; a similar abnormality occurs in several other primary neuronal degenerations. **Antibodies in CSF** from patients with MSA react specifically with rat **locus ceruleus,** suggesting an immunologic basis for the degenerative process. Compared to controls, patients with MSA have more exposures to a variety of toxins, contacted generally through occupational exposure.

Management

Treatment of autonomic insufficiency is discussed in another chapter of this book. However, several aspects of management are particularly relevant to MSA. Rigidity, bradykinesia, and tremor do respond to antiparkinsonian drugs, particularly early in the disease. Unfortunately, **dopaminergic drugs** should generally be avoided or used with extreme caution because they can exacerbate postural hypotension. **Anticholinergic drugs** have comparable efficacy without affecting the blood pressure. Patients view the urinary retention from anticholinergics as a benefit.

Anesthetic management is also important since most patients lack the adrenal medullary response that may be critical during surgery or traumatic injuries. In addition, abnormal physiologic and pharmacologic responses alter the clinical signs (e.g., respiration, pupils, temperature, blood pressure, heart rate) used to evaluate and monitor the patient during the peri- and postoperative period. If surgery is absolutely necessary, both surgeon and anesthetist must become familiar with the manifestations and management of autonomic and neurologic aspects of MSA.

References

1. Bannister R, Mathias C, Polinsky R. Clinical features of autonomic failure: a comparison between UK and US experience. In: Bannister R, ed. Autonomic failure. London: Oxford University Press, 1988:281–8.

2. Oppenheimer D. Neuropathology and neurochemistry of autonomic failure. A. Neuropathology of autonomic failure. In: Bannister R, ed. Autonomic failure. London: Oxford University Press, 1988:451–63.
3. Polinsky RJ. Shy-Drager syndrome. In: Jankovic J, Tolosa E, eds. Parkinson's disease and movement disorders, 2nd edition. Baltimore: Williams and Wilkins, 1993:191–204.
4. Polinsky RJ. Neurochemical and pharmacological abnormalities in chronic autonomic failure syndromes. In: Low P, ed. Evaluation and management of clinical autonomic disorders. Boston: Little Brown, 1992:537–49.
5. Tamaoka A, Mizusawa H, Mori H, Shoji S. Ubiquitinated αB-crystallin in glial cytoplasmic inclusions from the brain of a patient with multiple system atrophy. J Neurol Sci 1995; 129:192–8.

45   Central Nervous System Disorders

Eduardo E. Benarroch
Department of Neurology
Mayo Clinic
Rochester, Minnesota

The **central autonomic network** includes the insular and medial prefrontal cortex, amygdala, preoptic–hypothalamic unit, periaqueuctal gray matter, parabrachial region of the pons, nucleus of the solitary tract (NTS), the intermediate reticular zone of the medulla, and the ventrolateral and ventromedial medulla. Disorders involving any of these regions or their preganglionic sympathetic and parasympathetic effector mechanism may result in (1) **syndromes of autonomic failure,** characterized by orthostatic hypotension, anhidrosis, impotence, neurogenic bladder, gastrointestinal dysmotility, and Horner's syndrome; or (2) **syndromes of autonomic hyperactivity** resulting in cardiac arrhythmias, hypertension, hyper- or hypothermia, hyperhidrosis, myocardial damage, and "neurogenic" pulmonary edema, isolated or in various combinations.

Disorders in Telencephalic Autonomic Regions

Hemispheric stroke involving the insula or medial prefrontal cortex may produce cardiac arrhythmias; the side of lesion may determine the type of arrhythmia, reflecting the lateralizing influence of the cerebral hemispheres on autonomic control. Infarction of the **opercular cortex** may produce **transient hyperhidrosis** in the contralateral face and arm. Uni- or bilateral infarction of the **cingulate gyrus** can produce **urinary and fecal incontinence, fever, tachycardia,** and even **sudden death.** The mesial frontal lobe can also be affected by hydrocephalus and convexity tumors, such as meningiomas, which commonly produce uninhibited neurogenic bladder.

   Limbic seizures involving the amygdalo–hippocampal, cingulate, opercular, anterior frontopolar, and orbitofrontal regions commonly produce autonomic manifestations. Alterations of heart rate are the most common autonomic change during seizure activity; the most common is **ictal sinus tachycardia,** but **sinoatrial block, sinus arrest, atrial fibrillation, premature ventricular contractions,** and **supraventricular or ventricular tachycardia** may also occur. Syncope may be a manifestations of seizures, and their differentiation requires simultaneous EEG/ECG recording. Rhythm disturbances may be the primary cause of sudden death in epileptic patients. Temporo-limbic discharges may also produce thermoregulatory responses; **unilateral pilomotor seizures,** although rare, may be important as a manifestation of a malignant gliomas in the ipsilateral temporal lobe.

Disorders of the Hypothalamus

   Disorders involving the hypothalamus or its connections may produce complex autonomic disturbances, either in isolation or combined with disturbances of endocrine, thirst, caloric balance, or sexual function. **Disorders of thermoregulation** are an important manifestation of neoplastic, degenerative, or inflammatory hypothalamic disease. Continuous hypothermia has been described in **Wernicke's encephalopathy, head injury, multiple sclerosis, mesodiencephalic hematoma,** and **toluene toxicity.** Wernicke's encephalopathy should be suspected in alcoholics and malnourished patients presenting with unexplained hypothermia, and prompt, immediate treatment with **thiamine** should be pursued. Episodic hyperhidrosis and hypothermia may occur as a manifestation of **agenesis of the corpus callosum** and has been attributed to involvement of the medial preoptic–anterior hypothalamic region. The episodes may be associated with other manifestations of autonomic hyperactivity and alterations of level of consciousness; they may vary in duration and be associated with long-lasting spontaneous remissions. **Anticonvulsants, cyproheptadine, clonidine,** or **oxybutinin** may control both hyperhidrosis and hypothermia.

Acute Hydrocephalus

   The syndrome of **autonomic hyperactivity** is characterized by acute episodes of hypertension, tachycardia, diaphoresis, hypo- or hyperthermia, skin vasodilatation, lacrimation, pupillary changes, hyperventilation, shivering, and increased muscle tone, in various combinations. In 1929 Penfield first described this syndrome in a patient with a tumor at the level of the foramen of Monro with hydrocephalus; since then, several cases of episodic autonomic paroxysms have been reported, in general in association with lesions near the third ventricle. Acute hydrocephalus, typically after subarachnoid hemorrhage, may cause similar episodes, which may reverse completely after shunt treatment.

Head Injury

   The majority of cases of **autonomic hyperactivity** result from severe closed head injury, usually associated with a decorticate state and widespread axonal injury in the white matter; the proposed mechanism is a release of the hypothalamus from inhibitory cortical control, and these patients may respond to opioids or bromocriptine.

Fatal Familial Insomnia

Fatal familial insomnia (FFI) is an **autosomal dominant prion disease** linked to a mutation in the prion protein (PrP) gene. The main manifestations of FFI are progressive insomnia, motor dysfunction, and dysautonomia; this consists of sympathetic hyperactivity, manifested by hyperhidrosis, fever, tachycardia, and hypertension. The main pathological findings are severe atrophy of the anteroventral and dorsomedial nuclei of the **thalamus,** both involved in limbic circuits.

Neuroleptic Malignant Syndrome

The neuroleptic malignant syndrome is discussed in Chapter 25.

Disorders of the Brainstem

Involvement of reflex autonomic centers of the medulla oblongata, including the NTS, dorsal vagal and ambigual nuclei, intermediate reticular formation, and ventral medulla, by neoplastic, ischemic, inflammatory, or degenerative lesions commonly produce severe cardiorespiratory abnormalities, including excessive sympathoexcitation, baroreflex failure, orthostatic hypotension, and sleep apnea. Excessive sympathoexcitation may reflect hypoxemic activation of sympathoexcitatory neurons of the rostral ventrolateral medulla during ischemia or compression. Baroreflex failure reflects bilateral damage of the NTS, the first relay station of baroreceptor afferents; this resembles clinically a pheochromocytoma, with episodes of acute hypertension or excessive lability of arterial pressure.

Brainstem Ischemia and Stroke

Transient brainstem ischemia may produce hypertension that precedes other focal neurologic deficits. Bilateral pontomedullary strokes may produce persistent tachycardia, episodic bradycardia, orthostatic hypotension, cardiorespiratory arrest, Ondine's curse, vomiting, hiccups, dysphagia, aperistaltic esophagus, gastroesophageal reflux, gastric retention, recurrent unexplained fever, Horner's syndrome, urinary retention or generalized hyperhidrosis. **Lateral medullary strokes (Wallenberg's syndrome)** may also produce profound bradycardia, supine hypotension, or central hypoventilation.

Posterior Fossa Tumors

Orthostatic hypotension may be the presenting manifestation of posterior fossa tumors, or may develop after their surgical treatment. Paroxysmal hypertension has been reported in tumors involving the cerebellum or the cerebelopontine angle. **Pulsatile compression of the ventrolateral medulla** by a basilar artery aneurysm or vascular loops may also produce episodic hypertension.

Syringobulbia may affect the NTS or its connections with cardiovagal and vasomotor neurons of the ventrolateral medulla. This condition may produce orthostatic hypotension, abnormal cardiovagal function, or central baroreflex failure, as well as Horner's syndrome.

Inflammatory and Toxic Conditions

Bulbar poliomyelitis may produce hypertension and respiratory failure. Plaques of multiple sclerosis close to the region of the NTS may produce neurogenic pulmonary edema.

Disorders of the Spinal Cord

Traumatic spinal cord lesions above T5 level produce profound abnormalities in control of cardiovascular, thermoregulatory, bladder, bowel and sexual function, including the syndrome of autonomic dysreflexia. This is discussed in Chapter 46.

Syringomyelia produces partial interruption of descending autonomic pathways in the intermediolateral cell columns of the spinal cord, either directly by a cervical syrinx or by an associated Chiari malformation. The manifestations include Horner's syndrome, sweating abnormalities, and trophic and vasomotor changes in the limbs, especially the hands. Micturition and defecation may be affected, but at an advanced stage.

Multiple sclerosis can lead to neurogenic bladder with detrusor sphincter dyssynergia, and neurogenic bowel and sexual dysfunction. Nevertheless, there are subclinical abnormalities in cardiovascular tests including reduced heart rate response to deep breathing and sympathetic vasoconstrictor failure. Abnormal thermoregulatory sweating is frequently found in multiple sclerosis patients.

Tetanus may produce severe parasympathetic and sympathetic hyperactivity due to both disinhibition of preganglionic neurons and direct damage of autonomic brainstem nuclei. Parasympathetic hyperactivity produces sinus arrest, salivation, and increased bronchial secretion frequently observed in severe cases; sympathetic hyperactivity results in tachycardia, arrhythmias, labile hypertension, progressive and refractory hypotension, peripheral vasoconstriction, fever, and profuse sweating.

Amyotrophic lateral sclerosis (ALS) may produce subclinical involvement of autonomic function. In a recent study, 38% of 74 patients with classical ALS had abnormal autonomic function tests, particularly the sudomotor axon reflex responses in the foot and the heart rate responses to deep breathing.

References

1. Talman WT. Cardiovascular regulation and lesions of the central nervous system. Ann Neurol 1983;18:1–12.
2. Carmel PW. Vegetative dysfunctions of the hypothalamus. Acta Neurochir (Wien) 1985;75:113–21.

3. LeWitt PA, Newman RP, Greenberg HS, Rocher LL, Calne DB, Ehrenkranz JRL. Episodic hyperhidrosis, hypothermia, and agenesis of corpus callosum. **Neurology 1983;** 33:1122–9.
4. Ropper AH. Acute autonomic emergencies and autonomic storm. In: Low PA, ed. Clinical autonomic disorders: evaluation and management. Boston: Little Brown, 1992:747–65.
5. Mathias CJ. Role of the central nervous system in human secondary hypertension. J Cardiovasc Pharmacol 1987;10(suppl. 12):S93–9.

46 Autonomic Disturbances in Spinal Cord Injuries

Christopher J. Mathias
Department of Medicine
St. Mary's Hospital/Imperial College of Science, Technology and Medicine
University of London
London, United Kingdom

Normal functioning of the autonomic nervous system is critically dependent on integrity of the spinal cord, as the **entire sympathetic outflow** (T1–L2/3) and the **sacral parasympathetic outflow** travel and synapse within the spinal cord before supplying various target organs (Fig. 1). In spinal cord injuries, therefore, autonomic impairment usually occurs, and this depends upon the site and the extent of the lesion. In cervical and high thoracic transection, the entire or a large part of the sympathetic outflow, together with the sacral parasympathetic outflow, is separated from cerebral control. Autonomic malfunction may affect the cardiovascular, thermoregulatory, gastrointestinal, urinary, and reproductive systems. The problems are usually worse in those with higher lesions.

Soon after cord injury, there is a transient state of **hypoexcitability,** described as **spinal shock.** There is flaccid paralysis of muscles, lack of tendon reflexes, and impairment of **spinal autonomic function** with atony of the urinary bladder and large bowel, dilatation of blood vessels, and lack of spinal autonomic reflexes. This may last from a few days to a few weeks, following which activity in the isolated cord returns. In the chronic phase, with return of isolated spinal function, a different set of autonomic abnormalities occurs.

Cardiovascular System

In recent high injuries basal blood pressure, especially diastolic, is usually lower than normal. Plasma norepinephrine and epinephrine levels are low, as

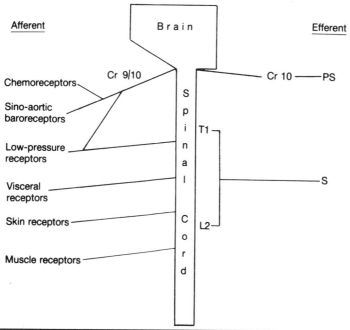

Figure 1.   Schematic outline of the major autonomic pathways controlling the circulation. The major afferent input into the central nervous system is through the glossopharyngeal (CR9) and vagus (CR10) nerves by activation of baroreceptors in the carotid sinus and aortic arch. Chemoreceptors and low-pressure receptors also influence the efferent outflow. The latter consists of the cranial parasympathetic (PS) outflow to the heart via the vagus nerves, and the sympathetic outflow from the thoracic and upper lumbar segments of the spinal cord. Activation of visceral, skin, and muscle receptors, in addition to cerebral stimulation, influences the efferent outflow. In high spinal cord lesions, therefore, the input from chemoreceptors and baroreceptors is preserved along with the vagal efferent outflow, but there is no connection between the brain and the rest of the sympathetic outflow. The spinal sympathetic outflow may be activated through a range of afferents (visual, skin, muscle). This occurs through isolated spinal cord reflexes, not controlled by cerebral pathways, as seen normally. Reprinted with permission from Mathias CJ and Frankel HL, Cardiovascular control in spinal man. Ann. Rev. Physiol. 1988, 50:577–592.

in the chronic phase. Basal heart rate is usually below normal. In patients with high cervical lesions, who need artificial ventilation because of diaphragmatic paralysis, severe **bradycardia** and **cardiac arrest** may occur during **tracheal stimulation** (Fig. 2). This results from increased vagal activity, as efferent muscarinic blockade with atropine prevents bradycardia. Vagal activity is increased by hypoxia and by the absence of sympathetic reflexes; furthermore, there is an inability to reduce vagal activity through the pulmonary inflation reflex because of the inability to breathe. It is necessary to prevent such episodes by adequate oxygenation, treatment of respiratory infection and pulmonary emboli (which contribute to hypoxia), avoidance of cholinomimetic agents such as neostigmine and carbachol, and, if necessary, the use of parenteral atropine or a demand cardiac pacemaker.

In the chronic stage, the levels of basal systolic and diastolic blood pressure are related closely to the level of the spinal lesion, being lower in the high

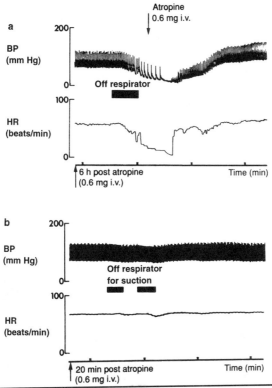

a

Atropine
0.6 mg i.v.

200

BP
(mm Hg)

0

Off respirator

100

HR
(beats/min)

0

6 h post atropine
(0.6 mg i.v.)   Time (min)

b

200

BP
(mm Hg)

0

Off respirator
for suction

100

HR
(beats/min)

0

20 min post atropine
(0.6 mg i.v.)   Time (min)

Figure 2.   (a) The effect of disconnecting the respirator (as required for aspirating the airways) on the blood pressure (BP) and heart rate (HR) of a recently injured tetraplegic patient (C4/5 lesion) in spinal shock, 6 hr after the last dose of intravenous atropine. Sinus bradycardia and cardiac arrest, also observed in the electrocardiograph, were reversed by reconnection, intravenous atropine, and external cardiac massage (reprinted with permission from Frankel HL, Mathias CJ and Spalding JMK. Mechanisms of reflex cardiac arrest in tetraplegic patients. Lancet, 1975 ii;1183–1185). (b) The effect of tracheal suction, 20 min after atropine in the same patient. Disconnection from the respiratory and tracheal suction did not lower either heart rate or blood pressure (reprinted with permission from Mathias CJ. Bradycardia and cardiac arrest during tracheal suction—mechanisms in tetraplegic patients. Eur. J. Int. Care Med. 1976, 2:147–156).

lesions and rising toward normal as the lesion descends. In tetraplegic subjects, plasma norepinephrine levels are about 25% of the levels observed in normal subjects, and they have reduced basal muscle sympathetic nerve activity, as measured by microneurography. Complicating factors, such as renal damage and failure, can elevate blood pressure, regardless of the lesion.

In high lesions the blood pressure is sensitive to a number of physiological stimuli. **Postural (orthostatic) hypotension** is a particular problem in the early stages (Fig. 3). Plasma norepinephrine levels are low and do not rise with head-up postural change, unlike normal subjects. There is a marked **rise in levels of plasma renin, aldosterone, and vasopressin.** The rise in vasopressin may contribute to reduced urine output when upright. Improvement in symptoms and in postural blood pressure follows **repeated head-up tilt,** which presumably improves cerebral autoregulation and releases the various hormones which

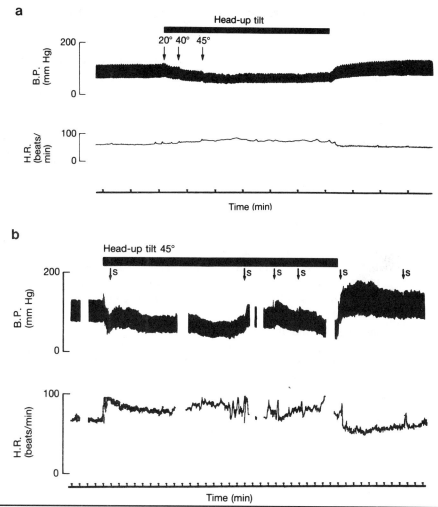

Figure 3. (a) Blood pressure (BP) and heart rate (HR) in a tetraplegic patient before and after head-up tilt, in the early stages of rehabilitation, where there were few muscle spasms and minimal autonomic dysreflexia (reprinted with permission from Mathias CJ and Frankel HL. The cardiovascular system in tetraplegia and paraplegia. In: Frankel HL, ed. Handbook of Clinical Neurology: Spinal Chord Trauma, Vol. 61. Elsevier, Netherlands, 1992: 435–56). (b) Blood pressure (BP) and heart rate (HR) in a chronic tetraplegic patient before, during and after head-up tilt to 45°. Blood pressure promptly falls but with partial recovery, which in this case is linked to skeletal muscle spasms (S) inducing spinal sympathetic activity. Some of the later oscillations may be due to the rise in plasma renin, which was measured where there were interruptions in the intraarterial record. In the later phases of head-up tilt, skeletal muscle spasms occur more frequently and further elevate the blood pressure. On return to the horizontal, blood pressure rises rapidly above the previous level and then returns slowly to the horizontal. Heart rate usually moves in the opposite direction, except during muscle spasms when there is an initial increase (reprinted with permission from Mathias CJ and Frankel HL. Cardiovascular control in spinal man. Annu. Rev. Phys. 1988, 50:577–92).

constrict blood vessels, raise intravascular volume, and thus reduce the postural blood pressure fall. Drugs such as the sympathomimetic **ephedrine** may need to be used.

The reverse, **severe hypertension,** may occur during **autonomic dysreflexia** following stimulation below the level of the lesion. This may occur through the skin (such as from complicating pressure sores), from abdominal and pelvic viscera (by contraction of the urinary bladder or irritation from a urethral catheter) (Fig. 4), or via skeletal muscles (during muscle spasms). The paroxysmal rise in blood pressure is the result of increased sympathetic neural activity causing constriction of both resistance and capacitance vessels. These changes occur below the level of the lesion, while above the lesion there may be sweating and dilatation of cutaneous vessels over the face and neck. Autonomic dysreflexia is accompanied by increased levels of plasma norepinephrine. Plasma norepinephrine levels, even at the height of hypertension, however, are increased only two- or threefold above the low basal levels, and are still within the range of basal levels in normal subjects; this differs markedly from the levels seen in hypertensive crises due to a **pheochromocytoma.**

During autonomic dysreflexia **muscle sympathetic nerve activity** measured by sympathetic microneurography shows only a modest increase, suggesting that the pressor response may be due to α-adrenergic receptor sensitivity. This also may explain the increased pressor response to intravenously infused norepinephrine. Other factors, such as impaired baroreflex activity, may be of importance as there is pressor hypersensitivity to a wide range of vasoactive agents of different chemical structures which act on a variety of receptors. Tetraplegic subjects also have an enhanced depressor response to vasodilator agents which, furthermore, favors baroreflex impairment.

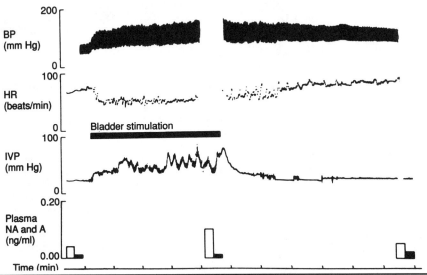

Figure 4.   Blood pressure (BP), heart rate (HR), intravesical pressure (IVP), plasma norepinephrine (NA) (open histograms) and plasma epinephrine (A) (filled histograms) in a tetraplegic patient before, during, and after urinary bladder stimulation induced by suprapubic percussion of the anterior abdominal wall. The rise in BP is accompanied by a fall in heart rate as a result of increased vagal activity in response to the elevated blood pressure. Plasma NE but not E levels rise, suggesting an increase in sympathetic neural activity, independent of adrenomedullary activation (reprinted with permission from Mathias CJ and Frankel HL. The neurological and hormonal control of blood vessels and heart in spinal man. J. Autonomic Nervous Syst. (suppl), 1986, 457–64).

Autonomic dysreflexia is a serious problem and may result in considerable morbidity, with severe sweating and a throbbing headache, and even mortality as a result of intracranial hemorrhage. The management consists of preventing the initiating factor caused by increased sympathoneuronal activity. If necessary, a variety of drugs to reduce sympathetic efferent activity can be used.

Cutaneous Circulation

In higher lesions, the skin below the lesion is usually warmer and veins appear dilated. There may be extravasation of fluid into subcutaneous tissue which could contribute to skin breakdown and pressure sores. Vasodilation often occurs in the nose (**Guttmann's sign**); similar changes occur after the adrenergic neuron depleting agents, **reserpine** and **guanethidine**, in hypertensive patients.

In spinal shock the cutaneous responses to the triple or **Lewis response** are exaggerated, hence the term **dermatographia rubra**. With the return of spinal cord reflex activity, in the chronic phase, there is sympathetic vasoconstriction and skin pallor, hence the term **dermatographia alba**.

Thermoregulation

Hypothermia may readily occur in high lesions as shivering is diminished and the individual may be unable to vasoconstrict the cutaneous circulation.

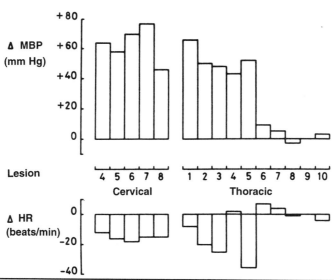

Figure 5. Changes in mean blood pressure (MBP) and heart rate (HR) in patients with spinal cord lesions at different levels (cervical and thoracic) after urinary bladder stimulation induced by suprapubic percussion of the anterior abdominal wall. In the cervical and high thoracic lesions, there is a marked elevation in blood pressure and a fall in heart rate. In patients with lesions below T5 there are minimal cardiovascular changes (reprinted with permission from Mathias CJ and Frankel HL. The neurological and hormonal control of blood vessels and heart in spinal man. J. Autonomic Nervous Syst. (suppl), 1986, 457–64).

The reverse may occur, causing **hyperthermia** because of the inability to sweat and to reflexly vasodilate in the periphery, as needed to lose heat.

Maintenance of environmental temperature therefore is of critical importance. With hyperthermia tepid sponging, increasing air flow with a fan to accelerate heat loss, and in severe cases ice-cooled saline by intravenous infusion or urinary bladder irrigation may be needed.

Gastrointestinal System

In the early stages of spinal cord injury, there is vagal hyperactivity which may contribute to acid hypersecretion, with gastric ulceration and hemorrhage. **H2 receptor antagonists,** or allied agents, need to be used prophylactically. In high lesions **paralytic ileus** may occur; the mechanisms are unclear and often follow ingestion of solid food, which should be avoided. Large bowel dysfunction is common and adequate training, together with the use of an appropriate diet, mild laxatives, and stool softeners may be needed.

Urinary System

In the early stages **bladder atony** occurs, with urinary retention, bladder distention, and urinary overflow. With recovery of isolated cord function, the bladder can be trained to be an automated reflex or **neurogenic bladder.** Catheters should ideally be used intermittently in the early stages. Urinary infection in skin, bone, and other tissues may cause **secondary amyloidosis,** with renal infiltration and serious sequelae.

Reproductive System

In the male, sexual function is affected, especially in the early stages, with both **erectile** and **ejaculatory failure.** In the chronic phase, **priapism** may occur during **autonomic dysreflexia.** Ejaculation, if it occurs, is often retrograde. Various approaches, which include electrical stimulation and collection of seminal fluid, have been used for artificial insemination.

In women, **menstrual cycle disruption** often occurs in the early stages. There is usually recovery within a year, and successful pregnancy has occurred in both tetraplegics and paraplegics. In high lesions, severe autonomic dysreflexia may accompany **uterine contractions.** Such patients are particularly prone, with the elevation of blood pressure, to epileptic seizures and cerebral hemorrhage. It is essential to lower their blood pressure. A combination of anticonvulsant (such as **phenytoin**) and agents to reduce spinal cord activity (such as **spinal anesthetics**) may be needed along with other agents to control blood pressure.

Reference

1. Mathias CJ, Frankel HL. Autonomic disturbances in spinal cord lesions. In: Bannister R, Mathias CJ, eds. Autonomic failure: Textbook of clinical disorders of the autonomic nervous system, 3rd edition. Oxford: Oxford University Press, 1992:839–81.

Peripheral Autonomic Disorders

47 Pure Autonomic Failure

Irwin J. Schatz
University of Hawaii John A. Burns School of Medicine
Department of Medicine
Honolulu, Hawaii

Clinical Description

Pure autonomic failure (PAF, idiopathic orthostatic hypotension, Bradbury–Eggleston syndrome), a form of **neurogenic orthostatic hypotension (OH)**, affects men slightly more often than women, usually in middle age. Its onset is slow and insidious; the patient will often recall that symptoms first came on several years prior to seeking help, but they were considered minor at the time. Unsteadiness, dizziness, or **faintness upon standing,** worse in the morning, after meals or exercise, or in hot weather usually causes the patient to seek advice. Close questioning often will reveal **aching in the neck or occiput** when dizzy; patients learn that lying down relieves these symptoms. A decreased ability to sweat may be apparent; this is noticed particularly in hot climates.

Men found to have PAF may have sought advice about **urinary tract symptoms,** including hesitancy, urgency, dribbling, and occasional incontinence. Other forms of autonomic disturbance may also be apparent: **impotence,** erectile and ejaculatory dysfunction, an inability to appreciate orgasm, and **retrograde ejaculation.** Women may experience **urinary retention** or **incontinence** as early symptoms. Evidence of normal sympathetic and parasympathetic activity, such as nausea and pallor, may not occur when expected, since these functions require an intact autonomic nervous system. Of significance are negative findings: there should be no indication from the history or physical examination of cerebellar, striatal, pyramidal, and extrapyramidal dysfunction. If present, **hoarseness** (due to vocal abductor cord paresis) and **sleep apnea** are two unusual symptoms highly suggestive of Multiple System Atrophy (MSA, Shy–Drager syndrome); they should point to that disorder and not PAF.

Definitive diagnosis of **hypotension** as the cause of orthostatic symptoms is usually made by the demonstration of a decline in systolic blood pressure of 20 mm Hg and diastolic blood pressure of 10 mm Hg after at least 1 min of standing. A tilt table may also be used for this purpose, but is not necessary. The diagnosis cannot be excluded on the basis of a single measurement of upright blood pressure which does not fulfill these criteria. Either the patient should be instructed to measure and record blood pressure at home accurately, or several measurements of orthostatic blood pressure should be made by the physician or other health personnel, preferably early in the morning or after a meal. The demonstration of a repeatedly normal blood pressure response to standing excludes OH; nonetheless, autonomic failure occasionally may be present in its early forms in the absence of a substantial drop in postural blood pressure. Although patients may present initially with autonomic dysfunction and no signs of a disturbance of blood pressure control, it is difficult to confirm a diagnosis of PAF in the absence of OH.

Differential Diagnosis

It is crucial that this syndrome be distinguished from two other important forms of neurogenic OH: MSA and idiopathic parkinsonism (IP) with OH. PAF is less progressive and generally induces less disabling symptoms than do these other syndromes. Accordingly, it is vital that the physician make a distinction among these three important neurogenic causes of OH, so that a correct prognosis is provided to the patient for appropriate lifestyle planning.

Patients with PAF most often will have a prolonged and sometimes stable course; accordingly, statements about their future from their caregivers should reflect that this is a chronic illness which may be characterized by periods of both stability and slow progression.

Clinical Distinctions

PAF is a disease of the peripheral sympathetic nervous system; the postganglionic neurons are affected. Accordingly, there should be no symptoms or signs of cerebellar, striatal, extrapyramidal, or pyramidal tract dysfunction. The presence of such signs may occasionally present some time after the initial manifestations of orthostatic hypotension and/or urinary bladder incompetence. In such patients, an initial diagnosis of PAF must be changed to MSA or IP when these newer manifestations of central nervous system disease become apparent. It is incumbent upon physicians to make a meticulous search for CNS disorders before diagnosing PAF. However, clinical evidence of IP preceded the initial manifestations of autonomic failure by 5 years in a group of representative patients studied in the United Kingdom.

Catecholamine Studies

PAF patients have extraordinarily low recumbent **plasma norepinephrine** levels, whereas these should be near normal in MSA or IP patients. This is a valuable and relatively commonplace method of laboratory confirmation of the diagnosis.

Upon standing, there should be little increase in plasma norepinephrine; this indicates an inability in PAF patients to stimulate the release of catecholamines. Patients with MSA or IP may have a somewhat decreased ability to elevate catecholamines upon standing but this is not as marked as is seen in PAF patients.

When norepinephrine is infused into PAF patients, there will be an abnormally exaggerated increase in blood pressure, reflecting an excessive sensitivity of **postsynaptic receptors** to exogenous catecholamines. Again, MSA and IP patients will have a slightly increased blood pressure response to infused norepinephrine (Table 1), but generally not as marked as that seen in PAF and not characterized by a leftward shift in the dose–response curve.

Table 1. Measurement of Plasma Norepinephrine (NE) and Response to Exogenous Catecholamines in PAF and SDS

	PAF	SDS
Plasma NE with patient recumbent	Very low	Normal
Plasma NE when patient stands	Minimal or no increase	Subnormal increase
NE infusion	Very marked increase in blood pressure	Modest increase in blood pressure

Note. Adapted from Schatz IJ. Orthostatic hypotension, 1st edition, p. 60. Philadelphia: F.A. Davis.

Recent data suggest that β-adrenergic receptor supersensitivity is present to a greater degree in PAF patients than in those with MSA. These conclusions were derived from a study of the use of intravenous **isoproterenol** in patients with various forms of autonomic failure and in control subjects. The slopes of the blood pressure dose–response relationships were more negative in patients with MSA and PAF than in controls, consistent with impaired baroreflex modulation. A further shift to the left in patients with PAF indicated β-adrenergic receptor supersensitivity.

Response to Food

IP patients will have a much less extensive and dramatic drop in blood pressure when given a measured food load compared to MSA and PAF patients. This may be a useful clinical tool in differentiating these syndromes, for occasional patients with mild parkinsonism and significant orthostatic hypotension are difficult to distinguish from MSA patients.

Diagnostic Imaging Techniques

The most accurate method of distinguishing between PAF and MSA patients consists of the use of computed tomography, magnetic resonance imaging, and positron emission tomography, as reported recently. MSA patients show **cerebellar atrophy, signal hypointensity,** and a generalized reduction in glucose utilization rate. Decreased glucose utilization indicates hypometabolism; this was seen most prominently in the cerebellum, brainstem, striatum, and frontal and motor cortices in the MSA patients. None of these findings were present in patients with PAF. Obviously, most clinicians will not utilize complex and expensive imaging techniques to make this distinction, since a clinical differentiation is usually possible. Occasionally, however, a patient may insist on accumulating as much information about his/her prognosis as is possible; in such instances, utilization of at least computer tomography and magnetic resonance imaging may be justified. Patients with PAF will have demonstrable disturbance in laboratory tests designed to detect autonomic dysfunction (see Chapter 20).

Management

An important aspect of treatment in these patients is patient education. There must be full understanding of the relatively benign nature of PAF, and the fact that although potentially disabling, it rarely will lead to death. As with all other chronic and disabling illnesses, patients should understand the likely natural course of their illness and learn to live within the limitations imparted by their disability. Strong reassurance and the presence of similarly afflicted patients in support groups will be of inestimable value in management.

See Chapters 65–68 for a discussion of nonpharmacologic and pharmacologic approaches to therapy.

References

1. Bradbury S, Eggleston C. Postural hypotension: A report of three cases. Am Heart J 1925;I:75–86.
2. Schatz IJ. Orthostatic hypotension. I. Functional and neurogenic causes. Arch Int Med 1984;144:773–7.
3. Bannister R. Chapter 15 in: Autonomic failure: clinical features of autonomic failure, 2nd edition. London: Oxford University Press, 1988: 281.
4. Polinsky RJ, *et al*. Pharmacologic distinction of different orthostatic hypotension syndromes. Neurology 1981;31:1–7.
5. Baser SM, Brown RT, Curras MT, Baucom CE, Hooper DR, Polinsky RJ: Beta receptor sensitivity in autonomic failure. Neurology 1991;41:1107–12.
6. Thomaides T, Bleasdale-Barr K, Chaudhuri K, Pavitt D. Cardiovascular and hormonal responses to liquid food challenge in idiopathic Parkinson's disease, multiple system atrophy, and pure autonomic failure. Neurology 1993;43(5):900–4.
7. Fulham MJ, Dubinsky RM, Polinsky RJ, Brooks RA. Computed tomography, magnetic resonance imaging and positron emission tomography with (18F) fluorodeoxyglucose in multiple system atrophy and pure autonomic failure. Clin Auton Res 1991;1:27–36.

48

Familial Dysautonomia

Felicia B. Axelrod
Pediatrics
New York University School of Medicine
New York, New York

Familial dysautonomia (FD, Riley–Day syndrome), is an inherited neurologic disease affecting the development and survival of sensory, sympathetic, and some parasympathetic neurons. FD is the best known of the group of disorders referred to as hereditary sensory and autonomic neuropathies

(HSAN), which are generally characterized by widespread sensory dysfunction and variable autonomic dysfunction.

The pervasive nature of the autonomic nervous system results in protean functional abnormalities. Signs of the disorder are present from birth, and neurologic function slowly deteriorates with age so that symptoms and problems vary with time. The disease process cannot be arrested. Treatment is preventative, symptomatic, and supportive. It must be directed toward specific problems which can vary considerably among patients and at different ages.

Genetics and Diagnosis

FD is an **autosomal recessive disorder** which currently appears confined to individuals of **Ashkenazi Jewish** extraction. In this population, the carrier rate has been estimated to be 1 in 30, with a disease frequency of 1 in 3600 live births. Utilizing genetic linkage, the gene has been localized to the distal long arm of chromosome 9 (q31) with sufficient DNA markers to permit prenatal diagnosis and carrier identification for families in which there has been an affected individual.

Although penetrance is complete, there is marked variability in expression of the disease. Diagnosis is based upon clinical recognition of both sensory and autonomic dysfunction. The combination of the five "cardinal" criteria, i.e., **alacrima, absent fungiform papillae** (Fig. 1), **depressed patellar reflexes, abnormal histamine test,** (Fig. 2) and **pupillary hypersensitivity** to parasympathomimetic agents (pilocarpine 0.0625%), in an individual of Ashkenazi Jewish extraction is usually sufficient to make the diagnosis. Further supportive evidence is provided by findings of decreased response to pain and temperature, orthostatic hypotension, periodic erythematous blotching of the skin, and increased sweating. In addition, cinesophagrams may reveal delay in cricopharyngeal closure, tertiary contractions of the esophagus, gastroesophageal reflux, and delayed gastric emptying. Sural nerve biopsy is rarely required unless one of the five "cardinal" criteria is not present or the patient is not of Jewish extraction.

Sural Nerve Pathology

The sural nerve fascicular area is reduced and contains markedly diminished numbers of nonmyelinated and small-diameter myelinated axons. Catecholamine-containing fibers are missing. Even in the youngest subject extensive pathology is evident.

Spinal Cord Pathology

Intrauterine development and postnatal maintenance of dorsal root ganglion neurons are abnormal. The **dorsal root ganglia** are grossly reduced in size due to decreased neuronal population. Within the spinal cord, lateral root entry

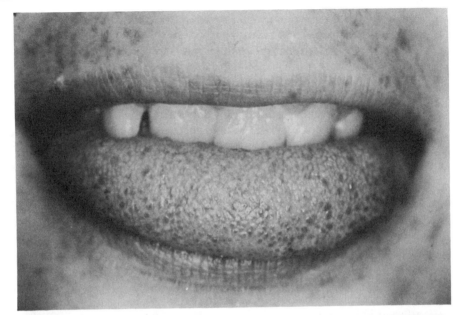

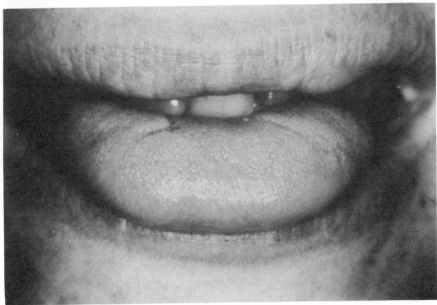

Figure 1. (A) Normal tongue with fungiform papillae present on the tip. (B) Dysautonomic tongue.

zones and **Lissauer's tracts** are severely depleted of axons. With increasing age, there is further depletion of neurons in dorsal root ganglia and an increase in residual **nodules of Nageotte.** In addition, loss of dorsal column myelinated axons becomes evident in older patients. Diminution of primary substance P axons in the **substantia gelatinosa** of spinal cord and medulla has been demonstrated using immunohistochemistry.

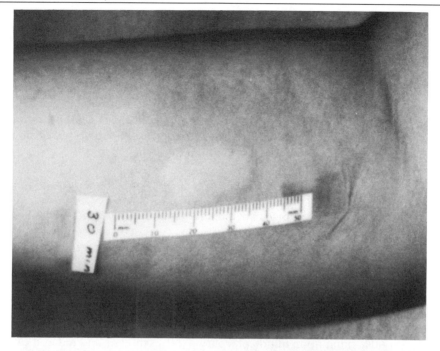

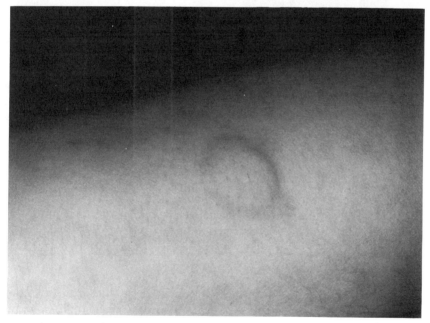

Figure 2. (A) Normal histamine test. Reaction displays diffuse axon flare around a central wheal. (B) Dysautonomic histamine test. Only a narrow areola surrounds the wheal.

Sympathetic Nervous System Pathology

In adult patients with FD, the mean volume of superior cervical sympathetic ganglia is reduced to 34% of the normal size reflecting severe decrease in number of neurons. The anatomical defect in the ganglion cells extends to preganglionic neurons as the intermediolateral gray columns of the spinal cord also contain low number of neurons. **Tyrosine hydroxylase,** as measured by immunocytochemical techniques, can identify catecholaminergic neurons which produce dopamine. Although clinical, anatomic, biochemical, and pharmacologic data suggest diminution in the numbers of sympathetic neurons in FD, staining for tyrosine hydroxylase is enhanced in FD neurons from sympathetic ganglia. Ultrastructural study of peripheral blood vessels demonstrates the absence of autonomic nerve terminals.

Parasympathetic Nervous System

Parasympathetic ganglia are minimally affected. The sphenopalatine ganglia are consistently reduced in sized with low total neuronal counts, but the neuronal population is only questionably reduced in other parasympathetic ganglia, such as the ciliary ganglia.

Biochemical Data

Consistent with the decrease in the sympathetic neuronal population, there is a 60% diminution in norepinephrine (NE) synthesis and reduced catabolite excretion. However, dopamine products continue to be excreted in normal amounts resulting in a reduced 3-methoxy-4-hydroxymandelic acid (VMA) to 3-methoxy-4-hydroxyphenylacetic acid (HVA) ratios. In addition, there is no appropriate increase in plasma levels of NE and dopamineβ-hydroxylase (DBH) when the FD patient goes from supine to standing position, but during **emotional crises** plasma NE and dopamine are markedly elevated. During such crises, **vomiting** usually coincides with high dopamine levels. The high NE may appear through peripheral conversion of dopamine by DBH. **Diazepam** sedates patients in crises and relieves vomiting, possibly by blocking the release of dopamine.

Supine early morning plasm renin activity is elevated in FD subjects and the release of renin and aldosterone is not coordinated. In FD individuals with supine hypertension, an increase in plasm atrial natriuretic peptide (ANP) occurs. The combination of these factors may explain the exaggerated nocturnal urine volume and increased excretion of salt in some FD individuals.

Clinical Symptoms and Treatment

There is a baseline neurological dysfunction and slow degeneration with age in FD (Table 1). In addition, the pervasive nature of the autonomic nervous system results in protean functional abnormalities involving other systems. FD patients also are susceptible to periodic autonomic storms, termed **dysautonomic crises** (Table 2). The crises are a systemic reaction to stress, either physical or emotional. At the present time, the disease process cannot be arrested. Treatment is preventative, symptomatic, and supportive. It must be directed toward specific problems within each system which vary considerably among patients and with different ages.

Table 1. Neurologic Abnormalities

Sensory system
    *Pain loss sparing hands, soles of feet, neck, and genital areas
    *Temperature appreciation abnormal on the trunk and lower extremities
    Patellar reflexes depressed
    Insensitivity to fractures/Charcot joints
Autonomic system
    Oropharyngeal incoordination (feeding problems, especially liquids)
    *Esophageal dysmotility, gastroesophageal reflux
    Insensitivity to hypercapnia and hypoxia
    Breath-holding
    *Postural hypotension without compensatory tachycardia
    *Supine hypertension
Motor system
    Hypotonia
    Mild/moderate development delay
    *Gait often broad based or mildly ataxic
    *Spinal curvature (95%, especially kyphosis)
Cranial nerves
    No overflow tears
    Taste deficient, especially sweet
    Corneal reflexes depressed/corneal ulcerations
    *Optic nerve atrophy
    Exotropia, myopia
    Speech frequently dysarthric and nasal
Intelligence/personality
    Usually normal intelligence (verbal skills better than motor)
    Tend to be concrete or literal
    Skin picking (especially fingers and nose)
    *Resistant to change (some patients are phobic)

    * Progressive neurologic abnormalities.

Signs of the disorder are present from birth with **oropharyngeal incoordination** as one of the earliest signs. Poor sucking or discoordinated swallowing is observed in 60% of infants in the neonatal period. Oropharyngeal incoordination often persists and puts the patient at risk for **aspiration pneumonia**, the major cause of lung infections. If thickening of formula and different nipples are ineffective, then gastrostomy may be necessary. If gastroesphageal reflux is

Table 2. Autonomic Crisis Features

Excessive sweating of head and trunk
Erythematous blotching of face and trunk
Mottling of peripheral extremities (cutis marmorata)
Hypertension and tachycardia
Nausea/vomiting
Severe dysphagia/drooling
Irritability
Insomnia
Worsening of tone

present, the risk for aspiration increases. If medical management with prokinetic agents, H2 antagonists, thickening of feeds, and position is not successful, then surgical intervention, **fundoplication**, is performed. Failure of medical management would result in persistence of pneumonia, hematemesis, or apnea.

Crises, associated with vomiting, occur in approximately 40% of the FD patients. They have been managed most effectively with a combination of intravenous or rectally administered diazepam (0.2 mg/kg q3h), chloral hydrate rectal suppositories (30 mg/kg q6h), and avoidance of dehydration and aspiration.

As FD patients have decreased sensitivity to hypoxia and hypercapnia, tachypnea is rarely seen with respiratory infections. Other frequent manifestations include hypotonia, delayed developmental milestones, labile body temperature and blood pressure, absence of overflow tears and corneal anesthesia, marked diaphoresis with excitement, breath-holding episodes, ataxia, spinal curvature, and intractable vomiting.

Clinical manifestations of **orthostatic hypotension** definitely worsen with age and include episodes of lightheadedness or dizzy spells. Some patients complain of "weak legs." Frequently, the low pressures are not appreciated by the patient although they will list forward when standing or walking. Infrequently there is syncope. Orthostatic hypotension is treated by maintaining adequate hydration as monitored by blood urea nitrogen levels. Lower extremity exercises are encouraged to increase muscle tone and promote venous return. Elastic stockings and fludrocortisone have also been of some benefit.

Renal function also appears to deteriorate with advancing age, as indicated by slowly rising serum urea and creatinine. Pathological studies reveal excess glomerulosclerosis. Although the cause of the progressive renal disease is not certain, hypoperfusion of the kidney seems a likely explanation. Hypoperfusion could occur because of dehydration, postural hypotension, or vasoconstriction of renal vessels as a result of sympathetic supersensitivity during vomiting crisis.

Sexual maturation is frequently delayed, but primary and secondary sex characteristics eventually develop in both sexes. Women with dysautonomia have conceived and delivered normal infants. Pregnancies were tolerated well. At time of delivery blood pressures were labile. One male has fathered six children.

Prognosis

With greater understanding of the disorder and development of treatment programs, survival statistics have markedly improved so that increasing numbers of patients are reaching adulthood. Survival statistics prior to 1960 reveal that 50% of patients died before 5 years of age. Current survival statistics indicate that a newborn with FD has a 50% probability of reaching 30 years of age. Many of the adults have been able to achieve independent function. Patients have even married and reproduced with all offspring being phenotypically normal despite their obligatory heterozygote state. Causes of death are less often related to pulmonary complications indicating that more aggressive treatment of aspirations has been beneficial. Of recent concern have been the patients who have succumbed to unexplained deaths which may have been the result of unopposed vagal stimulation or a sleep abnormality. A few adult patients have died of renal failure.

References

1. Axelrod FB, Nachtgall R, Dancis J. Familial dysautonomia: diagnosis, pathogenesis and management. In: Schulman I, ed. Advances in pediatrics, Vol. 21. Chicago: Yearbook, 1974:75–96.
2. Axelrod FB, Iyer K, Fish I, Pearson J, Stein ME, Spielholz N. Progressive sensory loss in familial dysautonomia. Pediatrics 1981;65:517–22.
3. Blumenfeld A, Slaugenhaupt SA, Axelrod FB, Lucente De, Maayan CH, Lieberg CB, Ozelius LJ, Trofatter JA, Haines JL, Breakefield XO, Gusella JF. Localization of the gene for familial dysautonomia on Chromosome 9 and definition of DNA markers for genetic diagnosis. Nature Genet 1993;4:160–4.
4. Pearson J, Axelrod FB, Dancis J. Current concepts of dysautonomia neurological defects. Ann NY Acad Sci 1974;228:288–300.
5. Ziegler MG, Lake RC, Kopin IJ. Deficient sympathetic nervous system response in familial dysautonomia. N Engl J Med 1976;294:630–3.

49 *Hereditary Autonomic Neuropathies*

Yadollah Harati
Baylor College of Medicine
Houston, Texas

Aziz Taher Shaibani
Department of Neurology
Baylor College of Medicine
Houston, Texas

There are few inherited peripheral neuropathies in which autonomic dysfunction, whether clinical or subclinical, is detected (Table 1). Autonomic abnormalities are frequent and prominent in **familial dysautonomia** and **amyloidosis**, reviewed separately in Chapters 48 and 50. In this chapter the remaining inherited neuropathies with autonomic involvement will be discussed.

Fabry's Disease

Fabry's disease or Anderson–Fabry's disease (**angiokeratoma corporis diffusum**) is an X-linked recessive, slowly progressive metabolic disorder with protean and nonspecific clinical manifestations. Although the skin, kidney, heart, and peripheral and central nervous system are the most frequently involved organs, autonomic dysfunction may also be present. The clinical manifestations of the disease in the affected hemizygous males result from progressive and widespread accumulation of neutral glycosphingolipids, due to α-galactosyl deficiency, in the lysosomes of vascular endothelial, smooth muscle and other

Table 1. **Inherited Peripheral Neuropathies with Dysautonomia**

1. Hereditary sensory and autonomic neuropathies type I, II, III[a] (see Chapter 48), IV, and V
2. Hereditary motor–sensory neuropathy type I and II (Charcot Marie Tooth disease 1,2)
3. **Fabry's disease**[a]
4. Multiple endocrine neoplasia type 2B (MEN 2B)
5. **Amyloidosis**[a] (see Chapter 50)
6. Porphyrias[a]

[a] Dysautonomia is prominent and clinically significant.

cells, ganglia, and body fluids. The classically affected males have no detectable α-galactosidase activity with the onset of disease manifestation in childhood or adolescence. Variants and milder forms of the disease in which residual enzyme activity may be detected have been reported. The gene for the enzyme has been mapped to the region between Xq21.33 and Xq22 of the long arm of the X-chromosome. Thus far, over 30 different small mutations in this gene have been reported.

Clinical Manifestations of Fabry's Disease

The most prominent and frequent clinical presentation of the disease includes bouts of **severe painful burning sensation** in the hands and feet, a reddish purple maculopapular rash (angiokeratoma) of lower abdomen, pelvic, genital, and upper thigh regions and, at times, in oral mucosa and conjunctive, hypohidrosis, and lenticular and corneal opacities. Any boy or young male who presents with severe painful sensory neuropathy should be suspected as having Fabry's disease and careful scrutiny for the skin lesions should be conducted as typical skin lesions are usually sparse and may be easily overlooked. Triggering factors for the episodic pain include fatigue, exercise, emotional stress, and rapid changes in temperature and humidity. The pathophysiological events leading to the incapacitating episodes of pain or acroparesthesias have not been clarified.

Early albuminuria, uremia, renal failure, cardiomyopathy, cardiac hypertrophy, conduction abnormalities, aortic degeneration, hypertension, and mitral valve thickening, atrioventricular block, and supraventricular arrhythmias may occur. Short P–R interval, ST–T changes, and left ventricular hypertrophy are common EKG abnormalities of Fabry's disease. Although cardiac involvement is a constant feature of Fabry's disease, most patients do not experience cardiac symptoms until late in the disease course. Cerebrovascular disease secondary to multifocal abnormalities of large and small vessels may also occur. In young male patients with unexplained cardiovascular abnormalities and a history of acroparesthesia, angiokeratoma, and ophthalmologic findings the diagnosis of Fabry's disease should always be considered. Ocular manifestations involving the cornea, lens, conjunctiva, and retina are early and prominent, but require slit lamp microscopic evaluation.

Involvement of many other tissues and organs results in a variety of symptoms and signs, including **gastrointestinal** (episodic diarrhea, abdominal cramps, achalasia), **musculoskeletal** (bony deformities), **hematopoietic** (anemia, foamy macrophages, iron deficiency), pulmonary, vestibular, and auditory symptoms.

Autonomic Involvement

Although there are many reports of structural abnormalities of the autonomic nervous system in Fabry's disease, overt clinical autonomic dysfunction is not commonly observed. The contribution of autonomic dysfunction to the overall morbidity of Fabry's disease is unknown.

Anhidrosis or hypohidrosis and possibly the episodic pain are probably caused by the involvement of sympathetic ganglion cells and degeneration of unmyelinated nerve fibers. Both glycosphingolipid accumulation and vascular ischemia appear to play a role in the abnormalities of autonomic ganglia. There is a preferential loss of small myelinated and unmyelinated fibers in the sural nerve biopsies. Detailed clinical autonomic testing has shown involvement of both sympathetic and parasympathetic systems, the latter being more readily demonstrated. Diminished pupillary responses to pilocarpine, impaired gastrointestinal motility, and reduced tear and saliva formation may be observed early. Sympathetic dysfunction is evident by the loss of the cutaneous flare response to scratch and histamine and the absence of thermal finger-tip wrinkling. Blood pressure and heart rate and plasma norepinephrine responses to tilt are usually intact. Accumulation of ceramide trihexose in the myenteric nerve plexi throughout the gut results in disturbances in peristalsis and gastrocolic reflexes in over 60% of hemizygous patients. Intestinal dysmotility may produce areas of high intraluminal pressure allowing the formation of diverticula. Intestinal stasis and bacterial overgrowth will produce diarrhea.

There is no effective treatment for the autonomic dysfunction observed in Fabry's disease. It has been suggested that carbamazepine used in the treatment of episodic pain may result in a dose-dependent aggravation of autonomic dysfunction including urinary retention, nausea, vomiting, and ileus.

A successful renal transplantation not only corrects the renal function but may also result in relief from acroparesthesia and pain and a partial restoration of sweating. Enzyme replacement, especially when obtained from human placenta, has been feasibly used in the treatment of Fabry's disease in a few patients in an experimental trial.

Porphyria

Acute hepatic porphyrias (**acute intermittent porphyria, variegate porphyria, and hereditary coproporphyria**) are a group of autosomal dominantly inherited metabolic disorders that manifest as acute or subacute, severe, life-threatening motor neuropathy, abdominal pain, autonomic dysfunction, and neuropsychiatric manifestations. Its gene is thought to be present in 1/80,000 people, though only 1/3 of affected persons ever manifest symptoms of the disease. The basic defect is a 50% reduction in **porphobilinogen deaminase** activity (acute intermittent porphyria), **protoporphyrinogen-IX oxidase** (variegate porphyria), and **coproporphyrinogen oxidase** (coproporphyria) resulting in abnormalities of heme synthesis. In the presence of sufficient endogenous or exogenous stimuli (e.g., drugs, hormones, menstruation, starvation), this partial deficiency may lead to clinical manifestations.

Clinical Manifestation of Porphyria

The neurologic manifestations of all forms of the acute porphyrias are identical. Symptoms of the acute attack include severe **abdominal pain, nausea, vomiting,** pain in limbs and back, constipation, urinary frequency and hesitancy, diarrhea, convulsions, and abnormal behavior. Abdominal pain and ileus may occur several days before neurological manifestations. Porphyria affects predominantly motor nerves, often leading to proximal, facial, and bulbar weakness. It usually develops within 2 to 3 days of the onset of abdominal pain and psychiatric symptoms and may begin in the upper limbs with wrist and finger extensor weakness or with cranial nerve dysfunction. The progression of weakness to trunk and respiratory muscles may resemble Guillain–Barré syndrome, but the ascending pattern of weakness is rare, cerebrospinal fluid is usually normal, and in some patients the reflexes remain intact. The nerve conduction velocities in porphyria are not slowed to the levels observed in demyelinating lesions. The mechanism of the neuropathic changes is poorly understood, although there is some evidence that heme pathway intermediates such as delta-aminolevulinic acid and porphyrins may be neurotoxic.

Autonomic Involvement in Porphyria

Autonomic disturbances are prevalent immediately before and during the attacks of porphyrias, suggesting a greater and earlier susceptibility of the autonomic nerves. Persistent **sinus tachycardia** invariably precedes the development of peripheral neuropathy and respiratory paralysis, and, along with **labile hypertension,** may be explained by damage to vagus or glossopharyngeal nerves, their nuclei, or central connections. Tachycardia and hypertension may be associated with increased catecholamine release and urinary excretion, suggesting increased peripheral sympathetic activity. Patients may have chronic hypertension between the attacks leading to renal function impairment. **Orthostatic hypotension** may occur in acute attacks of **variegate porphyria.** Employment of a battery of baroreflex tests during the acute attack reveals mostly reversible parasympathetic or sympathetic dysfunction. The parasympathetic tests, however, become abnormal earlier and more frequently than sympathetic tests. The immediate response of heart rate to standing (30:15 ratio) or the Valsalva maneuver may be mildly abnormal in asymptomatic subjects with **acute intermittent porphyria,** suggesting the occurrence of a subclinical autonomic neuropathy in latent porphyrics.

Gastrointestinal disturbances including abdominal pain, severe vomiting, obstinate constipation, intestinal dilatation, and stasis may be explained by the impaired gut motor activity due to autonomic and/or enteric nerve damage. Studies on impaired proximal gastrointestinal tract motility and reduced circulating gut peptides in a few patients with acute intermittent porphyria tend to support this hypothesis. Other autonomic dysfunctions observed in acute intermittent porphyrias include sweating disturbances, pupillary dilation, and hesitancy in micturition and bladder distention.

Limited pathologic studies of the autonomic nervous system in acute intermittent porphyrias have revealed lesions of vagus nerve including axonal degeneration and demyelination, and chromatolysis of dorsal nuclei and sympathetic chain as well as the splanchnic motor cells of the lateral horns and cells of the celiac ganglion.

Treatment of Porphyria

With modern intensive care techniques and the advent of **hematin** therapy the mortality rate for acute intermittent porphyrias is less than 10%. Porphyrogenic drug avoidance, very high glucose intake, vitamin B6, β blockers, analgesics, selective anticonvulsants, and hematin therapy (2–5 mg/kg/day intravenously for 3–14 days) are the mainstays of therapy. Recovery from psychiatric and autonomic dysfunction is usually rapid. All at-risk relatives should be screened for the latent disease.

Multiple Endocrine Neoplasia Type 2B (MEN 2B)

Multiple endocrine neoplasia type 2 syndromes are neural crest disorders. The MEN type 2 syndromes comprise clinically related autosomal dominant cancer syndromes. MEN type 2A (**Sipple syndrome**) is characterized by **medullary thyroid carcinoma, pheochromocytoma** in about 50% of cases, and **parathyroid hyperplasia** or adenoma in about 25%. MEN 2B is similar to MEN 2A but is characterized by earlier age of tumor onset and the developmental abnormalities, which include **intestinal ganglioneuromatosis, atypical facies** with mucosal neuromas of distal tongue and subconjunctiva, **marfanoid habitus, muscle underdevelopment,** and **bony deformities.**

Autonomic manifestations of MEN 2B are not prominent and are generally overshadowed by its other symptoms and signs. They include **impaired lacrimation, orthostatic hypotension, impaired reflex vasodilatation** of skin, and parasympathetic **denervation supersensitivity of pupils,** with intact sweating and salivary gland function. There are gross and microscopic abnormalities of the peripheral autonomic nervous system with both sympathetic and parasympathetic systems affected. There is disorganized hypertrophy and proliferation of autonomic nerves and ganglia (**ganglioneuromatosis**). Neural proliferation of the alimentary tract (**Auerbach** and **Meissner's** plexi), upper respiratory tract, bladder, prostate, and skin may also be seen. Nerve biopsy shows degeneration and regeneration of unmyelinated fibers.

Genetic linkage studies of MEN has mapped the gene responsible for this syndrome to the pericentromeric region of **chromosome 10**. This region also contains the RET proto- oncogene, which codes for a receptor tyrosine kinase.

Different missense mutation within RET proto-oncogene is thought to be responsible for MEN 2A and 2B.

The prognosis in the MEN 2B syndrome is generally poor as a result of an aggressive **medullary thyroid carcinoma,** that develops earlier in life than in patients with MEN 2A (5 years survival of 78% for MEN 2B and 86% for 2A). This can be improved by regular screening of patients at risk; early diagnosis allows thyroidectomy and/or adrenalectomy which are likely to be curative.

Hereditary Motor and Sensory Neuropathies Type I and II (Charcot Marie Tooth "CMT," 1 and 2)

Clinically significant autonomic dysfunction is not a common feature of CMT 1 and 2. When a battery of autonomic function tests is systematically employed in patients with well-established CMT abnormalities of sudomotor and local vasomotor responses, heart rate, and blood pressure changes, pupillary abnormalities and impaired tear production may be observed, suggesting involvement of postganglionic sympathetic and parasympathetic nerve fibers. Sural nerve biopsies may show abnormalities of unmyelinated nerve fibers, explaining the frequently observed abnormalities of sweat function tests.

Type I, II, IV, and V Hereditary Sensory and Autonomic Neuropathy (HSAN)

Type I HSAN with a dominant and type II with a probable autosomal recessive inheritance pattern exhibit no significant autonomic dysfunction except for hypohidrosis. Type IV shares some of the features of types II and III, but the patients may have episodes of fever, low IQ, severe hypohidrosis, and markedly reduced pain perception. The inheritance pattern is probably autosomal recessive. There is a marked loss of small myelinated and unmyelinated nerve fibers. Type V presents with selective loss of extremity pain perception and thermal discrimination and impaired sudomotor function. Sural nerve biopsy reveals selective loss of small myelinated fibers with only a slightly decreased number of larger myelinated fibers.

References

1. Desnick RJ, Ioannov YA, Eng CM. Alpha-galactosidase A deficiency: Fabry disease. In: Scriver CR, Beaudet AL, Sly WS, Valle D. eds. The metabolic basis of inherited disease New York: McGraw–Hill, 1995: 2741–84.
2. Cable WL, Kolodny EH, Adams RD. Fabry disease: impaired autonomic function. Neurology 1982;32:498–502.
3. Desnick RJ, Anderson K. Heme biosynthesis and its disorders; the porphyrias and sideroblastic anemias. In Hoffman R, Benz EJ, Shattil SJ, Furie B, Cohen H, eds. Hematology, basic principles and practice New York: Churchill Livingstone, 1991: 350–67.
4. Gorchein A. Autonomic neuropathy in porphyria. In: Bannister R, ed. Autonomic failure: a textbook of clinical disorders of autonomic nervous system, 2nd ed. Oxford: Oxford University Press, 1987: 715–32.
5. Dyck PJ, Carney JA, Sizemore GW, *et al.* Multiple endocrine neoplasia, type 2b: phenotype recognition, neurologic features, and their pathologic basis. Ann Neurol 1979;6:302.
6. Harati Y, Low PA. Autonomic peripheral neuropathies: diagnosis and clinical presentation. In: Appel SH, ed. Current neurology. Chicago: YearBook Medical Publishers, 1990: 105–76.

50   *Amyloidotic Autonomic Failure*

Aziz Taher Shaibani
Baylor College of Medicine
Houston, Texas

Yadollah Harati
Baylor College of Medicine
Houston, Texas

Amyloidosis is a multisystem disease caused by extracellular deposition of a homogeneous insoluble protein consisting of polypeptide fibrils arranged in β-pleated sheets which demonstrates **green birefringence** under polarized light after Congo red staining. In this condition, amyloid deposits may be widespread (**systemic amyloidosis**) or restricted to certain organs (**localized amyloidosis**). Unfortunately, previous classification of systemic amyloidosis has been confusing. Initially, cases were classified as primary amyloidosis, secondary amyloidosis, or familial amyloidosis. "Primary amyloidosis" was applied to cases without an identifiable etiology, while "secondary amyloidosis" described deposition in association with chronic inflammatory diseases. "Familial amyloidosis" was classified according to the initial region of body involvement (upper vs lower extremities), according to the geographical localization of the kindreds (Swedish, German, Japanese, etc.), and numerically (familial amyloid neuropathy type I, II, III, etc.). A recent, much clearer classification is based on the chemical composition of the deposits (Table 1).

The clinical presentation depends on the organs involved and the size of the amyloid fibrils. Involvement of the peripheral nervous system is an important feature of the systemic amyloidoses and typically presents with **the classical clinical triad** of: **small fiber neuropathy, autonomic neuropathy** (AN), and **carpal tunnel syndrome** (CTS). Autonomic failure is an important feature of immunoglobulin-derived amyloidosis and hereditary systemic amyloidosis, and must be considered in all patients with familial or paraproteinemic neuropathies having autonomic dysfunction (especially when CTS coexists). The mechanism of nerve injury is probably the same in all amyloidoses, and involves physical pressure exerted by amyloid deposits on dorsal root ganglia or autonomic ganglia, or directly on nerve fibers. Toxic, ischemic, and immunologic mechanisms have been suggested as alternatives.

The following amyloidoses may demonstrate autonomic involvement:

Immunoglobulin Amyloidosis (AL)

The amyloid fibrils in AL amyloidopathy are composed of immunoglobulin **light chain proteins** or their degradation products. AL is the most common form of systemic amyloidosis and occurs as both primary amyloidosis and amyloidosis associated with **multiple myeloma** (MM), **Waldenstrom's macroglobulinemia, non-Hodgkin's lymphoma,** and solid tumors like **hypernephroma.** In primary amyloidosis, the peripheral nervous system is involved in more than 50% of patients and is the presenting symptom in 40% of those

Table 1.   Classification of Amyloidosis

	Type	Previous name	Subunit protein	PNS involvement	% Total
Systemic amyloidosis	Ig derived (AL)	Primary/myeloma associated	Ig light chain	PN, AN, CTS	71
	Reactive (AA)	Secondary A	Amyloid A.	PN, AN	4
	Dialysis associated		B$_2$-microglobulin	CTS	?
	Hereditary	Heredofamilial			3
		FAP I, II	TTR (see Table 2)	PN, AN, CTS	
		FAP III	Apolipoprotein	PN	
		FAP IV	Gelsolin	PN, CN	
		—	Fibrinogen	None	
		—	Lysosome	None	
Localized amyloidosis					22
	Alzheimer's disease (H,A), HCHA (H), CAA(A), Genitourinary A (A), Lichen A (A), Cutaneous A (H,A), IBM (H,A), Medullary ca. thyroid (H), Bronchopulmonary A (A)				

Note. Ig, immunoglobulin; FAP, familial amyloid neuropathy; PNS, peripheral nervous system; PN, peripheral neuropathy; AN, autonomic neuropathy; CN, cranial neuropathy; CTS, carpal tunnel syndrome; HCHA, hereditary cerebral hemorrhage with amyloidosis; CAA, cerebral amyloid angiopathy; IBM, inclusion body myopathy; H, hereditary; A, acquired.

cases. In amyloidosis associated with multiple myeloma, 13% of patients develop clinical and 40% electrophysiological evidence of polyneuropathy.

The **peripheral neuropathy in AL** is axonal, distal, symmetrical, and sensory with impaired pinprick and temperature more than vibratory and proprioceptive sensations consistent with a **small fiber neuropathy.** As the disease progresses, large fiber involvement appears. Subtle autonomic abnormalities, as detected by autonomic function tests, seem to be prevalent even in asymptomatic patients. Both sympathetic and parasympathetic systems are affected to different extents. Signs of AN include: **orthostatic hypotension** (OH) with inappropriate heart rate response, impotence, dry mouth, and GI autonomic disturbances (dysphagia, early satiety, diarrhea, constipation), sluggish pupillary reaction, impairment of sweating, and bladder dysfunction. Autonomic dysfunction, rather than deposition of amyloid in the mucosa, seems to be a more frequent cause of GI symptoms in these patients. Target organs other than PNS include the heart, skeletal muscles, liver, intestine, spleen, kidney, tongue, and skin.

Pathogenesis

Pathological investigations have shown infiltration of dorsal root and sympathetic ganglia in patients with amyloidotic neuropathy early in the course of the disease. Intermediolateral cell column neurons at the T7 level of the spinal cord may also be reduced.

Diagnosis

Tests of autonomic function are often abnormal. Serum and urine protein electrophoresis detect a **monoclonal gammopathy** in 80% of cases. Erythrocyte sedimentation rate (ESR) is commonly elevated. Anemia and proteinuria are common. Electron microscopic examiantion of the amyloid-laden tissues is the most sensitive method of recognizing this disorder. **Abdominal fat aspiration** and **rectal biopsy** show amyloid in 80% of cases, and bone marrow stains positive for amyloid in 50% of cases. The bone marrow also provides an estimate of the number of the plasma cells. In AL without MM, 3–5% of the bone marrow cells typically are plasma cells with no malignant features. This is increased in AL with MM to more than 50% and many plasma cells display malignant features. Sural nerve biopsy provides another tissue source for diagnosis. In patients suspected of having amyloidosis, any tissue obtained during any surgery (e.g., flexor retinaculum during carpal tunnel surgery) may contain amyloid and should be specifically examined for amyloid deposit.

Treatment

There is no cure for AL. **Metoclopramide** has been used to treat early satiety while **octreotide**, a **somatostatin analog**, has been successfully used to treat amyloidosis-associated diarrhea. **Cisapride** was reported to be useful in intestinal pseudo-obstruction in AL associated with MM. Although **fludrocortisone** is the mainstay of treatment of OH, **midodrine, erythropoietin,** and l-threo-3,4-dihydroxyphenylserine (DOPS) are also reported to be helpful. Other therapies for OH include elastic support extending to the waist and instructions to the patients to rise slowly from the lying position and to sit on the edge of the bed for a few minutes before walking. In patients with syncope, investigation of cardiac arrhythmias or heart block can be life-saving. Treatment of the nonneurologic manifestations of this condition is also symptomatic (diuretics, antiarrhythmics, etc.).

Prognosis

The prognosis of AL remains poor. The 5-year survival rate is only 20%. Patients with MM have a particularly poor prognosis with a median survival of 24–36 months. AL amyloidosis presenting solely as neuropathy has a better prognosis with a median survival of more than 5 years. The influence of the autonomic neuropathy (AN) on the evolution of the disease has been evaluated recently. Median survival from the time of diagnosis of AL patients with AN was 7.3 months vs 14.8 months for those without AN. Patients with prolonged QT on EKG had even shorter survival. Whether the prolonged QT is due to a primary cardiac or autonomic disorder is not clear.

Reactive Amyloidosis (AA)

AA is associated with several chronic inflammatory diseases like rheumatoid arthritis, tuberculosis, leprosy, osteomyelitis, and suppurative infections. The amyloid in these conditions contains a degradation product of acute phase serum protein. AN has been reported only rarely in association with this type of amyloidosis, and no studies are available concerning its course and pathology.

Hereditary Amyloidosis

This variety is described in many kindreds from around the world and is often named after the primarily affected organs (renal, cardiac, cerebral, neuropathic, etc.). The most common type is **familial amyloidotic polyneuropathy** (FAP). All types of FAP are autosomal dominant and cause symptoms from the third to seventh decades of life. At least six types of protein variants have been described in association with FAP (Table 1), but autonomic dysfunction has been reported only with the largest group, **transthyretin amyloidosis** (TTR A).

Transthyretin (TTR) is a normal plasma protein composed of 127 amino acids, synthesized in the liver and choroid plexus, involved in the transport of vitamin A and thyroid hormones. It is coded by a single gene located on chromosome 18. Most patients with TTR amyloidosis are heterozygous for that gene. Thus far, 41 disease-causing mutations in the TTR gene have been identified, of which 20 have been reported to be associated with autonomic dysfunction of differing severity (Table 2).

Autonomic involvement in TTR A is common and occurs early with both sympathetic and parasympathetic systems being affected. The severity of auto-

Table 2.   Transthyretin Amyloidoses with Autonomic Involvement

Mutation	Organs involved	Geographic kindreds
Cys10Arg	Heart, eye, PN	U.S.A. (Hungarian)
Val30Met	PN, eye	U.S.A. Sweden, Japan, Portugal
Val30Ala	Heart	U.S.A. (German)
Val30Leu	PN	Japan
Phe33Ile	PN, eye	Israel
Phe33Leu	PN, heart	U.S.A. (Polish)
GGlu42Gly	PN, heart	Japan
Gly47Arg	PN	Japan, U.S.A.
Gly47Ala	Heart	Italy
Gly47Val	CTS, PN, heart	Sri Lanka
Thr49Ala	Heart, CTS	France, Italy
Ser50Arg	PN	Japan
Ser50Ile	Heart, PN	Japan
Ser52Pro	PN, heart, kidney	England
Leu55Pro	Heart, eye	U.S.A. (Dutch, France) Taiwan
Leu58Arg	CTS, eye	Japan
Thr60Ala	Heart, CTS	U.S.A.
Val171Ala	PN, eye, CTS	France, Majorca
Ser77Tyr	Kidney	U.S.A. (IL-German, Tx) France
Tyr114Cys	PN, eye	Japan

Note. CTS, carpal tunnel syndrome; PN, peripheral neuropathy.

nomic involvement generally correlates with the progression of the disease. Autonomic symptoms include: alternating diarrhea and constipation, palpitation due to cardiac dysrhythmias, anorexia, nausea and vomiting, OH, impotence, urinary and fecal incontinence, and hypohidrosis. Delayed gastric emptying may cause organ distension and anorexia with subsequent cachexia which may be an important factor in mortality. GI dysfunction is due to autonomic involvement as well as direct deposition of amyloid in the intestinal wall. The **scalloped pupil deformity** has been described in Portuguese and Swedish kindreds and is probably due to involvement of the ciliary nerves. AN may also cause severe urinary retention with secondary renal damage.

Although diagnosis should not be difficult in typical cases, other hereditary neuropathies like hereditary motor and sensory neuropathies and hereditary sensory and autonomic neuropathies should be excluded. The late onset, predominant sensory symptoms, prominent early autonomic involvement, and frequent association with CTS strongly favor the diagnosis of FAP. Nevertheless, nerve biopsy and DNA analysis may be required for confirmation of diagnosis.

Pathogenesis

Normal **transthyretin** is not amyloidogenic, but most of its mutants probably are. Met30 TTR, which is the most common mutation, demonstrated amyloidogenicity in transgenic mice. Amyloid deposits were eventually noted in intestine, kidney, and heart, but not in peripheral nerves (the most common site of involvement in humans). It is not clear how TTR point mutations convert TTR into an amyloidogenic substance, but they may do so by changing its surface topography. Demonstration of amyloid deposit in dorsal root ganglia and sympathetic chains in FAP is, perhaps, due to absence of blood–nerve barrier in these structures, allowing easy access of amyloidogenic protein. The mechanism of OH in patients with FAP is not fully understood. Low levels of plasma norepinephrine in patients with OH without significant plasma norepinephrine response to postural changes and low serum dopamine β-hydroxylase activity suggest depletion of peripheral norepinephrine secondary to adrenergic denervation.

Laboratory Data and Diagnosis

Autonomic function tests are abnormal frequently and early in the course of the disease. Amyloid tissue diagnosis is not different from AL. DNA analysis by PCR technology is now available for some protein variants and provides valuable information for genetic counseling of family members at risk. This test can be applied to chorionic villi samples for prenatal diagnosis.

Treatment

Definitive treatment of TTR A depends on further advances in gene therapy. Supportive treatments are the only option at this time, especially early in the course of the disease. Anecdotal reports suggest benefit from plasmapheresis, colchicine, and oral L-threo-3,4-dihydroxyphenylserine (a noradrenalin precursor). Recently, liver transplantation was shown to be successful in stopping clinical progression in patients with FAP (met30 variant) (2).

Prognosis

The natural history of autonomic invovlement in FAP and its effect on survival remains to be established. Generally, FAP has a better prognosis than AL, with a life-span of 5–20 years after tissue diagnosis. Death usually results from renal failure, cardiac failure, or malnutrition.

References

1. Benson MD. Amyloidosis. In: Scriver CR, Beaudet AL, *et al.* eds. The molecular and metabolic basis of inherited disease, 7th ed. New York: McGraw–Hill, 1995.
2. Kyle RA, Dyck PJ. Amyloidosis and neuropathy. In: Dyck, Thomas, Lambert, Runge, eds. Peripheral neuropathy, Vol. II, 3rd ed. Philadelphia: Saunders, 1993. 1294–1309.
3. Haan J, Peters WG. Amyloid and peripheral nervous system disease. Clin Neurol Neurosurg 1994;96:1–9.
4. Yazawa M, Ikeda S. Autonomic nerve disorders in generalized amyloidosis. Nippon-Rinsho: Japanese J Clin Med 1992;50(4):818–26.
5. Niklasson U, Olofsson BO, Bjerle P. Autonomic neuropathy in familial amyloidotic polyneuropathy. Acta Neurol Scand 1989;79:182–7.

51

Diabetic Autonomic Failure

Michael Pfeifer
Southern Illinois University
School of Medicine
Springfield, Illinois

All organ systems innervated by the autonomic nervous system may be impaired in diabetic patients. The extent of impairment is highly variable from patient to patient but is generally related to duration of diabetes as with other complications of diabetes. Nerve impairment is further complicated by a decline in function with age.

Currently the only preventative treatment for autonomic dysfunction is maintenance of near-normal blood glucose. Each affected system will be reviewed below, but in general, manifestations of autonomic dysfunction are treated symptomatically when appropriate; often, patient education can avoid many potential life-threatening problems.

Iris

Sympathetic nerves, which dilate the iris, show earlier and more extensive impairment than the parasympathetic nerves which constrict the iris. This imbalance between parasympathetic and sympathetic nerves causes an inability to respond quickly to a dark stimulus. Patients will complain of inability to see in dark places such as movie theaters and will have difficulty driving at night. On clinical exam, small, poorly dilated pupils in a dark room combined with the above complaints are indicative. Pupillometry also measures ability to dilate. Education about recognition of the problem, reassurance, and proper precautions when in darkness are adequate in most cases. Treatment with sympathetic stimulants or parasympathetic blockers is generally not necessary.

Esophagus

Dysphagia is the most common presenting symptom. This is often confused with cardiac pain and/or gastric atony. Diagnosis of esophageal and pharyngeal motility dysfunction via barium swallow is generally adequate. Other sources of pain should be ruled out. At present, there is no effective therapy.

Stomach

Signs and symptoms of gastric emptying abnormalities include early satiety, nausea, vomiting, "brittle" diabetes, large fluctuations in blood glucose, and weight loss. Some patients may be asymptomatic. The most effective diagnostic tool for evaluation of gastric emptying abnormality is nuclear medicine solid phase gastric emptying studies. These studies measure both liquid- and solid-phase emptying, unlike upper gastrointestinal x-ray series which measure only liquid-phase gastric emptying. The use of beef stew or chicken livers is a more adequate test of solid gastric emptying than oatmeal, scrambled eggs, or hard-boiled eggs which are commonly used. These measure semisolid gastric emptying.

Successful treatment of gastric emptying abnormalities may be complex. Hyperglycemia, *per se*, may result in atonic stomach. Improvement in glucose control has the potential to correct the problem. However, it is difficult, if not impossible, to improve glucose control due to the mismatch between caloric absorption and insulin action onset. Therefore, it may be necessary to initially improve gastric emptying with pharmacological agents, then attempt to improve glucose control. Once glucose control is within acceptable limits it is reasonable to discontinue pharmacological therapy and evaluate whether glucose control alone is adequate therapy.

Effective pharmacological therapies with prokinetic action include **metoclopramide, bethanechol, cisapride, erythromycin, octreotide,** and **famotidine.** Metoclopramide inhibits the dopaminergic pathway which inhibits gastric emptying. By inhibiting this pathway, endogenous peristalsis may occur uninhibited. Severe vagal impairment will obviate its efficacy. The usual dose is 10 mg, 30 min before meals. Side effects include extrapyramidal symptoms, drooling, and nystagmus.

Bethanechol directly stimulates the stomach via the **muscarinic receptors.** Thus, it is generally effective in increasing gastric emptying even in cases where metoclopramide is not effective. In order to overcome an atonic stomach, bethanechol is given subcutaneously for the first 2 weeks. Beginning dose is 2.5 mg subcutaneously 30 min before each meal for approximately 3–4 days. Subcutaneous bethanechol is increased to 5 mg before each meal and snack for the remainder of the 2 weeks. At the end of this period, patients are switched to 50 mg of oral bethanechol 30 min before each meal and snack. Side effects include urinary urgency, sweating, and occasional nausea. If given after or too soon before the meal, it may cause regurgitation.

Cisapride increases smooth muscle activity of the intestines and has some direct ganglionic activity. Ten to 20 mg is given before meals. **Erythromycin** works by mimicking **motilin.** Typically 250 mg is given every 6 hr. The drawback to this drug is that it often interferes with antibiotic coverage.

Octreotide decreases gut hormone motility inhibitors such as gastric inhibitory polypeptide. As a promotility drug, it is not as good as cisapride or bethanechol but is not worse than metoclopramide. Typically 100 μg is given every 6 hr subcutaneously. **Famotidine** is an unusual H_2 blocker in that it has a neutral effect or some prokinetic effect unlike other H_2 blockers. Doses of 20–40 mg are given every 12–24 hr. This drug must be adjusted for renal function.

It is recommended that gastric emptying studies be repeated after pharmacological therapy has begun to verify that, in fact, emptying has improved. If not, other pharmacological therapies should be considered. An efficient method to measure efficacy of therapy is to give the drug with the gastric emptying study and measure the response. If a patient is unresponsive to any of these therapies, frequent small meals, six times a day, with high calorie liquid food may be necessary to maintain adequate nutrition.

Gallbladder

Diarrhea and the development of gallstones are symptoms of gallbladder atony. Gallstones are much more likely to develop in patients with hypercholesterolemia as is often seen in patients with diabetes. Gallbladder disease is evaluated by observing the response of the gallbladder to a fatty meal or cholecystokinin (CCK). Cholecystectomy may be indicated in some cases.

Colon

The most common gastrointestinal symptom of autonomic neuropathy is constipation. It is evaluated by clinical history. Constipation is treated with a variety of medications including high-fiber products such as psyllium, which is bulk-forming fiber acting to encourage peristaltic activity. **Mineral oil** and **bisacodyl** may also be effective. Bisacodyl acts directly on the colonic mucosa to produce normal peristalsis throughout the large intestine.

Diabetic diarrhea is a common result of autonomic dysfunction. However, other causes need to be ruled out. Diabetic diarrhea is characterized by frequent (8–20 bowel movements/day, 300 g of stool/day), watery, persistent movements and is often nocturnal. Mild steatorrhea is common. Treatment is aimed at the cause. Initially a **broad-spectrum antibiotic** is used to eliminated bacterial over-growth. Inappropriate spillage of bile salts into the intestines is also a common cause of diarrhea occurring in diabetic patients. If spillage of bile salts is suspected **bile salt binders** should be tried. Pharmacologic therapies include **methycellulose, diphenoxylate** hydrochloride with **atropine** sulfate (10 cc, 6–24 hr), and **lopera-mide** hydrochloride (10 cc, 6–24 hr). **Octreotide** (100 μg, subcutaneously every 4–6 hr) has been effective when other treatments have failed.

Bladder

Both afferent and efferent nerves to the bladder may be affected in patients with diabetes. **Afferent neuropathy** results in the inability to feel the need to void. Therefore, there is a decrease in frequency of urination which may be misinterpreted as an improvement in glucose control. The decreased frequency causes bladder stasis and may lead to an increase in the occurrence of urinary tract infection (UTI). **Efferent neuropathy** generally occurs later in the course of diabetes causing incomplete voiding, dribbling, and frequent urinary tract infections. Incontinence is a late finding and is very rare. Evaluation for bladder dysfunction is considered in males with >2 UTI/year and in females with >3 UTI/year. Cystometrogram effectively evaluates both afferent and efferent neuropathy. Afferent neuropathy can generally be treated by having the patient schedule urination every 4 hrs. Efferent neuropathy is treated with **bethanechol** given orally at a dosage of 30–50 mg four times a day. Incontinence may require placement of a suprapubic catheter and/or permanent catheterization.

Penis

The incidence of impotence, which may result from autonomic neuropathy, is nearly three times more common in diabetic males than in nondiabetic, age-matched males. Signs and symptoms include decreased tumescence and rigidity. **Retrograde ejaculation** occurs rarely and may be related to sympathetic dysfunc-tion. The diagnosis of neuropathic impotence is one of exclusion. (Fig. 1).

Treatment is aimed at the cause. Alternative medications for antihypertensive and psychotropic therapy should always be initiated before pharmacological or mechanical measures are used. If the cause is neuropathic, **yohimbine** is occasionally helpful for patients with early loss of penile rigidity or with pelvic steal syndrome. Suction devices or injections with **phentolamine, prostaglan-dins,** or **papaverine** can be useful. If the above methods fail or are unacceptable, penile prostheses may be useful. Complications with yohimbine include hyper-tension. Injections may cause bruising, pain, and priapism. Prostheses often fail to meet the patient's expectations and may be painful.

Vagina

A dry, thin, atrophic vaginal wall and lack of lubrication characterize vaginal autonomic neuropathy resulting in painful intercourse. Over-the-counter lubri-cants help decrease pain during intercourse. However, an estrogen cream not only adds moisture but also helps thicken the vaginal wall, thus preventing tearing.

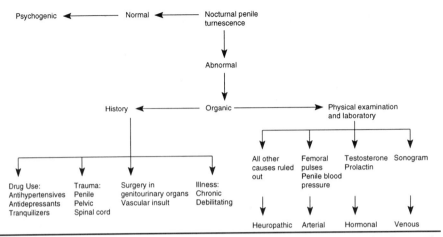

Figure 1.   The diagnosis of impotence secondary to diabetic autonomic neuropathy is one of exclusion. The above algorithm is suggested to evaluate the other possible etiologies of impotence.

Adrenal Medulla

In patients with severe autonomic neuropathy, there is a loss of both the adrenal output of epinephrine and probably of the sympathetic tone to the liver resulting in a decreased couterregulatory response to hypoglycemia. Without the adrenergic signs and symptoms, hypoglycemia may become severe before it is treated. Diagnosis of hypoglycemic unawareness is based on the lack of adrenergic responses such as tachycardia and blood pressure when blood glucose is <40 mg/dl. Effective management of this condition requires that the patient, family members, and co-workers be taught to recognize the subtle signs and symptoms of hypoglycemia (mood changes, confusion, slurred speech, fugue-like state, and memory lapses) and how to treat it with glucagon injections and glucose.

Sudomotor

Abnormal sweating patterns are commonly found in people with diabetes. Both upper and lower extremities fail to sweat while the trunk overcompensates. Eventually complete anhidrosis may occur. The patient generally complains of excessive sweating in the trunk area. Abnormal temperature regulation predisposes to heat stroke and heat exhaustion. Treatment is limited to education. Patients should be warned that they are at increased risk of heat stroke and heat exhaustion and informed of the necessary precautions.

Cardiovascular

Clinical manifestations of cardiovascular autonomic neuropathy include **exercise intolerance** and **painless myocardial ischemia. Postural hypotension** as a result of vascular autonomic dysfunction is characterized by postural dizziness, nausea, vertigo, weakness, and/or syncope. These signs and symptoms can be misinterpreted as hypoglycemia. Measurement of change in heart rate and blood pressure when moving form sitting or lying to a standing position provides evidence of this condition. This is a diagnosis of exclusion (Fig. 2). Treatment of postural hypotension resulting from autonomic neuropathy can be complex as supine hypertension and upright hypotension often occur concurrently. Both supine hypertension and upright hypotension cannot be treated in the same patient as treatment of one may aggravate the other and vice versa. Keeping the head of the bed in an upright position during sleep often helps the patient adjust to change in position and lessens supine hypertension. The most simple and efficacious treatment is an atomized spray of 10% **phenylephrine** hydrochloride (Neo-synephrine). The spray is used approximately every 2–4 hr, three or four sprays per nostril at each dosing. This nearly always results in an improvement in upright hypotension. Rare complications include septum perforation and ulceration. **Fludrocortisone** (0.1 to 0.5 mg) increases plasma volume and catecholamine sensitivity and is often effective. Sympathetic stimulants (**ephedrine** and **midodrine**) are also useful.

Cardiac denervation syndrome, a total loss of innervation to the heart, results in exercise intolerance, poor anesthesia outcome, pregnancy complications, sudden death, and probably cardiomyopathy and painless myocardial ischemia. This syndrome may be evaluated with simple, noninvasive tests such as R–R variation and Valsalva maneuver. Awareness of this condition may decrease long-term morbidity and mortality. There is no evidence that the occurrence of sudden death and cardiomyopathy can be prevented.

Painless myocardial ischemia, associated with increased morbidity and mortality is more common in diabetic patients, than in the nondiabetic population. An algorithm to identify those at risk for painless ischemia is in Fig. 3. A study in a small number of patients has shown that approximately 66% of patients screened via this algorithm had ischemia confirmed by a stress thallium test.

Cardiac denervation may also cause **exercise intolerance** in patients with diabetes. Symptoms may be vague and the patient may present with only

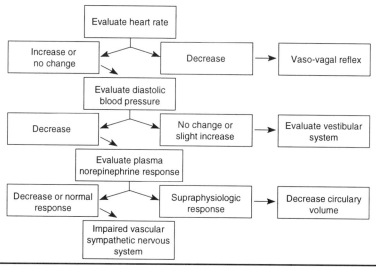

Figure 2. Postural hypotension as a result of vascular autonomic dysfunction is characterized by symptoms that may be misinterpreted as hypoglycemia. The above algorithm may be used to evaluate the etiology of postural hypotension.

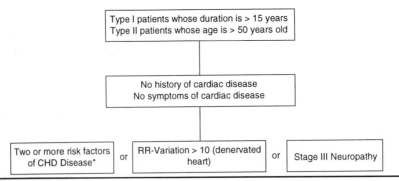

Figure 3.   The above criteria are used to identify the patients at risk for painless myocardial ischemia. *, series of risk factors.

fatigue as a complaint. The American Diabetes Association recommends that all diabetic patients who are new to an exercise program and are type II diabetics over the age of 40 or type I patients with a duration of diabetes >15 years should have an exercise tolerance test prior to initiating an exercise program. There is no known treatment for exercise intolerance, although one study has shown that aldose reductase inhibitors may improve intolerance.

References

1. Ward J, Goto Y, eds. Diabetic neuropathy. New York: Wiley, 1990.
2. Kirby RS, Carson CC, Webster GD, eds. Impotence: diagnosis and management of male erectile dysfunction. Oxford: Butterworth Heinemann, 1991.
3. Low PA, ed. Clinical autonomic disorders: evaluation and management. Boston: Little, Brown, 1993.

52   *Paraneoplastic Autonomic Dysfunction*

Ramesh K. Khurana
University of Maryland School of Medicine
Division of Neurology
The Union Memorial Hospital
Baltimore, Maryland

Paraneoplastic autonomic dysfunction (PAD), as a result of the tumor's remote effect upon the autonomic nervous system, is rare but it is extremely important to recognize because: (i) it may be the initial manifestation of an underlying malignancy; (ii) it is usually progressive and more devastating than the tumor itself; (iii) it may simulate metastatic disease or other conditions such as B_{12} deficiency and Shy–Drager syndrome; (iv) it may be confirmed with serologic tests; and (v) early treatment of the tumor may arrest the progression or even improve the autonomic dysfunction. Three syndromes have so far been delineated: autonomic neuropathy, enteric neuronopathy, and subacute sensory neuronopathy.

Autonomic Neuropathy

Autonomic dysfunction may occur with minimal or no somatic involvement. There is subacute onset of orthostatic, gastrointestinal, and genitourinary symptoms. Autonomic tests show widespread sympathetic and parasympathetic abnormalities but cardiovagal reflexes may be spared. It has been reported in temporal association with small cell lung cancer (SCLC), adenocarcinoma of pancreas or Hodgkin's disease, and carcinoma of the prostate.

Enteric Neuronopathy

Pseudo-obstruction of the bowels is the distinguishing feature of this illness. Symptoms of pseudo-obstruction—constipation, crampy abdominal pain, and vomiting—usually precede other autonomic symptoms. Postural dizziness, syncope, and other autonomic symptoms follow soon afterwards. Somatic neurologic findings are variable and include peripheral or central nervous system involvement. When the central nervous system is affected, this syndrome may mimic Shy–Drager syndrome.

Patients with true Shy–Drager syndrome may develop severe constipation, but pseudo-obstruction of the bowels is rare. There may be infiltration of myenteric plexus neurons with mononuclear cells, and progressive loss of enteric neurons. **Cytotoxic T cells** have been incriminated as effectors of the pathological lesions and **enteric neuronal autoantibodies,** as well as **Anti-Hu antibody,** have been reported. It occurs mostly in patients with SCLC, but rarely associates itself with **pulmonary carcinoid** and **undifferentiated epithelioma.**

Subacute Sensory Neuronopathy

First described by Denny-Brown in 1948, it is characterized by subacute onset and rapid progression of dysesthesias, paresthesias, lancinating pains, and numbness affecting the limbs, face, and tongue. Loss of joint and position sense, sensory ataxia, pseudoathetosis, and areflexia are common while motor strength is usually preserved. This syndrome may mimic subacute combined degeneration or tabes dorsalis. Autonomic dysfunction as a presenting manifestation occurs in 10% of cases but it may affect 28% of the patients during the course of illness.

Autonomic tests show sympathetic and parasympathetic insufficiency. It is usually associated with SCLC, but may occur in adenocarcinoma of lung, carcinoma of the prostate, neuroblastoma, testicular seminoma, and embryonal carcinoma; T-cell-mediated immune attack on the ganglionic neurons has been postulated. Anti-Hu antibody is found in the majority of these patients.

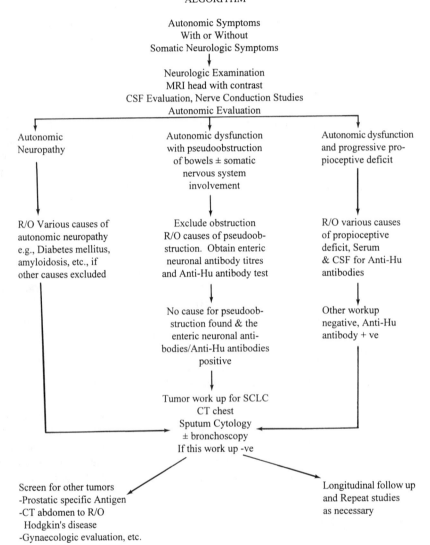

ALGORITHM

Autonomic Symptoms
With or Without
Somatic Neurologic Symptoms

Neurologic Examination
MRI head with contrast
CSF Evaluation, Nerve Conduction Studies
Autonomic Evaluation

Autonomic
Neuropathy

Autonomic dysfunction
with pseudoobstruction
of bowels ± somatic
nervous system
involvement

Autonomic dysfunction
and progressive pro-
pioceptive deficit

R/O Various causes of
autonomic neuropathy
e.g., Diabetes mellitus,
amyloidosis, etc., if
other causes excluded

Exclude obstruction
R/O causes of pseudoob-
struction. Obtain enteric
neuronal antibody titres
and Anti-Hu antibody test

R/O various causes
of propioceptive
deficit, Serum
& CSF for Anti-Hu
antibodies

No cause for pseudoob-
struction found & the
enteric neuronal anti-
bodies/Anti-Hu antibodies
positive

Other workup
negative, Anti-Hu
antibody + ve

Tumor work up for SCLC
CT chest
Sputum Cytology
± bronchoscopy
If this work up -ve

Screen for other tumors
-Prostatic specific Antigen
-CT abdomen to R/O
 Hodgkin's disease
-Gynaecologic evaluation, etc.

Longitudinal follow up
and Repeat studies
as necessary

Diagnosis

Paraneoplastic disorder should be suspected in patients presenting with progressive autonomic symptoms such as orthostatic hypotension, dry mouth, urinary retention, constipation, sweat disturbance, and impotence (see algorithm). Occurrence of pseudo-obstruction of bowels or progressive propriocep-tive deficit should strengthen this suspicion. The diagnosis is made by exclusion of other causes of autonomic neuropathy and the finding of a malignancy, typically SCLC. Serologic studies, searching for anti-Hu or enteric neuronal antibodies are helpful. Since tumors producing paraneoplastic manifestations are usually small, a close longitudinal follow-up and repeat studies may be necessary to diagnose the tumor.

Treatment

A proper diagnosis can spare the patients unnecessary surgery in cases of pseudo-obstruction of the bowels. Treatment may be directed at the tumor, the antibodies, and the symptoms. An early surgical or cytotoxic reduction of the tumor may diminish autonomic dysfunction in some patients. Use of steroids, plasmapheresis, or immunosuppression with cyclophosphamide to reduce the antibody so far have not affected the outcome of the patients. Symptomatic improvement of orthostatic hypotension with **fludrocortisone,** dry mouth with **artificial saliva,** etc., can temporarily improve the quality of life of these patients.

References

1. Khurana RK. Paraneoplastic autonomic dysfunction. In: Low PA, ed. Clinical autonomic disorders evaluation and management. Boston: Little Brown, 1993: 505–15.
2. Khurana RK. Cholinergic dysfunction in Shy-Drager syndrome: effect of the parasympathomimetic agent, bethanechol. Clin Autonom Res 1994;4:5–13.
3. Lennon VA, Sas DF, Busk MF, Scheithauer B, Malagelada J-R., Camilleri M, Miler LJ. Enteric neuronal antibodies in pseudoobstruction with small-cell lung carcinoma. Gastroenterology 1991;100:137–42.
4. Panegyres PK, Reading MC, Eriri MM. The inflammatory reaction of paraneoplastic ganglionitis and encephalitis: an immunohistochemical study. J Neurol 1993;240:93–7.
5. Dalmau J, Graus F, Rosenblum MK, Posner JB. Anti-Hu-associated paraneoplastic encephalomyelitis/Sensory Neuronopathy. A clinical study of 71 patients. Medicine 1992;71:59–72.

53

Guillain–Barré Syndrome

James G. McLeod
The University of Sydney
Department of Medicine
Sydney, N.S.W., Australia

Autonomic complications are relatively common in the **Guillain–Barré syndrome** (GBS), 65% of patients in one large retrospective series having had some dysautonomia. The most common manifestations are sinus tachycardia, postural hypostension, hypertension, arrhythmias, abnormal responses to drugs, and bladder dysfunction. Other causes of cardiovascular disturbances such as hypoxia, electrolyte disturbances, pulmonary embolus, gastrointestinal bleeding, and heart disease must be excluded before a diagnosis of autonomic dysfunction is made. Autonomic dysfunction may be a significant cause of mortality in GBS, 7% of patients having died with arrhythmias in one series.

Arrhythmias

Sustained sinus tachycardia is common, being present in approximately 30–60% of cases. It is most likely caused by vagal nerve damage that has been demonstrated in a number of separate studies. No specific treatment is required.

More serious arrhythmias (**bradycardia, atrial fibrillation, atrial flutter, paroxysmal tachycardia, ventricular fibrillation,** and EKG abnormalities have been noted in a number of series. These are probably due to excessive vagal activity.

Vagal spells are episodes of bradycardia or asystole that may occur spontaneously or during tracheal suction or Valsalva-like maneuvers and have been reported in up to 30% of cases in some series.

Hypertension

Intermittent or **paroxysmal hypertension** occurs in about 30% of cases and less commonly the hypertension is sustained. Paroxysmal hypertension is nearly always associated with quadriplegia and respiratory failure and often occurs in combination with orthostatic hypotension. The mechanism is most likely sympathetic overactivity and abnormalities of the afferent **baroreflex** pathways. Hypertension requires treatment only if it is sustained or severe and is best managed with β-adrenergic drugs.

Hypotension

Supine hypotension may be paroxysmal and alternating with episodes of hypertension. It is usually associated with reduced cardiac output and may be precipitated by reflex stimulation from intubation or tracheal suction resulting in a vasodepressor response. Postural hypotension occurs in about 30% of patients. The mechanism is **demyelination of peripheral sympathetic pathways** and mechanical factors such as paralysis of muscles resulting in impaired venous return to the heart. In management of patients with GBS, it is important to be aware of the possibility of postural hypotension in order to avoid possibly life-threatening falls of blood pressure on sitting or attempting to stand patients. Supine hypotension may respond to plasma expansion and agents such as **phenylephrine.**

Bladder Dysfunction

Urinary retention occurs in about 20% of patients with GBS. Urinary incontinence is uncommon and usually due to overflow from a distended bladder. The mechanism of retention is most likely demyelination of the sacral outflow to the bladder. Abdominal muscle paralysis may play a part. Management is with intermittent catheterization.

Other abnormalities inlcude **gastrointestinal dysfunction** (constipation, paralytic ileus, and gastric distension) and **abnormal drug responses.** Denervation supersensitivity to sympathomimetic drugs such as phenylephrine, ephedrine, dopamine, and isoproterenol has been reported as has severe hypotension with phentolamine, nitroglycerin, thiopental, and morphine.

Autonomic function studies have demonstrated abnormal sympathetic activity manifested by impaired sweating and reduced blood pressure response to sustained handgrip; excessive sympathetic outflow has been documented with microneurography. Impaired baroreflex sensitivity, abnormal heart-rate response to breathing, and abnormal Valsalva ratio reflect parasympathetic pathway involvement.

Pathology

Demyelination of fibers in the vagus and glossopharyngeal nerve and the preganglionic sympathetic efferent fibers have been demonstrated at autopsy. In animals with experimental allergic neuritis, there is demyelination and impaired conduction in the splanchnic and vagus nerves.

References

1. Ropper AH, Widjdick ESM, Truax BT. Guillain-Barré syndrome. Philadelphia: F.A. Davies, 1991.
2. Zochodne DW. Autonomic involvement in Guillain-Barré syndrome. A review. Muscle Nerve 1994;17:1154–5.
3. Winer JB, Hugher RAC. Identification of patients at risk of arrhythmia in the Guillain-Barré syndrome. Q J Med 1988;68:735–9.
4. Tuck RR, McLeod JG. Autonomic dysfunction in Guillain-Barré syndrome. J Neurol Neurosurg Psychiatry 1981;44:983–90.

54

Chagas' Disease

Mario Medici
*Department of
Neurology
School of Medicine
Montevideo 11300,
Uruguay*

Daniel Bulla
*School of Medicine
Montevideo 11300,
Uruguay*

Alba Larre Borges
*School of Medicine
Montevideo 11300,
Uruguay*

Raquel Ponce De Leon
*Department of
Neurology
School of Medicine
Montevideo 11300,
Uruguay*

Chagas' disease is a trypanosomiasis caused by *Trypanosoma cruzi* (*T. cruzi*), occurring almost exclusively in Latin America. The World Health Organization has recently estimated that 16 million people have been infected by *T. cruzi*, 50,000 of whom die every year of Chagas' disease.

There are three transmission courses of epidemiological importance: **vectorial, transfusional,** and **maternofetal,** the former being the most important in Latin American countries, while the transfusional course acquires greater importance in countries such as the United States and Canada due to the high immigration from endemic regions.

Vectorial transmission occurs through an insect belonging to the *Hemiptera* order, the *Reduviidae* family, and the *Triatominae* subfamily, of which there are 118 classified species, a few of which (those in the domestic habitat) are mainly responsible for transmission to humans.

Practically all autonomic structures may be affected, and there is an acute and chronic stage. The acute stage is characterized by a high parasitemia with tissue invasion and a distinct neurotropism of *T. cruzi*. There is inflammatory infiltration of many tissues, especially the heart and autonomic ganglia.

A month or two after the acute stage, *T. cruzi* practically disappears from the blood and tissue and the diagnosis subsequently is serologic. Approximately 25–30% of infected patents eventually become chronically symptomatic, usually after an interval of decades. Chronic Chagas cardiopathy is produced by destruction of the muscle fiber followed by fibrosis resulting in a dilated **cardiomyopathy.**

Autonomic function tests have demonstrated a predominantly **parasympathetic** neuropathy. Studies have included heart rate variability, the Valsalva ratio, BP response to sustained handgrip, and cardiovascular response to nor-epinephrine, atropine, and β blockers. There can be mild sympathetic involvement but orthostatic hypotension is uncommon.

The gastrointestinal tract is affected in over 90% but is symptomatic in fewer patients. There is denervation of Auerbach and Meissner parasympathetic plexi, results in **megaesophagus** and **megacolon.** Other levels can be also affected.

Symptoms consist of **dysphagia, constipation,** and diarrhea. Motor dysfunction precedes dilatation. By assessing esophageal transit with radionuclide studies, these alterations can be found in a high percentage of patients. Unlike **Hirschsprung's disease,** Chagas' disease is associated with a hypersensitivity of the colon to the administration of **methacholine.**

Autonomic alterations have been found in other structures, including the urinary tract, the central nervous system, iris, and bronchia.

References

1. Wendel S, Brener Z, Camargo ME, Rassi A. Chagas disease (American trypanosomiasis): its impact on transfusion and clinical medicine. Sao Paulo: ISBT Brazil, 1992.
2. Bannister R, Mathias C. Autonomic failure, 3rd ed. Oxford: Oxford University Press, 1992.
3. Amorin DS. Cardiopatía chagásica. Modelos experimentales. Arq Bras Cardiologia 1984;42:243–7.
4. Ponce de Leon R, Bulla D, Lago G, *et al*. Compromiso del sistema nervioso autónomo en la Enfermedad de Chagas. Acta Neurol Latinoam 1986;30:123–31.
5. X Congresso Latinoamericano de Parasitologia. Montevideo, 1991.

55 *Other Peripheral Neuropathies*

James G. McLeod
*The University of Sydney
Department of Medicine
Sydney, N.S.W., Australia*

The autonomic nervous system is affected to some extent in most peripheral neuropathies. In many of these the manifestations are only of minor importance, but in some conditions, (e.g., diabetes, primary and familial amyloidosis, Guillain–Barré syndrome, and Riley–Day syndrome), there may be profound disturbances of autonomic function such as orthostatic hypotension, impairment of heart-rate control, bladder dysfunction, and impotence. These conditions have been discussed in other chapters.

Hereditary Neuropathies

Hereditary sensory and autonomic neuropathies and **Charcot Marie Tooth disease** may manifest mild autonomic disturbances, mainly impairment of sweating. Other tests of autonomic function are not significantly impaired. This sort of autonomic dysfunction has also been described in **Fabry's disease** (see Chapter 49) and some **spinocerebellar degenerations** but not in **Friedreich's ataxia.**

Chronic Inflammatory Demyelinating Polyradiculoneuropathy (CIDP)

Autonomic function has been investigated in CIDP and the only significant abnormalities were in the 30 : 15 ratio and thermoregulatory sweat tests. These mild abnormalities of autonomic function contrast with the more severe abnormalities seen in **Guillain–Barré syndrome** in which there is probably more extensive conduction block and involvement of unmyelinated fibers.

Leprosy

Autonomic neuropathy is described in leprosy, particularly sweating of the skin supplied by diseased nerves, **cardiac denervation, postural hypotension,** and impairment of other autonomic reflexes. Abnormalities of the finger tip vasomotor reflexes recorded with a laser Doppler flowmeter in response to inspiratory gasp and the cold pressor tests may be an early sign of nerve damage.

Lyme Disease

Autonomic dysfunction manifested by resting tachycardia in a patient with a **Guillain–Barré-like syndrome** associated with Lyme disease has been described.

Chronic Renal Failure

Abnormalities of baroreflex function and other disturbances of sympathetic and parasympathetic function have been demonstrated. Improvement in autonomic function follows renal transplantation.

Vitamin B_{12} Deficiency

Orthostatic hypotension may occasionally be the initial manifestation of **pernicious anemia.** The pathological changes in the peripheral nerves are those of axonal degeneration. Postural hypotension may be caused by impairment of central mechanisms as well as damage to peripheral autonomic nerves.

Chronic Liver Disease

Autonomic dysfunction, predominantly involving the **parasympathetic nervous system,** is present in patients with both alcoholic and nonalcoholic liver disease, the latter including **primary biliary cirrhosis,** and **chronic active hepatitis.** Disordered autonomic function is present in some patients without evidence of peripheral neuropathy. The mechanism of the autonomic neuropathy is uncertain but it may result from nutritional and metabolic disturbances of the autonomic nerves.

Alcoholism

Clinical manifestations of autonomic dysfunction except for **distal impairment of sweating** are unusual in uncomplicated alcohol peripheral neuropathy although postural hypotension may be present in patients who are severely affected and those with **Wernicke's encephalopathy.** Parasympathetic function is usually affected before sympathetic function. Morphometric studies have demonstrated reduction of myelinated fibers in distal parts of the vagus and carotid sinus nerves but the splanchnic nerves are relatively spared.

Connective Tissue Diseases

Impairment of sweating of the extremities is common in **rheumatoid arthritis** and is probably related in most cases to damage of postganglionic efferent fibers in the peripheral nerve. In some cases there may be more extensive autonomic involvement since the heart-rate response to standing, Valsalva maneuver, and respiration may be impaired, particularly in patients with peripheral neuropathy. **Systemic lupus erythematosus** may occasionally be complicated by autonomic neuropathy and it has also been described in association with mixed connective tissue diseases. In **Sjögren's syndrome** there may be anhidrosis, pupillary abnormalities, and cardioparasympathetic dysfunction.

Drugs and Toxins

Vincristine can cause autonomic neuropathy manifested by constipation, abdominal pain, paralytic ileus, urinary retention, and other bladder disturbances. **Perhexiline maleate, amiodarone,** and **cisplatinum** may all cause peripheral neuropathy associated with postural hypotension and other features of autonomic failure. **Vacor rodenticide** poisoning causes orthostatic hypotension and gastrointestinal hypermotility. **Thallium** and **inorganic mercury** cause peripheral neuropathy which may be associated with tachycardia and hypertension. **Pain and redness** of the extremities and **profuse sweating** are associated with mercury poisoning in children giving rise to the name **pink disease.** In **arsenic** poisoning, excessive sweating and impairment of sweating in the extremities are described. **Acrylamide** is neurotoxic in its monomeric form and causes a peripheral neuropathy in which excessive sweating in the extremities due to disturbance of sympathetic function is a feature.

Autonomic function has been shown to be disturbed in some workers exposed to **organic solvents** contained in mainly aliphatic, aromatic, and other hydrocarbons, alcohol, ketones, esters, and ethers as well as **carbon disulfide** and **toluene.** Patients show a significantly impaired heart-rate variation on respiration and Valsalva ratio compared to controls. The most severely affected patients are those exposed to carbon disulfide. **Hexacarbon** neuropathy occurs through industrial exposure or inhalant abuse. Inhalation of **N-hexane** and **methyl-N-butyl-ketone** may result in a rapidly progressive polyneuropathy associated with autonomic features of excessive or impaired sweating, vasomotor alterations on the extremities, postural hypotension, and impotence.

References

1 Low PA, McLeod JG. The autonomic neuropathies. In: Low PA, ed. Clinical autonomic disorders. Boston: Little Brown, 1993: 395–422.
2. McLeod JG. Autonomic dysfunction in peripheral nerve disease. J. Clin. Neurophysiol. 1993;10:51–60.

PART XI

Orthostatic
Intolerance Syndromes

56 Postural Tachycardia Syndrome

Phillip A. Low
Department of Neurology
Mayo Clinic
Rochester, Minnesota

Ronald Schondorf
McGill University
Jewis General Hospital
Montreal, Quebec, Canada

Orthostatic hypotension (OH) occurs when orthostatic defenses, including neural reflexes, have failed, and generally occurs in the setting of widespread autonomic failure. The causes of OH are well-known and include **multiple-system atrophy** (MSA), **pure autonomic failure** (PAF), and the **autonomic neuropathies**. More common but less well-known are **disorders of reduced orthostatic tolerance,** the topic of this chapter.

Definition

Postural tachycardia syndrome (POTS) is defined as a syndrome of orthostatic symptoms associated with a heart rate increment of 30 bpm or greater (Table 1). We arbitrarily separate our patients into mild and florid POTS. Those whose heart rates do not exceed 120 bpm within 5 min of tilt are considered mild. Those whose heart rate persistently exceeds 120 bpm are considered florid.

Clinical Features

The age of presentation is between 15 and 50 years. The female : male ratio is 4 : 1. Most patients have had symptoms for about 1 year when first evaluated. The orthostatic symptoms consist of lightheadedness, visual blurring or tunneling, palpitations, tremulousness, and weakness (especially of the legs). Less frequent symptoms are hyperventilation, anxiety, chest wall pain, acral coldness or pain, and headaches. The symptoms are different than those of neurogenic OH (Table 2). The symptoms in POTS are due in part to **impaired cerebral perfusion** and in part to **compensatory autonomic mechanisms.** There may be an overrepresentation of migraine and sleep disorders.

Approximately 50% of patients have had an antecedent, presumed **viral illness.** Some patients have significant **cyclical variation** of the symptoms, sometimes related to their menstrual cycle. Others have cycles of **several days of intense orthostatic intolerance** (requiring up to 4 liters of saline for resuscitation of orthostatic tolerance), followed by a similar period when their symptoms are less. Some patients have episodic symptoms at rest associated with changes in BP and HR that are unrelated to arrhythmias.

POTS is **heterogenous,** and several categories are recognizable although their presumed mechanisms are not proven. Recognizable entities are shown in Table 3. Patients with a **length-dependent neuropathy** with sparing of cardiac autonomic innervation can develop this syndrome. Denervation of the limbs

Primer on the Autonomic Nervous System

Table 1. **Criteria for POTS**

1. Heart rate increment $\geq$ 30 bpm within 5 min
   of standing or tilt-up
2. Orthostatic symptoms consistently develop
3. Heart rate $\geq$ 120 bpm within 5 min of standing
   or tilt-up

results in reduced peripheral vascular tone, but OH is prevented by an increase in heart rate. This can occur for instance in a phase of diabetic or amyloid neuropathy. A second category of neuropathic POTS is idiopathic, often **immune-mediated**, occurring after a *viral infection* in half the cases. Some patients with POTS develop syncope, diagnosed as neurocardiogenic syncope. Some POTS patients have **mitral valve prolapse**. Some patients have long-standing **orthostatic intolerance**, and with **deconditioning** develop POTS. This category is recognizable by the long history and mild orthostatic tachycardia (<120 bpm). Some patients develop **orthostatic hypertension** and large oscillations in BP. These patients are assumed to have a brainstem origin of POTS.

Autonomic Function Tests

One-half to two-thirds of patients have a restricted autonomic neuropathy on autonomic function tests. These patients have peripheral sympathetic denervation, demonstrable on sudomotor or vasomotor tests. Cardiovascular heart-rate tests are normal. The cardiovascular responses to tilt-up are abnormal. The heart-rate response varies from 120 to 170 bpm on tilt-up, and typically attain these values by 2 min. There may be excessive BP and heart-rate oscillations.

Plasma norepinephrine is normal supine and is normal or increased with the patient erect. Considering the increased orthostatic stress the response is not excessive.

Table 2. **Comparison of POTS with Neurogenic OH**

Parameter	POTS	Neurogenic OH
Orthostatic symptoms		
Dizziness	+++	+
Tremulousness	++−+++	—
Palpitations	++−+++	—
Nausea	+−+++	—
Skin vasoconstr.	++−+++	—
Hyperhidrosis	+−+++	—
Chest wall pain	±−+++	—
Orthostatic hypotension	±	+++
Orthostatic tachycardia	+++	—
Standing norepinephrine	Increased or normal	Reduced

Table 3. Categories of POTS

1. Autonomic neuropathy of recognized type, e.g.,
   diabetes
2. Idiopathic restricted autonomic neuropathy
3. Neurocardiogenic syncope
4. Mitral valve prolapse
5. Deconditioning
6. Presumed brainstem dysfunction (oscillating BP;
   orthostatic hypertension)
7. Prolonged spaceflight

Diagnosis and Differential Diagnosis

The diagnosis of POTS is made by the presence of orthostatic symptoms associated with an excessive HR increment. The differential diagnosis is from panic disorder, chronic fatigue syndrome, somatization disorder, deconditioning, and neurogenic orthostatic hypotension.

When a patient develops the abrupt onset of orthostatic symptoms that include hyperventilation, dizziness, tremulousness, anxiety, excessive sweating, and nausea, and when orthostatic hypotension is not found on examination, an anxiety state or panic disorder is often made. Differentiation is made by the lack of prior symptoms, precipitation by the upright posture only, and the cessation of symptoms on assuming the recumbent posture, as well as the laboratory findings of dysautonomia. Chronic fatigue syndrome or somatization disorder is not associated with autonomic laboratory abnormalities; symptoms are also not confined to the standing posture.

The correct diagnosis of POTS is made by the criteria of POTS, evidence of an antecedent viral infection, and the presence of a restricted autonomic neuropathy. Difficulties can occur when patients with a psychiatric disorder or chronic fatigue syndrome become deconditioned and develop mild POTS. They should not have florid POTS. The differentiation from neurogenic OH is straightforward, since patients with POTS are younger and do not have OH. For the POTS patient with OH, additional points of difference are shown in Table 2.

Mechanisms of POTS

Some suggested **mechanisms of orthostatic intolerance** in POTS are shown in Table 4. These include impaired vasomotor tone, especially **venomotor tone**, as part of a **length-dependent autonomic neuropathy**. Another mechanism is **β-receptor supersensitivity**, manifested as an excessive response to standing and to isoproterenol infusion. The tachycardic response to tilt, tremulousness, and anxiety likely represent β-receptor supersensitivity. **Hypovolemia** has been reported in a few patients. Hyper- or hyposensitivity of vascular α adrenoreceptors has been suggested. **Excessive venous pooling** is seen in some patients. These patients may have a slightly bluish discoloration of their feet on standing.

Table 4.   **Some Suggested Mechanisms of POTS**

1. Length-dependent autonomic neuropathy
2. Beta-receptor supersensitivity
3. Alpha receptor hyper- or hyposensitivity
4. Altered sympathetic–parasympathetic balance
5. Brainstem dysregulation
6. Excessive venous pooling

Management

The management of POTS is still being defined. The evaluation of a patient needs to be individualized. Not all patients require treatment. The patient with symptomatic severe POTS without an identifiable etiology will need a combined cardiologic and autonomic laboratory evaluation. The cardiologic evaluation will include an EKG and 24-hr Holter monitor and cardiac echo study. Electrophysiologic testing is usually not required; it is most useful in patients with heart disease or an abnormal EKG. The neurologic evaluation is focused on seeking evidence for an autonomic neuropathy. Specialized laboratory studies seeking evidence of reduced plasma or red cell volume, peripheral autonomic failure, altered α- or β-receptor sensitivities, or altered baroreflex gain may be needed in some patients.

The **deconditioned hypovolemic patient** will do well with sleeping with the head of the bed elevated and plasma volume expanded with generous **salt** intake and **fludrocortisone.**

The patient with venous pooling needs a different approach to treatment. Body stockings may help as a temporary measure, but is inconvenient and unphysiological for long-term use. Several approaches appear to work in some patients. **Midodrine** is efficacious in some patients. In others, supplemental **octreotide** helps during periods of orthostatic decompensation. **Physical countermaneuvers** appear to be especially efficacious in the venous poolers. Some patients seem to benefit with a 3-month program of graduated **resistance training.**

The patient with peripheral adrenergic failure, manifest as a loss of late phase II, or frank OH, is best treated with **fludrocortisone** and an **α-agonist. Midodrine** appears to work best in terms of absorption, predictable duration of action, and lack of CNS side-effects, but is still an investigational drug.

The patient with florid POTS is likely β-receptor supersensitive. These patients respond to, but are sometimes exquisitely sensitive to, **β antagonists.**

A particularly difficult subset of patients have unstable hypertensive responses to tilt. Some of these patients have **BP responses up to 250/150** on standing. Some of these patients with autonomic instability respond to oral **phenobarbital.** An alternative treatment is **clonidine** or another **α2 agonist.**

References

1. Hoeldtke RD, Dworkin GE, Gaspar SR, Israel BC. Sympathotonic orthostatic orthostatic hypotension: a report of 4 cases. Neurology 1989;39:34–40.

2. Low PA, ed. Laboratory evaluation of autonomic failure. In Clinical autonomic disorders: evaluation and management. Boston: Little Brown, 1993: 169–96.
3. Low PA, Opfer-Gehrking TL, Textor S, Schondorf R, Suarez G, Fealey RD, Camilleri M. Comparison of the postural tachycardia syndrome (POTS) with neurogenic orthostatic hypotension. J Auton Nerv Syst 1994;50:181–8.
4. Schondorf R, Low PA. Idiopathic postural tachycardia syndrome. In: Clinical autonomic disorders: evaluation and management. Boston: Little Brown, 1993: 641–52.
5. Streeten DHP, Anderson GH Jr., Richardson R, Thomas FD. Abnormal orthostatic changes in blood pressure and heart rate in subjects with intact sympathetic nervous function: evidence for excessive venous pooling. J Lab Clin Med 1988;111:326–35

57 Orthostatic Intolerance: Mitral Valve Prolapse

H. Cecil Coghlan
Division of Cardiovascular Diseases
Uihlein Autonomic Research Laboratory
The University of Alabama at Birmingham
Birmingham, Alabama

Autonomic dysregulation in **mitral valve prolapse** (MVP) was first reported from our laboratory in 1976. Comparing responses to autonomic stimuli in 78 patients with MVP and 40 without MVP "referred because of presyncope, syncope or orthostatic tachycardia" and 23 normal volunteers, Taylor and co-workers found no abnormality of circulatory regulation pathognomonic of MVP and concluded that it was important to characterize the pattern of altered autonomic regulation of cardiovascular function in each patient to guide therapeutic decisions. This led to the concept of β_2-**adrenoreceptor supercoupling** as the cause of adrenergic hypersensitivity in symptomatic MVP patients later elaborated by Anwar. Hyperadrenergic responsiveness of these patients was also clearly documented by Boudoulas, Wooley, Pasternac and other researchers.

Ascertainment bias, inclusion of patients with echocardiographically diagnosed MVP based on bowing of leaflets that are not redundant or thickened and often not accompanied by carefully elucidated auscultatory features, and differences in echocardiographic criteria have all confused the problem without necessarily stimulating the desirable in-depth study of autonomic function in symptomatic MVP patients. This has led to psychiatric therapy that generally has failed to ameliorate or reverse the physiologic abnormalities that incapacitate patients.

The unexpected and frequent decline in cardiac output and left ventricular end-diastolic pressure during coronary sinus pacing in the supine position in a subset of patients with angina-like chest pain and normal coronary arteriograms led to our initial studies of autonomic function in 1974. We concluded that these patients, none of whom had even been suspected of having MVP, thus excluding ascertainment bias, with normal systolic and diastolic left ventricular function, would necessarily have a condition that impaired their venous return. Autonomic reflex testing with postural, Valsalva, handgrip, and cold pressor tests and assessment of heart rate variation on quiet and deep breathing showed significant differences between the patients who, on meticulous echocardiography and review of left ventricular cine angiograms, proved to have MVP and those who did not, in spite of similar symptomatic presentation. The Wooley and Boudoulas text (1) includes two comprehensive reviews of autonomic function in MVP patients (2, 3). Similar symptoms were observed in patients with MVP and their relatives and spouses without MVP.

Pathogenesis of symptoms remains incompletely defined. Abnormal renal excretion of **magnesium** and abnormal retention of a standard intravenous magnesium load (4) and discovery by Coghlan (5) of low intracellular magnesium in 62% of MVP patients diagnosed by rigorous clinical and echocardiographic criteria led to **magnesium supplementation** that dramatically improved chest pain in half the patients. Further research similar to this is needed before conclusions are drawn regarding the etiology of symptoms in MVP patients.

In the course of studies of more than 3000 symptomatic MVP patients, we have observed light headedness, fuzziness of the head, visual disturbance with difficult focusing or blurring of vision, fatigue, effort intolerance and occipital headache after being upright for a period of time, and even decreased attention and memory deficit with upright activity in carefully taken history. Cold hands and feet, as well as exaggerated vasoconstriction of the skin of hands, feet, legs, and even forearms, have often occurred upon standing. Twenty-one percent of our patients had syncope or near syncope and 34% had dizziness. Orthostatic hypotension, defined by a fall in blood pressure of 20 mm Hg systolic and 10 mm Hg diastolic upon standing that produced symptoms of inadequate end organ perfusion (brain, skeletal muscles, and heart (6)), was found in 25% of patients. Another 15% of symptomatic patients has maintained a systolic blood pressure of 100 mm Hg or more but has shown abnormal narrowing of pulse pressure to less than 18 mm Hg by Streeten's criteria (7) accompanied by excessive vasoconstriction of the skin and orthostatic symptoms.

Analysis of autonomic function has been based on simultaneous heart-rate and blood-pressure response to standardized challenges. Ten percent of patients had predominantly **cardioexcitatory** or "hyperadrenergic" responsiveness, 33% exhibited predominantly **cardioinhibitory** or "hyperparasympathetic" responses, and 54% had a **mixed** pattern.

Orthostatic intolerance is the salient and most incapacitating abnormality of cardiovascular regulation in our symptomatic MVP patients. In addition to **orthostatic hypotension** it presents as **neurocardiogenic syncope** and as **orthostatic tachycardia** (8) or postural orthostatic tachycardia syndrome (POTS) with symptoms similar to those described by Schondorf and Low (9). **Excessive venous pooling,** which our research suggests occurs mainly in the splanchnic venous bed during upright posture (even sitting in some patients), is a key cause of postural intolerance.

In a study of 129 consecutive MVP patients without a diagnosis of **orthostatic intolerance,** 30 patients (23%) met the criteria for POTS, and 64% had adrenergic or mixed autonomic dysregulation. Catecholamine values were more than two standard deviations greater than our normals for **norepinephrine** in 7/30, **epinephrine** in 8/30, and **dopamine** in 12/30 patients. While 69% of patients with POTS had normal systemic vascular resistance, 31% had values in excess of normal plus two standard deviations. Many of the patients developed symptoms after an apparent viral infection.

Incapacitating fatigue is another frequent symptom. About a third of patients met the criteria of POTS syndrome. Others had lesser degrees of tachycardia with clinical signs of venous pooling and abnormal skin vasoconstriction. **Arterial lactate** determination during upright exercise on a treadmill revealed levels far greater than controls, even at low levels of calculated external work. A stress protocol on a special bicycle that allowed a stable and reproducible apical echocardiographic assessment of left ventricular volume and mitral regurgitation, performed in 15 of those patients, showed a greater decline in left ventricular end-diastolic volume on assuming the sitting position and a failure to increase the volume during exercise (3). This impaired venous capacitance adjustment to the gravitational stress limits exercise cardiac output and may be the fundamental cause of the incapacitating fatigue and the effort intolerance of symptomatic MVP patients. Chronic vasoconstriction due to exaggerated adrenergic tone may further limit muscle blood flow as in patients with chronic heart failure. Gaffney and Blomqvist have postulated that chronic excessive adrenergic stimulation may cause reduction of circulating blood volume that may contribute to orthostatic intolerance, which they have reversed with low-dose clonidine (2).

Orthostatic intolerance has responded to oral **clonidine** (0.1 mg, half a tablet bid or tid) combined with **phenobarbital** if unstable autonomic regulation or significant "hyperparasympathetic responsiveness" was present. In many patients, **fludrocortisone** (0.1 mg, half or one tablet every 12 hr) has been required. A minority of patients have only improved with midodrine, a selective α-adrenergic agent. An elastic abdominal support has been helpful. We do not recommend waist-high elastic garments.

References

1. Boudoulas H, Wooley CF, eds. Mitral valve prolapse and the mitral valve prolapse syndrome. Mount Kisko, NY: Futura, 1988.
2. Gaffney AF, Blomqvist CG. Mitral valve prolapse and autonomic nervous system dysfunction: a pathophysiologic link. In: Boudoulas H, Wooley CF, eds. Mitral valve prolapse and the mitral valve prolapse syndrome. Mount Kisko, NY: Futura, 1988: 427–43.
3. Coghlan HC. Autonomic dysfunction in the mitral valve prolapse syndrome: the brain-heart connection and interaction. In: Boudoulas H, Wooley CF, eds. Mitral valve prolapse and the mitral valve prolapse syndrome. Mount Kisko, NY: Futura, 1988: 389–426 .
4. Cohen L, Laor A, Shnaider H, Palant A. Renal excretion of lactate and magnesium in mitral valve prolapse. Magnesium Res 1988;1:75–8.

5. Coghlan HC, Natello G. Erythrocyte magnesium in symptomatic patients with primary mitral valve prolapse: relationship to symptoms, mitral leaflet thickness, joint hypermobility and autonomic regulation. Magnesium Trace Elements, 1991–92;10:205–14.
6. Fealey RD, Robertson D. Management of orthostatic hypotension. In Low, PA. ed. Clinical autonomic disorders. Boston: Little, Brown, 1993: 731–43.
7. Streeten DHP. Orthostatic disorders of the circulation: mechanisms, manifestations and treatment. New York: Plenum, 1987.
8. Coghlan HC. Autonomic dysfunction and the heart. In: Rapaport E, ed. Cardiology and coexisting disease. New York: Churchill Livingstone, 1994: 293–347.
9. Schondorf R, Low PA. Idiopathic postural tachycardia syndromes. In: Low PA, ed. Clinical autonomic disorders. Boston: Little, Brown, 1993: 641–52.

58

Idiopathic Hypovolemia

Fetnat M. Fouad-Tarazi
Department of Cardiology
The Cleveland Clinic
Cleveland, Ohio

Circulatory volume depletion is usually considered a secondary phenomenon that occurs as a result of fluid loss via the kidney, the gastrointestinal tract, or the skin. Acute circulatory volume depletion may be also due to hemorrhagic blood loss. Contrary to acute volume depletion, which is characterized by hypotension and compensatory tachycardia, **chronic volume depletion** presents with clinical features related to the **associated hemodynamic and compensatory neurohumoral mechanisms.**

Chronic intravascular volume depletion is usually thought to be "secondary" to an underlying event. Patients are interrogated about their dietary habits, salt intake, diuretic use, gastrointestinal losses, excessive diuresis, and nocturia, as well as paroxysmal tachycardia. Search is usually pursued for surreptitious intake of medications, and urine toxicity screening tests are often performed. When no cause can be found, the hypovolemia is labeled **idiopathic.**

The syndrome of **idiopathic hypovolemia** is important to recognize because its normal clinical picture may lead to delays in diagnosis and use of appropriate therapy.

Clinical Features

Orthostatic intolerance is a common symptom in patients with chronic idiopathic hypovolemia. However, in contrast with other types of orthostatic intolerance, these patients frequently have **episodic clinical manifestations sug-**

gestive of **adrenergic hyperactivity** even in the supine resting posture (1). Extreme **elevations in blood pressure** have been reported previously in patients with idiopathic hypovolemia. However, hypertension has been described as labile (1). The episodic rise of blood pressure has been reported to be associated with symptoms of apprehension and perspiration, simulating pheochromocytoma (1). The plasma and urinary catecholamines are typically not elevated.

Our initial clinical impression was of an increased prevalence of vasovagal syncope in patients suffering from severe idiopathic hypovolemia. However, this impression was not substantiated by data analysis in 11 such patients (1); only 1 of the 11 patients developed vasovagal syncope during head-up tilt, while another had vasodepressor syncope without slowing of heart rate. Some patients with documented vasovagal response to tilt are hypovolemic.

Marked reduction of pulse pressure may occur in hypovolemic patients due to the elevation of diastolic blood pressure and the accompanying reduction of systolic blood pressure secondary to the reduction of cardiac output. The peripheral radial pulse may be difficult to palpate in such patients. The clinical importance of this phenomenon is to be stressed because it can be misleading clinically and give a false impression of hypotension unless the femoral arterial pulse is palpated or an intraarterial blood-pressure recording is obtained (1).

Hemodynamic Profile

Intense vasoconstriction is the most important systemic hemodynamic finding even when blood pressure is normal at rest (Tables 1 and 2). In our experience, cardiac index was in the low range of normal whereas left ventricular ejection fraction was normal. The intravascular blood volume was normally distributed between the cardiopulmonary and peripheral segments of the circulation but **the absolute value of the cardiopulmonary volume was reduced** compared with that of normal subjects.

Neurohumoral Indices

Patients with severe idiopathic hypovolemia typically have normal baroreceptor reflexes as well as a normal response of the autonomic nervous system

Table 1.   Blood Volume in Patients with Idiopathic Hypovolemia[a]

	Patients with idiopathic hypovolemia (n = 11)	Normal subjects[b] (n = 24)
TBV (ml/cm)	73 ± 2.3% of normal	29.4 ± 0.81 (male)
		23.7 ± 0.54 (female)
CPV (Ml/m²)	277 ± 14*	413 ± 13
CPV/TBV (%)	14.5 ± 0.14*	16.5 ± 0.5
Hemotocrit	42 ± 1.0	41 ± 0.6

Note. Data from Ref. (1).
[a] All values were obtained during normal salt intake and are given as mean ± SE. TBV, total blood volume; CPV, cardiopulmonary volume.
[b] Normal values taken from 12 men and 12 women.
* $P < 0.05$.

Table 2. **Systemic Hemodynamics in Patients with Idiopathic Hypovolemia and Normal Subjects**[a]

	Patients (n = 11)	Normal subjects (n = 45)
Age (years)	23–50	18–66
Systolic blood pressure (mm Hg)	129 ± 7.0	117 ± 1.6
Diastolic blood pressure (mm Hg)	85 ± 3.0*	78 ± 1.2
Heart rate (beats/min)	76 ± 3.3*	65 ± 1.3
Cardiac index (liters/min/m²)	2.7 ± 0.1**	2.9 ± 0.07
Total peripheral resistance (U. m²)	38 ± 1.3***	32 ± 0.8
Mean transit time (sec)	6.4 ± 0.4***	8.2 ± 0.3
Ejection fraction (%)	55 ± 1.5	55 ± 1.0

Note. Data from Ref. (1).
[a] All values are given as mean ± SE.
* $P < 0.02$ from normal subjects.
** $P < 0.05$ from normal subjects.
*** $P < 0.01$ from normal subjects.

to Valsalva maneuver, cold pressor test, and hyperventilation (1). Furthermore, supine plasma catecholamines were normal at rest and stimulated adequately during head-up tilt. The heart-rate response to graded isoproterenol infusion was increased; however, contrary to patients with hyper-β-adrenergic state (6–8), there was no excessive anxiety reaction and the only symptomatology was mild palpitation without chest discomfort. Serum electrolytes are normal in patients with idiopathic hypovolemia and unrestricted sodium intake. Supine plasma aldosterone was at the upper limit of normal and morning plasma cortisol was normal. Twenty-four-hour urinary sodium excretion ranged from 22 to 236 mEq without correlation to the aldosterone excretion rate.

Possible Mechanisms

The mechanism of volume depletion in patients with idiopathic hypovolemia is difficult to explain. It remains unclear whether **intravascular blood volume contraction** induces the **reflex hyperadrenergic response** or is secondary to **increased vasoconstriction** induced by a primary accentuation of sympathetic activity. Sympathetic overactivity accentuates hypovolemia because of the effects of catecholamine on the venous circulation. The **venoconstrictive effect** of catecholamines **increases capillary hydrostatic pressure** and results in transudation of fluid out of the vascular space (3). On the other hand, hypovolemia induces reflex sympathoadrenergic vasoconstriction so that a vicious circle is created. It has also been postulated that the intense vasoconstriction observed in patients with idiopathic hypovolemia could be due to vascular hyperreaction to a normal adrenergic stimulus affecting both arterial and venous circulation. In our experience, there was no evidence of adrenocortical hypofunction: although no strict metabolic studies were done, there was no clinical or laboratory evidence of sodium wasting in these patients.

Response to Therapy

The syndrome of **idiopathic hypovolemia** is important to recognize because of its important therapeutic implications. Unlike patients with hyper-β-adrenergic state, patients with idiopathic hypovolemia did not manifest improvement of symptoms when treated with β blockers. On the other hand, **acute expansion of blood volume** using human serum albumin led to obvious improvement of symptoms; the increase in blood volume was associated with an increase in cardiac output and a reduction of systemic vascular resistance as well as an attenuation of the tilt-induced accentuated tachycardic response.

Chronic blood volume expansion was difficult to maintain in our patients. Treatment with **fludrocortisone** and a high-sodium diet lead to some relief of symptoms in four of six patients who received this treatment (2). Addition of **clonidine** proved helpful in three of four patients, probably by toning down the sympathetic nervous system activity and buffering heart rate response to upright posture. Another mechanism of action of clonidine could be an **increase of transcapillary transfer of fluid into the venous system** (5).

Contrary to what would be generally conceived, the episodic hypertension in patients with idiopathic hypovolemia has been treated primarily with volume expansion which shuts off the excessive hyperreactive sympathoadrenal and/ or vascular mechanisms induced by the hypovolemic state. Indeed, antihypertensive treatment with a parenteral α-adrenergic blocker, **phentolamine**, given before blood volume expansion was reported to cause circulatory collapse (1) attributed to sudden inhibition of venoconstriction (6) and a marked decrease of venous return when hypovolemia was still uncorrected.

Thus, **idiopathic hypovolemia** is a definite syndrome characterized by **orthostatic intolerance,** disabling **orthostatic tachycardia,** and episodes of **paroxysmal supine hypertension**. The pathophysiologic mechanism of the syndrome is still unclear. Favorable clinical response has been observed when patients are treated with blood volume expansion, either alone or in combination with clonidine therapy.

References

1. Fouad FM, Tadena-Thome T, Bravo EL, Tarazi RC. Idiopathic hypovolemia. Ann Int Med 1986;104:298–303.
2. Frohlich ED, Tarazi RC, Dustan P. Hyperdynamic β-adrenergic circulatory state. Arch Int Med 1969;117:614–9.
3. Cohn JN. Relationship of plasm volume changes to resistance and capacitance vessel effects of sympathomimetic amines and angiotensin in man. Clin Sci 1966;30:267–78.
4. von Baumgarten R, Gupta PD, Henry JP, Sinclair R. Comparison of changes in vagal impulse traffic from venous and arterial systems during moderate hemorrhage. Fed Proc 1965;24:587.
5. Onesti G, Schwartz AB, Kim KE, Paz-Martinez V, Swartz D. Antihypertensive effect of clonidine. Circ Res 1971;28(Suppl II):53–69.
6. Fletcher GF. Hypotensive reactions after small doses of reserpine given parenterally. N Engl J Med 1963;268:309.

PART XII

Other Clinical Conditions

59

Disorders of Sweating

Robert Fealey
Department of Neurology
Mayo Medical Center
Rochester, Minnesota

Hyperhidrosis is defined as sweating that is excessive for a given stimulus. Some of the physiologic factors that increase the sweat response normally are mentioned in Table 1. When these physiologic considerations are exceeded pathologic responses or conditions need to be considered. Hyperhidrosis can be generalized or localized presenting the physician a challenging differential diagnosis. **Generalized hyperhidrosis** can be **primary** (many cases of essential hyperhidrosis) or **secondary** and due to general medical disorders. The hyperhidrosis is usually **episodic** rather than continuous with the neuroendocrine disorders. In **pheochromocyoma,** high circulating levels of catecholamines may stimulate normal thermoregulatory structures to produce cholinergic sudomotor activity as it can be blocked by local hyoscine administration. In **hyperthyroidism,** inappropriate heat production and increased autonomic nerve sensitivity to circulating epinephrine are causative and β-adrenergic blockade can be effective treatment. **Essential hyperhidrosis** with excessive, socially disabling palmar sweating is the most common disorder encountered. Treatment is only partially successful. These include anticholinergic medication, clonidine, and surgical excision (thoracic sympathectomy).

Localized hyperhidrosis is usually the result of autonomic nervous system lesions which are associated with **compensatory or perilesional hyperhidrosis;** not uncommonly the patient's attention is given to the excessive sweating area when **the abnormality is the widespread anhidrosis elsewhere.** Diabetic autonomic failure, pure autonomic failure, and chronic idiopathic anhidrosis are examples in which the phenomenon may occur. Both **gustatory sweating** and the **auriculotemporal (Frey's) syndrome** represent examples of localized hyperhidrosis due to aberrant regeneration of autonomic nerves damaged either surgically or by neuropathy. Rare cases of essential hyperhidrosis occur where the acral (distal) parts sweat heavily while other body parts do not sweat. **Contralateral hyperhidrosis** following cerebral infarction has been described as an uncommon complication possibly due to interruption of descending inhibitory pathways. Patients with cervical and upper thoracic **complete spinal cord traumatic transections** are frequently troubled with **localized hyperhidrosis of the head and upper trunk** when noxious stimuli below the level of their lesion cause autonomic hyperreflexia. When accompanied by paroxysmal hypertension this syndrome can be confused with pheochromocytoma. Often the causative stimulus is a **distended bladder or rectum. In syringomyelia** the excessive sweating is segmental and often appears in dermatomes where sensation is later disturbed. Hyperhidrosis with partial nerve trunk injury occurs as part of a **causalgia pain syndrome** and may be due to an obvious lesion or an

Table 1.   Normal (Physiologic) Factors Affecting Sweating

Parameter	Comments
Age and sex effects	Threshold higher and gland output lower in women; both sexes tend to reduce output at >70 years of age
Acclimatization	Increased output with endurance training or chronic heat exposure or higher humidity
Circadian rhythm	Threshold to sweat varies, often lowest in early morning hours
Posture	Lying on side can produce a contralateral hyperhidrosis and ipsolateral hypohidrosis
Stress and eating	Stress can augment sweating in palms, axillae, feet, forehead; some normals have symmetrical gustatory sweating with spicy foods

occult problem such as paraspinal metastatic deposits affecting the sympathetic chain or white rami.

Hypohidrosis and Anhidrosis

Hypohidrosis is reduction in sweating and **anhidrosis** is the absence of sweating as determined by an established test such as the thermoregualtory sweat test and the quantitative sudomotor axon reflex test (QSART).

Sweating discussed here primarily is thermoregulatory sweating, i.e., that providing man's principal route of excess body heat dissipation and regulated by the autonomic nervous system. **Physiologic hypohidrosis** occurs in skin over bony prominences, in proximal extremities in the elderly, and in dehydrated states where generalized hypohidrosis is observed. Pathologic hypohidrosis and anhidrosis may produce symptoms of **heat intolerance** and dry skin; for example a patient may recognize loss of sweating in the feet (stockings no longer wet at day's end), or that exercise in hot weather causes exhaustion but not sweating. **More often, patients are unaware** of specific symptoms and a high index of suspicion and careful observation for trophic skin changes or other signs

Table 2A.   Pathologic Hyperhidrosis: Differential Diagnosis—Some Causes of Generalized Hyperhidrosis

Condition	Pathophysiologic mechanism of sweating
Pheochromocytoma	Physiological response to inappropriate catecholamine-induced thermogenesis; inhibited by anticholinergics
Thyrotoxicosis	Physiological response to inappropriate catecholamine-induced thermogenesis; inhibited by β blockers
Acromegaly	? Due to excess growth hormone and prolactin, blocked by bromocryptine
Malignancy, chronic infection carcinoid syndrome	Night sweats; ? related to altered hypothalamic set point and effects of prostaglandin E_2
Episodic hypothermia	Developmental abnormalities of central thermoregulatory nucleii and corpus callosum; oxybutinin, clonidine, cyproheptadine, and anticonvulsants may be effective Rx

Table 2B. Pathologic Hyperhidrosis: Differential Diagnosis—Some Causes of Localized Hyperhidrosis

Condition	Pathophysiologic mechanism of sweating
Perilesional and compensatory hyperhidrosis	Central and/or peripheral denervation of large numbers of sweat glands produces increased sweat secretion in those remaining innervated
Gustatory sweating	Resprouting of secremotor axons to supply denervated sweat glands
Postcerebral infarct	Loss of contralateral inhibition with cortical and upper brainstem infarction
Autonomic dysreflexia	Uninhibited segmental somatosympathetic reflex
Causalgia	Damaged peripheral nerve with spontaneous activity of sudomotor axons

and symptoms of autonomic neuropathy has to be developed. Pathologic sweat loss is often best discussed in terms of abnormal patterns noted on direct testing and these are discussed next. Examples are shown in Fig. 1.

Distal Anhidrosis

This refers to sweat loss affecting the peripheral (acral) portions of the extremities, the lower anterior abdomen, and the central forehead. The feet

Table 3. Treatment Measures for Primary Hyperhidrosis

Treatment	Details of treatment	Side effects/complications
Topical Rx	Aluminum chloride hexahydrate in anhydrous ethyl alcohol (Drysol). Apply to dry skin qd or qod hs. Wash off, am. Occlusive technique (covering with Saran Wrap) may be needed	Irritation of skin; less effect on palms and soles
Tanning Rx	Glutaraldehyde (2–10%) solution, from chemical supply mfg. Apply 2–4 times a week prn.	Stains skin brown; for soles of feet only
Iontophoresis	For palms/soles; 15–30 mAmp current, 20 min @ start. Drionic battery run unit or galvanic generator needed. 3–6 rx's/week initially.	Shocks, tingling may occur; difficult to use in axilla; drionic unit not effective when batteries low
Anticholinergic	Glycopyrrolate (Robinual/Robinual Forte) @ 1–2 mg p.o., t.i.d. prn. For intermittent/adjunctive Rx.	Dry mouth, blurred vision. Contraindicated: glaucoma, GI or GU tract obstruction
Clonidine	Useful for paroxysmal, localized (e.g., hemibody) hyperhidrosis 0.1 to 0.3 mg p.o. t.i.d. or as TTS patch (0.1 to 0.3 mg/day) weekly	Somnolence, hypotension, constipation, nausea, rash, impotence, agitation
Excision	2nd and 3rd thoracic ganglionic sympathectomy (palmar hyperhidrosis) sweat glands (axilla)	Horner's syndrome, dry skin, transient dysesthetic pain; post-op scar or infection

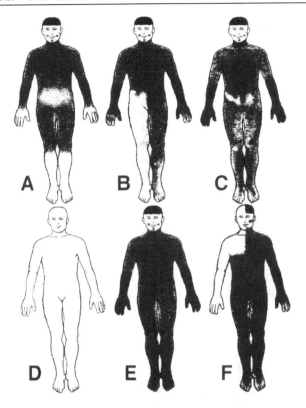

Figure 1.   Sweat distribution patterns. Examples from patients having diabetes mellitus (A through E); patient F had Pancoast's Syndrome (apical lung tumor) on the right. Shown are Distal (A), Segmental (B and F), Distal + Multifocal (Mixed) (C), Global (D), and Normal (E). Sweating in dark shaded areas. Note how the patterns of anhidrosis often suggest the pathophysiology: the glove and stocking loss (patient A) in peripheral neuropathy; the unilateral limb loss (patients B and F) when lesions of the sympathetic chain are encountered; the curvilinear, anterior dermatomal anhidrosis in diabetic truncal radiculopathy (patient C). Table 5 depicts the usual patterns of anhidrosis and likely site of the lesion noted in the disorders with potential sweating abnormalities.

by far are the most commonly affected and the lesion is usually a postganglionic denervation as occurs in peripheral neuropathy.

Global Anhidrosis

This refers to whole body (>80%) sweat loss. It can occur in central lesions (i.e., **Shy–Drager syndrome** (SDS), hypothalamic tumor, cervical spinal cord transsection); at times residual acral sweating will be present in SDS. Global anhidrosis combined with minute islands of preserved sweating is most often due to a widespread postganglionic lesion (i.e., **panautonomic neuropathy**).

Dermatomal, Focal, or Multifocal Anhidrosis

This is sweat loss within the distribution of a peripheral nerve(s) or its branches or root(s) of origin (T1 to L2 or L3 ventral roots). **Mononeuritis**

Table 4. Some Tests of Sympathetic Sudomotor Function

Test	Method	Use
Thermoregulatory sweat test	Whole body heating; Alizarin Red indicator of sweating and nonsweating skin	Good screen for focal or generalized lesions; determine pre- vs postganglionic when used with a postganglionic tests; body surface anhidrosis can be quantitated
QSART (quantitative sudomotor axon reflex)	Ionotphoresis of Ach; recording of indirect axon reflex response	Quantitative response from one or more sites; determine sweat volume and latency of response; test for postganglionic lesions
Silastic imprint method	Iontophoresis of pilocardpine; count of active sweat glands directly activated	Quantitative response from one or more sites; determine sweat drop size, density and is a test for postganglionic lesions
Q-TST (quantitative thermoregulatory sweat test)	Analyzes frequency sweat expulsion and local sweat rate	Quantitative response from one or more sites; determine sweat volume and latency response; test for postganglionic lesions, frequency of sweat expulsions with TRH and heating tests central control
PASP (peripheral autonomic skin potential)	Measures change in sweating indirectly by change in skin resistance	Dynamic, semiquantitative; adaptable to EMG equipment; complex, multisynaptic somatosympathetic loop with CNS and PNS components

Note. Ach, acetylcholine; TRH, thyrotropin-releasing hormone; EMG, electromyography; CNS, central nervous system; PNS, peripheral nervous system.

multiplex produces a multifocal pattern. Focal abnormalities can occur with skin disorders that damage sweat glands or plug their ducts.

Segmental Anhidrosis

This refers to large, contiguous body areas of sweat loss with sharply demarcated borders conforming to sympathetic dermatomes; sympathectomy produces such a pattern. When borders are not well defined and anhidrosis not contiguous a **regional pattern** is said to exist. Both postganglionic and preganglionic lesions may produce these distributions. (Figure 1F shows a patient with an apical lung tumor producing a segmental sweat defect and the patient's chief complaint of a dry right hand.)

Table 5. Sweating Disorders: Pattern and Site of Anhidrosis

Pattern/site of lesion (based on QSART and TST together)	Sweating disorder (selected examples)
Global segmental without acral sparing/pre- and postganglionic sympathetic cyton	Pure autonomic failure (PAF); chronic (idiopathic anhidrosis; Ross syndrome)
Global, segmental, or regional with or without acral sparing/preganglionic and later postganglionic sympathetic cyton	Multiple system atrophy with progressive autonomic failure (Shy–Drager syndrome)
Segmental or distal without acral sparing (often mixed), scattered "islands" of sweat, global at time/postganglionic sympathetic cyton or axon	Acute pandysautonomia (panautonomic neuropathy); idiopathic and acute cholinergic neuropathies
Regional global with or without acral sparing; can be normal/central sympathetic projections, pre- or postganglionic cyton or axon	Neurogenic chronic idiopathic intestinal pseudoobstruction (CIIP); paraneoplastic autonomic neuropathy; postural orthostatic tachycardia syndrome
	Central nervous system lesions
Global with or without acral sparing, hemianhidrosis/central sympathetic projections or preganglionic cytons	Tumors: hypothalamic, parasellar, posterior fossa (brainstem), spinal cord
Contralateral hyperhidrosis occurs with cortical lesions and ipsolateral anhidrosis with brainstem stroke/preganglionic	Cerebral infarction
Global anhidrosis with lesions above first thoracic level; segmental loss below cord level with thoracic lesions; little or no anhidrosis with lumbar cord lesions; perilesional hyperhidrosis with SCI and syrinx/preganglionic acute; pre- and/or postganglionic (chronically)	Spinal cord injury (SCI); syringomyelia; demyelinating myelopathy (i.e., M.S.)
Normal most often; distal common; regional loss in legs and lower abdomen central, pre- and/ or postganglionic	Parkinson's disease; hereditary system degenerations
Regional affecting trunk, proximal limbs; distal/pre- and postganglionic	Dysautonomia of advanced age
Distal most common; dermatomal, focal, segmental (head, leg) even global occur/postganglionic mostly (see Fig. 1)	Diabetic neuropathy, primary systemic amyloidosis
Global without acral sparing; distal regional and segmental; rarely normal/pre- and postganglionic	Guillain–Barré syndrome; Lambert–Eaton myasthenic syndrome; paraneoplastic autonomic neuropathy
Distal loss/postganglionic	Vincristine, heavy metal, uremic, nutritional, idiopathic small fiber neuropathy
Focal, multifocal, dermatomal/postganglionic axon, sweat gland (skin)	Connective tissue diseases
Distal, focal/multifocal, mixed; segmental affecting head and upper extremity postganglionic except preganglionic in Tangier's and sweat gland in Fabry's	Tangier and Fabry's disease
Multifocal affecting cooler areas of body; isolated islands of anhidrosis to widespread distal loss/postganglionic	Leprosy
	Iatrogenic causes
Block muscarinic receptors; reduce postganglionic (i.e., QSART) response for 48 hr; reduced sweating proximal extremities primarily with TST	Psychotropic drugs (phenothiazines, butyrophenones, tricyclic antidepressants), antiparkinsonian drugs (anticholinergics, i.e., Artane, Cogentin)
Segmental loss/ pre and postganglionic compensatory hyperhidrosis can occur	Surgical sympathectomy
	Anhidrosis due to skin disorders
Focal loss/postganglionic or sweat gland	Cholinergic urticaria
Plugging of sweat gland openings	Psoriasis and milia
Scattered areas to global anhidrosis; absence of sweat glands	Hypohidrotic ectodermal dysplasia
Sharp rectangular areas that define the radiation port/postganglionic, sweat gland	Radiation injury

Table 6. Heat Intolerance and Heat Stroke Management

Treatment of heat intolerance	Heat stroke treatment
1. Avoid hot/humid environments	1. Establish Dx criteria: (a) core temp. >41°C or 105.8°F; (b) impaired CNS state; (c) dry, hot ashen or pink skin
2. Be outdoors early am or late pm	2. Immediately remove from hot environment
3. Avoid strenuous activity in heat	3. Surface cool to core temp of 39°C
4. Set house thermostat lower	4. Correct hypovolemia with isotonic saline
5. Wear head covering but loose, light breathable clothing	5. Treat possible complications; DIC, shock rhabdomyolysis, renal failure, seizures
6. Keep well hydrated (2–3 liters/day)	6. Use diazepam to control shivering and seizures
7. Avoid alcohol, diuretics, anticholinergic, and neuroleptic drugs if possible	7. Use of dantrolene is controversial
8. Lower sweat set point with aspirin	

Hemianhidrosis

Sweat loss occurs over one half of the body due to a lesion of the descending sympathetic efferents in the brainstem or upper cervical cord. **Mixed** patterns of anhidrosis (i.e., distal with focal) often occur. Examples of most of the distributions just described are shown in Fig. 1.

Hyperthermia, heat intolerance, heat prostration, and **heat stroke** may occur with widespread failure of thermoregulatory sweating, whereas local skin trophic changes occur with chronic postganglionic sudomotor neuropathy. Heat prostration can be lessened by observing some preventative guidelines and dangerous hyperthermia can be successfully treated. Tables 2–6 provide the therapeutic measures for these clinical situations.

References

1. Quinton PM. Sweating and its disorders. Ann Rev Med 1983;34:429–52.
2. Fealey RD, Low PA , Thomas JE. Thermoregulatory sweating abnormalites in diabetes mellitus. Mayo Clin Proc 1989;64:617–28.
3. Khurana RK. Acral sympathetic dysfunctions and hyperhidrosis. In: Low PA, ed. Clinical autonomic disorders (Evaluation and Management). Boston: Little Brown, 1993: 767–75.
4. Fealey RD. The thermoregulatory sweat test. In: Low PA, ed. Clinical autonomic disorders (Evaluation and Management). Boston: Little Brown, 1993: 217–29.
5. Kihara M, Fealey R, Takahashi A, Schmelzer J. Sudomotor dysfunction and its investigation. In: Korczyn A, ed. Handbook of autonomic nervous system dysfunction. New York: Marcel Dekker, 1995: 523–33.
6. Ingall TJ. Hyperthermia and hypothermia. In: Low PA, ed. Clinical autonomic disorders (Evaluation and Management). Boston: Little Brown, 1993: 713–729.

60

Impotence

Douglas F. Milam
Department of Urology
Vanderbilt University
Nashville, Tennessee

Impotence, a condition defined by insufficient penile rigidity for vaginal penetration, is a frequent symptom of autonomic nervous system dysfunction. The wide spectrum of severity of impotence has led many investigators in the field to label all the variations of this disorder with the term **erectile dysfunction.** Approximately **10 million Americans** have erectile dysfunction. Table 1 illustrates the prevalence of erectile dysfunction in the United States measured by two prospective longitudinal studies. As one can see, at age 40 approximately 5% of men never have penile rigidity sufficient for vaginal penetration. By age 70, at least 15% of American men experience complete impotence while **approximately 50% have varying degrees of erectile dysfunction.** Age and physical health are the most important predictors of the onset of impotence.

The substantial prevalence of erectile dysfunction in the general population complicates identification of true neurogenic impotence due to autonomic nervous system disease. The population distributions characterizing the age of onset of many autonomic dysfunction syndromes overlaps that of nonneurologic impotence. Also, at this point, tests to conclusively identify the neurologic mediation of erectile dysfunction lack sufficient sensitivity and specificity for definitive diagnosis. Identification of neurologic impotence is in part a diagnosis of exclusion.

Etiology of Erectile Dysfunction

Psychogenic impotence was formerly felt to be the most common etiology of erectile dysfunction. Progressive advances in the understanding of the mechanics and neurophysiology of erectile function have identified many other causes of impotence. Psychogenic impotence is now felt to represent **less than 15%** of patients seen by impotence specialists. Other causes include **endocrine** disorders, **vascular** disease, **central and peripheral nerve** disorders, **neuromuscular junction** disorders, **drug-induced** impotence and **venogenic erectile dysfunction.**

Endocrine Disorders

Endocrine disorders play an important role in the etiology of impotence (see Fig. 1). The most obvious, but one of the least prevalent endocrine causes of erectile dysfunction, is **hypogonadism.** Erectile ability is partially **androgen-dependent.** Any disease process which disrupts the hypothalamic–gonadal axis may decrease or even eliminate androgen production by the testes. These

300

Table 1. Prevalence of Impotence

Age (years)	Mild impotence (%)	Moderate impotence (%)	Complete impotence (%)
40	16.5	17.4	4.9
70	18	34	15

	Affected (%)
55	8
65	25
75	55
80	65

Note. MMAS did not correlate testosterone level with impotence (1). Adapted from Baltimore Longitudinal Study of Aging (2).

patients usually complain of **decreased libido** in addition to loss of rigidity. Physical examination of the testes in patients afflicted with primary or secondary hypogonadism often demonstrates **soft, atrophic gonads.** Androgen replacement (**testosterone** cipionate 200 mg q2-3 weeks) generally induces return of erectile function in patients with very low or undetectable serum testosterone concentrations due to hypogonadism. These patients are relatively uncommon, however. More commonly, the impotent patient will have normal or mildly decreased levels of circulating androgens. Testosterone replacement uncommonly restores erectile function in patients with mildly decreased serum testosterone levels. Testosterone supplementation is never indicated for patients with normal circulating androgen levels.

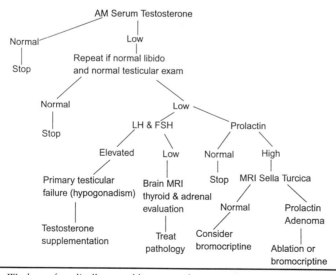

Figure 1. Workup of medically treatable causes of impotence.

The **most common endocrine disorder** affecting erectile ability is **diabetes mellitus.** Diabetes affects both the autonomic and somatic nervous systems in addition to causing atherosclerotic vascular disease. The most important effect diabetes has on erectile ability appears to relate to loss of function of **long autonomic nerves.** Erection is mediated by **efferent parasympathetic cholinergic** neural stimuli. Loss of long cholinergic neurons results in interruption of the efferent side of the erectile reflex arc. Diabetes also appears to produce dysfunction of the neuromuscular junction at the level of arterial smooth muscle in the **penile corpora cavernosa.** Studies have indicated markedly decreased acetylcholine concentration in the trabecular tissue of the corpora cavernosa in diabetics. These findings probably represent a combination of neural loss and neuromuscular junction dysfunction.

Other endocrine disorders including **hypothyroidism, hyperthyroidism,** and **adrenal dysfunction** may uncommonly cause impotence. Due to the rare occurrence of thyroid and adrenal conditions causing impotence, however, testing of those axes is not a part of the routine workup of erectile dysfunction.

Vascular Disease

Vascular disease is a major cause of impotence in the United States. This is primarily due to the prevalent and often severe nature of peripheral vascular disease. Penile erection is obtained by a combination of **relaxation of arteriolar smooth muscle** and increasing **venous outflow resistance distal to the trabecular corpora cavernosa.** This process leads to complete filling of the corpora cavernosa with blood at systemic blood pressure. The principal blood vessels supplying the corpora cavernosa are the **cavernosal arteries.** These vessels are terminal branches of the **pudendal artery** which itself is the terminal branch of the **internal iliac artery.** Either large- or small-vessel arterial disease may decrease corporal blood pressure, leading to failure to achieve penile lengthening and rigidity.

Veno-occlusive disease in the penis is also a significant cause of impotence. These patients typically experience normal initial rigidity, but lose their erection within a brief period of time. This disorder does not play an important role in the differential diagnosis of impotence in the autonomic dysfunction patient and will not be discussed further.

Neurogenic Impotence

Pure neurogenic impotence is a frequent cause of erectile failure. Interruption of either somatic or autonomic nerves or their end units may cause impotence. These nerves control the flow of blood into and likely out of the corpora cavernosa. Afferent somatic sensory signals are carried from the penis via the pudendal nerve to **sacral segments 2–4.** This information is routed both to the brain and to spinal cord autonomic centers. Parasympathetic autonomic nerves originate in the **interomediolateral gray matter** of sacral segments 2–4. These preganglionic fibers exit the anterior nerve roots to join with the sympathetic fibers of the **hypogastric nerve** to form the **pelvic plexus** and **cavernosal nerves.**

The paired nerves penetrate the **corpora cavernosa** and innervate the cavernous artery and vein. Parasympathetic ganglia are located distally near the end organ.

Sympathetic innervation also originates in the **intermediolateral lateral gray matter** but at **thoracolumbar levels T10–L2**. Sympathetic efferents course through the retroperitoneum and condense into the **hypogastric plexus** located anterior and slightly distal to the aortic bifurcation. A concentration of **postganglionic sympathetic fibers** forms the **hypogastric nerve** which is joined by parasympathetic efferents. Adrenergic innervation appears to play a role in the process of **detumescence**. High concentrations of norepinephrine have been demonstrated in the tissue of the corpora cavernosa and tributary arterioles. Additionally, the α-adrenergic antagonist phentolamine is routinely utilized for intracorporal injection therapy to produce erection.

Interestingly, other noncholinergic and nonadrenergic substances appear to play important roles in both induction of erection and detumescence. The two most important groups of substances appear to be **prostaglandins** and **endothelium-derived relaxing factor**. The mechanism of control of these substances by higher centers is only now being investigated.

Afferent signals capable of initiating erection can either originate within the brain, as is the case with psychogenic erections, or result from tactile stimulation. Patients with spinal cord lesions below the thoracolumbar level do not experience tactile reflexive erections but do experience psychogenic erections. There is no discrete center for psychogenic erections. The **temporal lobe** appears to be important; however, other locations such as the gyrus rectus, the cingulate gyrus, the hypothalamus, and the mammillary bodies also appear to be important.

Neurologic testing can often identify the location of autonomic neuropathy. Somatosensory evoked potentials measure pudendal nerve conduction velocity. Conduction is delayed in **multiple sclerosis** and **Shy–Drager syndrome**. These tests can be used to confirm physical examination findings or to identify subtle changes. The **bulbocavernosus reflex** is also useful in identifying potential interruption of the sacral reflex arc. This test is performed by glans stimulation and EMG measurement of bulbocavernosus muscle activity. This test, however, principally examines somatic sensory pathways and is not a good test for the pathways of erection.

Urinary sphincter electromyogram can often be useful in the workup of **multiple-system atrophy** (MSA). The striated urinary sphincter is innervated by Onuf's nucleus and anterior horn cells. These cells are selectively lost in MSA. Prolongation of motor units of urethral and anal sphincters are demonstrable in MSA but not Parkinson's disease. Normal latencies are on the order of 8 msec. MSA patients typically show latencies greater than 20 msec. Other testing methods including measurement of cavernous smooth muscle activity and sympathetic skin responses and acetylcholine sweatspot testing have been utilized with varying results.

References

1. Feldman HA, Goldstein I, Hatzichristou DG, *et al*. Impotence and its medical and psychosocial correlates in Massachusetts male aging study. In press.

2. Morley JE. Baltimore longitudinal study of aging: Impotence. Am J Med 1986;80:897.
3. Blanco R, Saenz de Tejada I, Goldstein I, Krave RJ, Wotiz HH, Cohen RH. Dysfunctional penile cholinergic nerves in diabetic impotent men. J Urol 1990;44:278–80.
4. Benson GS, McConnell JA, Lipschultz LI, *et al.* Neuromorphology and neuropharmacology of the human penis. J Clin Invest 1980;65:506.
5. Eardley I, Quinn NP, Fowler CJ, *et al.* The value of urethral sphincter electromyography in the differential diagnosis of parkinsonism. Br J Urol 1989;64:360.

61 Sleep Apnea and Autonomic Failure

Sudhansu Chokroverty
VA Medical Center
Lyons, New Jersey
St. Vincent's Hospital and Medical Center
of New York
Robert Wood Johnson Medical School
Piscataway, New Jersey
New York Medical College
Valhalla, New York

Sleep, breathing and the autonomic nervous system (ANS) are closely interrelated. **The nucleus tractus solitarius (NTS)**, located in the medulla, not only is the most important structure of the **central autonomic network** but also contains medullary **respiratory neurons** and lower brainstem **hypnogenic neurons.** Through its reciprocally connected ascending projections to the hypothalamus, the limbic system, and other supramedullary regions as well as the descending projections to the ventral medulla and intermediolateral neurons of the spinal cord, the NTS integrates autonomic, respiratory, and hypnogenic neurons. The peripheral respiratory receptors and central respiratory and lower brainstem hypnogenic neurons are also intimately linked by the ANS. Disorders of the ANS may thus implicate breathing during sleep causing a variety of **respiratory dysrhythmias** including sleep apnea. This chapter briefly summarizes such respiratory dysrhythmias in autonomic failure (AF).

Respiration is controlled by independent systems: **automatic** (autonomic or metabolic) and **voluntary** (or behavioral). These two systems behave differently during wakefulness and two states of sleep [e.g., non-rapid eye movement (NREM) and rapid eye movement (REM) sleep determined on the basis of EEG criteria]. During NREM sleep, respiration is controlled entirely by the metabolic controlling system, whereas during wakefulness both the voluntary and the metabolic systems remain active and during REM sleep, the voluntary system is also partly active. Therefore, a failure of the metabolic controlling system in the medulla as a result of pathology in the ascending, descending, or afferent projections of the central autonomic network or brainstem lesions will cause sleep apnea and other respiratory dysrhythmias during sleep (**Ondine's curse**). During normal sleep, there is mild hypoventilation as a result of decreased number of functioning respiratory units, decreased sensitivity of the medullary chemoreceptors, and increased upper airway resistance. This **physiological sleep-related hypoventilation** becomes prolonged during pathological alteration.

Sleep Apnea in Autonomic Failure

Sleep apnea and other respiratory dysrhythmias have been described in many patients with AF. AF can be primary or secondary to a variety of central or peripheral neurological or other medical disorders and familial dysautonomia. The best known condition with primary AF is the **Shy–Drager syndrome** (**multiple-system atrophy** with progressive autonomic failure). The Shy–Drager syndrome (SDS) is a multisystem neurodegenerative disease characterized initially by dysautonomic manifestations (e.g., four most important manifestations consist of **orthostatic hypotension, urinary sphincter dysfunction, hypo- or anhidrosis,** and **impotence** in men) followed by a parkinsonian-cerebellar syndrome and upper motor neuron and lower neuron dysfunction. A number of sleep-related respiratory dysrhythmias have been noted in most of these patients (Fig. 1) in the intermediate stage of the illness which lasts on an average about

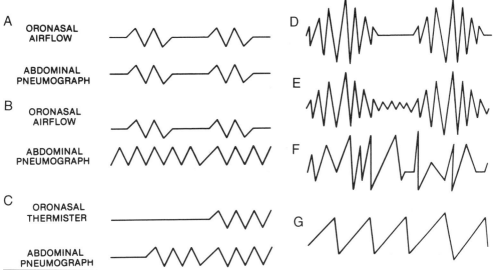

Figure 1. Schematic diagram to show different respiratory patterns in the Shy–Drager syndrome. (A) Central apnea, (B) upper airway obstructive apnea, (C) mixed apnea, (D) Cheyne–Stokes breathing, (E) Cheyne–Stokes variant pattern, (F) dysrhythmic breathing, (G) apneustic breathing. Reproduced, with permission, from Bannister R, Mathias CJ. Clinical features and investigation of the primary autonomic failure syndromes. In: Autonomic failure: a textbook of clinical disorders of the autonomic nervous system. Oxford: Oxford University Press, 1992:531–47.

9 years. Polysomnographic (PSG) recordings confirmed the presence of sleep apnea (Fig. 2) and other respiratory dysrhythmias in many reports.

The most common respiratory disturbances in SDS are **sleep apnea** or **hypopnea, dysrhythmic breathing,** and **nocturnal stridor.** Sleep apnea can be three types: **central (CA), upper airway obstructive (OA)** and **mixed type (MA).** During CA, there is cessation of both airflow and effort (i.e., no diaphragmatic or intercostal muscle activities), whereas during OA there is no airflow but the effort continues (Fig. 1). MA is characterized by an initial period of CA followed by OA (Fig. 2). Hypopnea has the same significance as apnea and is manifested by a reduction of the tidal volume by one-half of the value of the preceding respiratory cycle. To be significant, apnea or hypopnea must last **at least 10 sec;** apnea or hypopnea index (number of episodes per hour of sleep) or **respiratory disturbance index** (total number of apneas and hypopneas per hour of sleep) should be five or more.

Apneic–hypopneic episodes are accompanied by oxygen desaturation, repeated arousals throughout the night causing a reduction of slow wave and REM sleep, and increased wakefulness after sleep onset. These nocturnal episodes of repeated oxygen desaturation and arousals may cause **daytime somnolence, early morning headache,** daytime fatigue, intellectual deterioration, and impotence in men, and may lead to systemic or pulmonary hypertension,

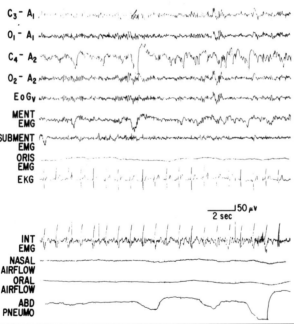

Figure 2.   Polygraphic recording in a patient with the Shy–Drager syndrome showing electroencephalogram (top four channels), electrooculogram (vertical), electromyograms of mentalis (MENT), submental (subment), oris, and intercostal (INT) muscles, electrocardiogram (EKG), nasal and oral airflow, abdominal pneumogram (ABD PNEUMO). The recording shows a portion of an episode of mixed apnea associated with oxygen desaturation during stage 2 NREM sleep. (Reproduced, with permission, from Chokroverty S. Sleep and breathing in neurological disorders. In: Edelman NH, Santiago TV, eds. Breathing disorders of sleep. New York: Churchill Livingstone, 1986: 225–264.)

congestive cardiac failure, or cardiac arrhythmias. Hypercapnic ventilatory responses may be impaired in some of these patients, suggesting impairment of central respiratory chemoreceptors in the brainstem. **Dysrhythmic breathing,** characterized by a pattern of nonrhythmic respirations of irregular rate, rhythm, and amplitude (Fig. 1), more apparent during sleep than during wakefulness and often accompanied by short periods of apneas or hypopneas, is very common in SDS. Hypercapnic ventilatory responses may be normal in such patients, implying a defect in the respiratory pattern generators in the brainstem. In many patients with SDS, **nocturnal stridor** is a common feature causing marked inspiratory breathing difficulty and is associated with laryngeal abductor paralysis, severe snoring, and upper airway obstruction. Less commonly, the patients with SDS may have other respiratory disturbances which may include **apneustic breathing** with a prolonged inspiration and an increase in the ratio of inspiratory to expiratory time, inspiratory gasps, **Cheyne–Stokes** or Cheyne–Stokes variant breathing (Fig. 1), which is a type of central apnea, and sudden respiratory arrest, often during sleep at night leading to sudden death.

Neuropathologic findings in SDS comprise those noted in striatonigral and olivopontocerebellar degeneration, and **oligondendroglial inclusions and neuronal loss** in the intermediolateral column of the spinal cord. Respiratory dysrhythmias probably result in part from direct involvement of the brainstem region containing respiratory neurons in addition to other mechanisms.

Sleep apneas accompanied by oxygen desaturation have also been noted in patients with **familial dysautonomia (Riley–Day syndrome)** and acquired polyneuropathies, particularly **diabetic autonomic neuropathies,** occasionally also in **amyloidosis** and **Guillain–Barré syndrome.** Familial dysautonomia is a recessively inherited disorder confined to the Jewish population. In addition to the dysautonomic manifestations of fluctuating postural hypotension and paroxysmal hypertension, defective lacrimation, impaired sweating, and vasomotor instability, the patient presents a variety of cardiovascular, skeletal, renal, neuromuscular, and respiratory abnormalities. PSG recordings in several reports of familial dysautonomia documented central and upper airway obstructive sleep apneas. In diabetic autonomic neuropathies, PSG recordings have also documented central and obstructive apneas in addition to respiratory irregularities associated with esophageal reflux during sleep causing frequent awakenings.

Diagnosis

First and foremost in the diagnosis of AF is the clinical manifestation of dysautonomia followed by autonomic function tests. For secondary AF, appropriate tests to establish the primary cause should be performed. To document the presence, type, and severity of sleep apnea, it is essential to perform **overnight PSG** consisting of simultaneous recording of electroencephalogram, electrooculogram, electromyogram, electrocardiogram, recording of respiration by oronasal thermistors and thoraco-abdominal respiratory bands (Respitrace), and oxygen saturation by finger oximetry. All patients with complaints of excessive daytime sleepiness should have a PSG preformed. Daytime nap studies are not adequate as REM sleep is usually not recorded and the severity and presence of sleep apnea are difficult to assess.

Multiple sleep latency test during daytime may be obtained to document pathological sleepiness. A mean sleep latency of less than 5 min is consistent with excessive sleepiness. Pulmonary function tests including assessment of chemical control of breathing by determining hypercapnic and hypoxic ventilatory responses and mouth occlusion pressure ($P_{.01}$) are important to exclude intrinsic pulmonary diseases and to identify impairment of chemical control of breathing. EMG of the upper airway, diaphragmatic, and intercostal muscles may be indicated in selected patients with SDS. In patients with nocturnal stridor upper airway endoscopy and laryngoscopy may be needed to detect laryngeal paralysis.

Treatment

Only symptomatic measures for sleep apnea or other respiratory dysrhythmias and treatment of the primary condition causing secondary AF are available. SDS is an inexorably progressive neurological disease pursuing a relentless course despite improvement of orthostatic hypotension and other dysautonomic manifestations following symptomatic treatment which may improve the quality of life temporarily.

General measures and medical treatment. General measures include avoidance of alcohol and sedative-hypnotics which may depress respiration. Medical treatment of sleep apnea is not generally satisfactory, but **protriptyline,** a nonsedative tricyclic antidepressant, and **medroxyprogesterone** in mild cases of central and obstructive apneas, and **acetazolamide** in central apnea, may have some limited usefulness.

Mechanical treatment. In moderate to severe cases of upper airway obstructive apnea, nasal **continuous positive airway pressure** (CPAP) by using a nasal mask throughout the night is useful. Following such treatment, often sleep quality will improve and daytime somnolence will be eliminated due to reduction or elimination of sleep-related obstructive or mixed apneas or oxygen desaturation. However, the natural history of SDS will not be altered by such treatment. The benefit of nasal CPAP in SDS has not been as dramatic as in patients with primary obstructive sleep apnea syndrome because of the natural history of inexorable progression of the illness despite all symptomatic measures. A sufficient number of studies have not been made in such disorders using CPAP treatment. In acquired autonomic neuropathies, CPAP treatment is an excellent therapy for obstructive apneas. Several types of home CPAP units are available.

Surgical treatment. Tracheostomy remains the only effective emergency treatment for severe respiratory dysfunction in patients with laryngeal stridor due to laryngeal abductor paralysis and in patients who have been resuscitated from respiratory arrest. However, a decision to preform tracheostomy in a progressive neurodegenerative disease with AF with an overall unfavorable prognosis must be carefully weighed before pursuing this therapy.

References

1. Chokroverty S. Sleep, breathing and neurological disorders. In: Chokroverty S, ed. Sleep disorders medicine: basic science, technical consideration and clinical aspects. Boston: Butterworth-Heinemann, 1994: 295–335.
2. Chokroverty S. Sleep apnea and autonomic failure. In: Low PA, ed. Clinical Autonomic Disorders. Boston: Little Brown, 1993: 589–603.
3. Shy GM, Drager GA. A neurological syndrome associated with orthostatic hypotension. Arch Neurol 1960;2,511–27.
4. Bannister R, Mathias CJ. Clinical features and investigation of the primary autonomic failure syndromes. Bannister R, Mathias CJ, eds. Autonomic failure: a textbook of clinical disorders of the autonomic nervous system, 3rd ed. Oxford: Oxford University Press, 1992: 531–47.
5. Low PA. Laboratory evaluation of autonomic failure. Low PA, ed. Clinical autonomic disorders. Boston: Little Brown, 1993: 169–95.

62

Hypoadrenocorticism

David H. P. Streeten
SUNY Health Science Center
Syracuse, New York

The autonomic nervous system has important relationships with the function of the adrenal cortex both (a) in the actions of sympathetic nervous function on adrenocortical secretion, and (b) in the profound effects of cortisol and aldosterone deficiency on the efficacy of sympathetic nervous activity in maintaining the blood pressure, especially during stress.

Effects of Autonomic Activity on Adrenocortical Secretion

There is convincing evidence from animal studies that the hypothalamic-pituitary–adrenal (HPA) system is stimulated at various central sites, resulting in an increase in **corticotropin-releasing hormone** (CRH) secretion and the release of ACTH from pituitary corticotropes *in vitro*. On the other hand, measurements in the human subject have shown that increasing plasma norepinephrine (NE) levels by NE infusions, into the range seen in moderate stress, had no effect on the ACTH or cortisol response to CRH administration. While these observations fail to show any direct action of NE on the pituitary response to CRH, they do not rule out the possibility that autonomic neuronal activity within the hypothalamus might increase CRH or vasopressin release and consequently cortisol secretion in human subjects. In patients with **multiple system** atrophy (MSA) and **pure autonomic failure,** insulin-induced hypoglycemia, normally a potent stimulus to the sympathetic nervous system, frequently fails to stimulate epinephrine release from the adrenal medulla, yet does not fail to increase HPA function, as indicated by a normal increase in cortisol secretion. These important observations strongly suggest that diffuse autonomic insufficiency has little if any effect on adrenocortical secretion in response to hypoglycemic stress in mankind.

In contrast with the findings related to the release of cortisol, there is little doubt that autonomic failure, through the loss of β-adrenergic stimulation of renin release from the juxtaglomerular apparatus, which it induces, profoundly reduces the adrenocortical section of aldosterone. **Hyporeninemic hypoaldosteronism** may arise either centrally in patients with MSA or peripherally in patients with diabetic or other forms of peripheral neuropathy. It may cause **hyperkalemia** and **hypovolemia,** which are reversible with fludrocortisone administration. It also contributes to the severity of the orthostatic hypotension that results predominantly from the direct effect of autonomic failure on vascular contractility, and this is somewhat ameliorated but not completely corrected by fludrocortisone in these patients.

Effects of Hypoadrenocorticism on Autonomic Failure

Cortisol, secreted by the cells of the zona fasciculata, reaches the zona medullaris via the adrenal portal venous circulation to create an unusually high concentration of the steroid within the adrenal medulla. This **elevated cortisol** concentration is required for induction of the enzyme **phenylethanolamine N-methyltransferase** which normally methylates **norepinephrine** to form **epinephrine.** The deficiency of epinephrine production which one would, therefore, expect to result from adrenocortical insufficiency may play an important role in the excessive susceptibility of patients with primary or secondary hypocortisolism to fasting or insulin-induced hypoglycemia. There is no clear evidence that adrenocortical deficiency has other direct effects on the function of autonomic neurons.

Cortisol and other glucocorticoids do have an essential function in **sensitizing** the vasoconstrictive response of the peripheral vasculature to norepinephrine. This phenomenon was first demonstrated in the experiments of Fritz and Levine who found that the sensitivity of the mesoappendicular arterial supply of the rat to locally applied NE was strikingly reduced *in vivo* by previous bilateral adrenalectomy. This requirement of the vasculature for adequate concentrations of glucocorticoid is of great clinical importance. It probably underlies the **orthostatic hypotension** that is so reliable an early clinical manifestation of **cortisol deficiency,** and it causes recumbent hypotension and shock in patients with adrenocortical deficiency during stress. The common stress-induced hypotension that is unresponsive to intravenous infusions of phenylephrine, norepinephrine, epinephrine, and dopamine is certainly due to hypocortisolism in many patients. In these individuals glucocorticoid administration rapidly restores normal vascular responsiveness to sympathomimetic drugs and is followed by restoration of normotension.

References

1. Vale W, Vaughan J, Smith M, Yamamoto G, Rivier J, Rivier C. Effects of synthetic bovine corticotropin-releasing factor, glucocorticoids, catecholamines, neurohypophyseal peptides, and other substances on cultured corticotropic cells. Endocrinology 1983;113:1121.
2. Milson SR, Donald RA, Espiner EA, Nichols MG, Livesey JH. The effect of peripheral catecholamine concentrations on the pituitary-adrenal response to corticotrophin releasing factor in man. Clin Endocrinol 1986;25:241–6.
3. Polinsky RJ, Kopin IJ, Ebert MH, Weisse V, Recant L. Hormonal responses to hypoglycemia in orthostatic hypotension patients with adrenergic insufficiency. Life Sci 1981;29:417–25.
4. Fritz I, Levine R. Action of adrenal cortical steroids and norepinephrine on vascular responses to stress in adrenalectomized rats. Am J Physiol 1951;165:456–65.

63

Surgical Sympathectomy

Peter R. Wilson
Department of Anesthesiology
Mayo Clinic
Rochester, Minnesota

Surgical sympathectomy (Table 1) includes all physical techniques for interrupting the continuity of the sympathetic ganglia or peripheral sympathetic nerves. The most common sites for sympathectomy are at the upper thoracic ganglia, stellate ganglion, and lumbar sympathetic chain. Operative techniques involve cutting or thermocoagulation at open operation or via thoracoscopy. A variation of surgical sympathectomy involves stripping of the adventitia (including the sympathetic nerves) of arteries to reverse sympathetically mediated vasoconstriction.

Chemical sympathectomy involves the injection of neurolytic agents such as phenol or alcohol near the sympathetic chain and ganglia to coagulate the tissues. This is achieved by blind needle techniques or under fluoroscopic, CT, or MRI guidance. There are few studies comparing the relative efficacies of surgical and chemical sympathectomies. However, advantages claimed for chemical sympathectomy in the lumbar region include simplicity (injection versus major abdominal surgery), lower mortality and morbidity, lower cost and inconvenience (outpatient versus inpatient procedure), and ability to perform the procedure on patients too physiologically unstable for open operation.

Pharmacologic sympathectomy involves the use of drugs to interfere with central control of sympathetic tone, block transmission at the sympathetic ganglia, produce false transmitters, and deplete or block the synthesis, release, action, or effect of sympathetic transmitters on the presynaptic terminal or end-organ receptors (usually blood vessels).

Table 1.   Surgical Sympathectomy

Surgical (cervico) thoracic sympathectomy

Indications
 Primary palmar hyperhidrosis
 Sympathetically maintained pain of the upper extremity (RSD/CRPS)
 Peripheral vascular insufficiency of the upper extremities
   Buerger's, Raynaud's, scleroderma, frostbite, plastic/reconstructive surgical free flaps
 Thoracic outlet syndrome
 Prolonged QT syndrome
Complications
 Pneumothorax
 Branchial plexus injury
 Edema and pain of the upper extremity
 Horner's syndrome

Surgical lumbar sympathectomy

Indications
 Peripheral vascular insufficiency of the lower extremities
   Atherosclerotic disease (large- or small-vessel)
 Demarcation/improvement in stump healing after amputation for ischemia
 Sympathetically maintained pain (RSD/CRPS)
Complications
 All those of abdominal surgery
 Ureteric damage (rare)
 Postural hypotension
 Impotence (rare, especially bilateral)
 Nerve damage/neuralgias
 Edema and pain of the lower extremity

Although the function of the peripheral sympathetic system has been studied intensively, it is clear that all aspects are not understood. While the role in regulation of circulation is relatively well understood, the role of the sympathetic nervous system in inflammatory processes or in pain states such as reflex sympathetic dystrophy (complex regional pain syndrome type I), causalgia (complex regional pain syndrome, type II), or neuropathic pain conditions such as postherpetic neuralgia or phantom limb pain remains controversial and incompletely understood.

The long-term clinical effects of surgical, chemical, or pharmacologic sympathectomy have not been studied in detail. For example, many clinical papers describe the failure of surgical sympathectomy in some cases after 2 weeks–6 months (i.e., the return to the presurgical vasomotor tone or compensatory hyperhidrosis). However, there are no good data for the incidence of this occurrence or the time course of return of sympathetic function. Similarly, there are no data regarding the relative role of two potential mechanisms: "reinnervation" and development of denervated receptor supersensitivity to circulating catecholamines.

Surgical sympathectomy is a procedure with a long history, but with a decreasing place in the medical armamentarium because of inadequate information about its long-term effects and the improvements in pharmacological methods of sympathectomy.

References

1. Jones NF. Acute and chronic ischemia of the hand: pathophysiology, treatment and prognosis. J Hand Surg (AM) 1991;16:1074–83.
2. Shepherd JT. The evolving knowledge of the physiopathology of the circulation in human limbs. From sympathectomy to molecular biology. Int Angiol 1992;11:8–13.
3. Schwartz PJ, Locati EH, Moss AJ, Crampton RS, Trazzi R, Ruberti U. Left cardiac sympathetic denervation in the therapy of congenital long Q-T syndrome. A worldwide report. Circulation 1991;84:503–11.
4. Schott GD. Visceral afferents: their contribution to "sympathetic dependent" pain. Brain 1994;117(2):397–413.
5. O'Riordain DS, Maher M, Waldron DJ, O'Donovan B, Brady MP. Limiting the anatomic extent of upper thoracic sympathectomy for primary palmar hyperhidrosis. Surg Gynaecol Obstet 1993;176:151–4.

64

Mastocytosis

L. Jackson Roberts II
Vanderbilt University
Nashville, Tennessee

Although **mastocytosis** is not a disorder of the autonomic nervous system, some of the symptoms and signs of the disease may be interpreted as consistent with autonomic dysfunction. Thus, it is important for physicians involved in the evaluation of patients suspected of having disorders of the autonomic nervous system to recognize the hallmarks of the disease.

Mastocytosis and Allied Activation Disorders of the Mast Cell

Mastocytosis is characterized by an abnormal proliferation of **tissue mast cells.** The cause of the overproliferation of mast cells remains unknown. Although unusual forms of the disease can occur primarily in children, e.g., a localized **mastocytoma,** the disease in adults exists primarily in two forms; one in which the abnormal proliferation of mast cells either appears to be limited to the skin (**cutaneous mastocytosis**) or involves multiple tissues throughout the body (**systemic mastocytosis**).

In recent years, an allied activation idiopathic disorder(s) of mast cells has also been identified in which patients experience episodes of systemic mast cell activation in the absence of any evidence of abnormal mast cell proliferation. An allergic basis for the activation of mast cells may be suspected in some patients, while in others the cause remains unclear. Whereas mastocytosis is an uncommon disease, idiopathic activation disorders of the mast cell are encountered more frequently.

The **symptoms** of both mastocytosis and systemic activation disorders of the mast cell are attributed primarily to **episodic release of mast cell mediators.** The episodes of mastocyte activation can be brief, lasting several minutes, or protracted, lasting a few hours. These episodes frequently occur without any identifiable inciting cause. However, **exposure to heat, exertion,** and **emotional upset** are commonly identified as **precipitating factors** by many patients. The major symptoms experienced by these patients are listed in Table 1. Probably the most important clinical clue which should lead one to suspect a diagnosis of systemic mast cell disease is flushing. In some patients, cutaneous vasodilation is not appreciated but patients will usually note that they feel very warm. Unlike allergic anaphylaxis, bronchospasm, angioedema, and urticaria are uncommon manifestations. Characteristically, following an episode of mastocyte activation, patients experience **extreme fatigue and lethargy,** which can last for hours.

Hemodynamic alterations frequently occur during episodes of systemic mast cell activation. Characteristically, the **blood pressure falls** and the **heart rate increases.** At times the reduction in blood pressure can be profound, resulting in severe **lightheadedness** or frank **syncope.** The reduction in blood pressure in accentuated in the upright position and patients note that lightheadedness is improved upon assuming the supine position. However, in occasional patients the **blood pressure increases,** at times dramatically, during episodes of mast cell activation. The elevation in blood pressure is also accompanied by an **increase in heart rate.** The basis for the rise in blood pressure in some patients remains speculative.

Mast Cell Mediators Responsible for the Symptoms and Signs

The hemodynamic alterations and symptoms experienced by patients with mastocytosis had previously been attributed to the release of excessive quantities of **histamine** from mast cells. However, treatment with antagonists of histamine H1 and H2 receptors had not been found to prevent episodes of vasodilation in these patients. In 1980, the discovery of marked overproducion

Table 1.   **Symptoms of Systemic Mast Cell Activation**

1. Flushing (and/or a feeling of warmth)
2. Palpitations
3. Dyspnea (usually without wheezing)
4. Chest discomfort
5. Headache
6. Lightheadedness and occasionally syncope
7. Gastrointestinal symptoms
   A. Nausea and occasionally vomiting
   B. Abdominal cramps and occasionally diarrhea
8. Profound lethargy after the attack

of **prostaglandin D$_2$**, a potent vasodilator, in patients with mastocytosis was reported. Subsequently, it was found that treatment of patients with mastocytosis with inhibitors of prostaglandin biosynthesis in addition to antihistamines can be effective in ameliorating episodes of vasodilation in these patients. However, a subset of patients with disorders of systemic mast cell activation are **aspirin hypersensitive** and administration of any prostaglandin inhibitor, even in small doses, can provoke a severe episode of mastocyte activation. Thus, great caution must be exercised in treating patients with disorders of systemic mast cell activation with inhibitors of prostaglandin biosynthesis. The pathogenesis of aspirin hypersensitivity remains poorly understood.

Diagnosis

The diagnosis of systemic disorders of the mast cell is not always straightforward. Patients with mastocytosis frequently have small **pigmented cutaneous lesions,** termed **urticaria pigmentosa.** Urticaria pigmentosa lesions characteristically urticate when stroked (**Darier's sign**). When visible cutaneous clues to the diagnosis are absent, the diagnosis relies on the recognition of a compatible clinical history. In patients with mastocytosis, a diagnosis may be made histologically by demonstrating abnormal mast cell proliferation in the skin or bone marrow. In patients with activation disorders of the mast cell in the absence of abnormal mast cell proliferation, the diagnosis relies entirely on demonstrating a release of increased quantities of **histamine and prostaglandin D$_2$** during episodes of suspected mastocyte activation. In patients with systemic mastocytosis, increased urinary excretion of metabolites of histamine and prostaglandin D$_2$ can usually be demonstrated even at quiescent times. On the other hand, in patients with idiopathic activation disorders of the mast cell, **increased excretion of metabolites of histamine and prostaglandin D$_2$** can only be demonstrated in fractional urines collected during episodes of mastocyte activation.

Patients with disorders of systemic mast cell activation may be encountered more frequently than previously thought and some of the symptoms and signs manifested by these patients, e.g., **orthostatic intolerance and orthostatic hypotension,** are not unlike some of those experienced by patients with autonomic dysfunction. Specifically, a patient with "spells" characterized by flushing that may be precipated by heat, exertion, or emotional upset accompanied by lightheadedness and either a reduction or an increase in blood pressure and tachycardia should lead the astute clinician to consider the possiblity of a disorder of systemic mast cell activation.

References

1. Metcalfe DD. Classification and diagnosis of mastocytosis: current status. J Invest Dermatol 1991; 96:S2–4.
2. Soter NN. The skin in mastocytosis. J Invest Dermatol 1991;96:S32–9.
3. Roberts LJ, II, Oates JA. Disorders of vasodilator hormones: the cardinoid syndrome and mastocytosis. In: Wilson JD, Foster DW, eds. Williams textbook of endocrinology, 8th ed. Philadelphia: W. B. Saunders, 1992: 1619–33.
4. Roberts LJ, Oates JA. The biochemical diagnosis of systemic mast cell disorders. J Invest Dermatol 1991;96:S19–25.

65 Nonpharmacological Management of Autonomic Disorders

Wouter Wieling
Department of Medicine
Academic Medical Center
Amsterdam
The Netherlands

External Support and Physical Counter-Maneuvers

Applying **external pressure** to the lower half of the body substantially reduces venous pooling when upright, and consequently arterial pressure and cerebral perfusion are better maintained. External support can be applied by bandages firmly wrapped around the legs, or a snugly fitted abdominal binder, but is best accomplished by a custom- fitted counterpressure support garment, made of elastic mesh, which forms a single unit extending from the metatarsals to the costal margin. The design of the garment creates a gradient of counterpressure maximal at the ankles and minimal at the waist. The gradient compensates for height-dependent gravitational pooling in the legs and has an effect comparable to being submersed to the waist in water.

External support garments are helpful in the treatment of a patient with incapacitating orthostatic hypotension, but have several disadvantages. First, the motivation of the patient must be strong, since they are uncomfortable to wear. Second, they **disrupt normal physiology,** in that they attenuate compensatory neurohumoral responses and diminish adaptation of autoregulatory mechanisms of the cerebral blood vessels to low systemic pressure. In addition, support garments prevent the formation of **peripheral edema** in the legs, which is considered to be an essential factor for effective therapy of orthostatic hypotension by acting as a perivascular **water jacket** that limits the vascular volume available for orthostatic pooling. We, therefore, only use an abdominal binder as a temporary expedient to achieve mobility in our most severely affected patients.

It is important to realize that specific treatment of the underlying disease in patients with autonomic failure is usually not possible and that the goal in management consequently is to obtain symptomatic improvement by other means. Physical maneuvers that are both easy to apply and effective in combating orthostatic dizziness in daily life are, therefore, of obvious importance. Patients with autonomic failure have discovered several such maneuvers themselves. The beneficial effects of **leg-crossing, squatting, abdominal compression, bending forward,** and **placing one foot on a chair** have been described. A great advantage of these maneuvers is that they can be applied instantaneously at the moment of symptomatic low upright pressure. The subtle but significant effects of physical maneuvers on a low standing blood pressure are difficult to monitor by sphygmomanometric readings, but a Finapres device, which tracks the blood pressure signal continuously and noninvasively, enables quantification of their effects in great detail (Fig. 1). In daily practice the effectiveness of physical maneuvers in an individual patient can be assessed by the length of time a patient can stand in place before experiencing orthostatic symptoms (**standing time**). An increase in the standing time from only 1 min to 3–5 min implies a substantial improvement in functional capacity.

Leg-Crossing

Leg-crossing is the simplest maneuver to increase the standing time in a patient with autonomic failure. It has the advantage that it can be performed without much effort and without bringing attention to the patient's problem. The maneuver is performed by crossing one leg in direct contact with the other while actively standing on both legs (Fig. 2). Crossing ones legs is often applied unintentionally also by healthy humans when standing for prolonged periods (cocktail party posture). The increase in mean arterial pressure and pulse pressure induced by leg-crossing (Figs. 1 and 3A) can be attributed to tensing and compression of the muscles in the upper legs and abdomen with mechanical squeezing of venous vessels. The result is an increase in central blood volume and thereby in cardiac filling pressures, cardiac output, and arterial pressure.

Although the increase in upright blood pressure induced by leg-crossing is relatively small with an increase in mean arterial pressure of 10–15 mm Hg (Figs. 1 and 3A), one should realize that medical treatment with **fludrocortisone, erythropoietin,** and **midodrine** results in similarly small blood pressure increases. Despite these small increases the standing time improves markedly by all four, because they shift mean arterial pressure from just below to just above the critical level of perfusion of the brain. A driving pressure of about 40 mm Hg is needed to maintain cerebral blood flow in young adult subjects in supine posture. Normal humans in the **upright position** need a mean arterial pressure of about **70 mm Hg** measured at heart level in order to compensate for the effects of gravity on the circulation. Patients with orthostatic hypotension tolerate a much lower standing mean pressure occasionally as low as 50 mm Hg, probably by adaption of autoregulatory mechanisms of the blood vessels in the brain.

Preliminary data suggest that leg-crossing is also effective in combating episodes of orthostatic hypotension in otherwise healthy subjects with a postural tachycardia syndrome or under fainting conditions. The maneuver can also be used for the prevention of orthostatic dizziness in the sitting position. Importantly, the rise in arterial pressure during leg-crossing is additive to that induced by volume expansion by **fludrocortisone** and **head-up tilted sleeping** and, presumably, to other treatment modalities as well. It is our experience that after proper instruction and training patients automatically apply leg-crossing in daily life.

Squatting

Squatting increases arterial mean pressure and pulse pressure (Figs. 1 and 3B) by two mechanisms. First, blood is squeezed from the veins of the legs and of the

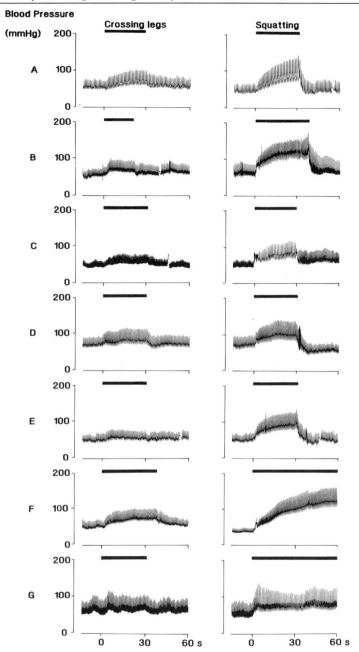

Figure 1.   Effects on arterial blood pressure of leg-crossing and squatting in 7 patients with hypoadrenergic orthostatic hypotension. Subjects are standing quietly prior to the maneuvers. Bars indicate periods of standing with legs crossed and squatting. Note the instantaneous increase both in absolute arterial pressure and pulse pressure. Reprinted with permission from Van Lieshout JJ, Ten Harkel ADJ, Weiling W. Combating orthostatic dizziness in autonomic failure by physical maneuvers. 339:897–8, © by The Lancet Ltd., 1992.

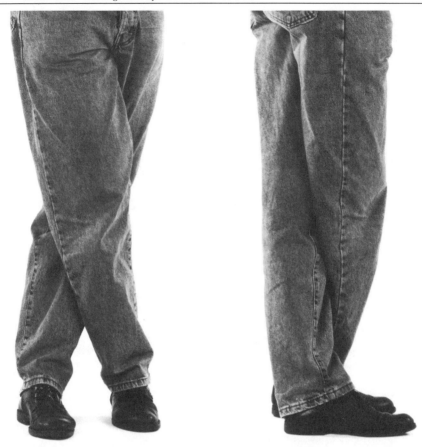

Figure 2.   Legs in the crossed position; from the front and from the side (cocktail party posture). Used with permission from Ten Harkel (unpublished).

splanchnic vascular bed, which **increases cardiac filling pressures** and cardiac output. Second, the mechanical impediment of the circulation to the legs **increases systemic vascular resistance.** Squatting is an effective emergency mechanism to prevent a loss of consciousness when presyncopal symptoms develop rapidly. Bending over as if to tie ones shoes has similar effects and is simpler to perform by elderly patients. The beneficial effects of **sitting in knee–chest position** or **placing one foot on a chair** while standing are comparable to squatting. The effects of placing a foot in a chair on the level of blood pressure are stronger than those induced by leg-crossing (Fig. 3A and 3C), but evidently more difficult to apply in daily life.

Abdominal Compression and Bending Forward

The arterial pressure-raising effect of abdominal compression (Fig. 3D) can again be attributed to the squeezing of blood from the compliant splanchnic venous pool and results in an increased central blood volume and left ventricular filling. Bending forward shortens the hydrostatic height difference between the

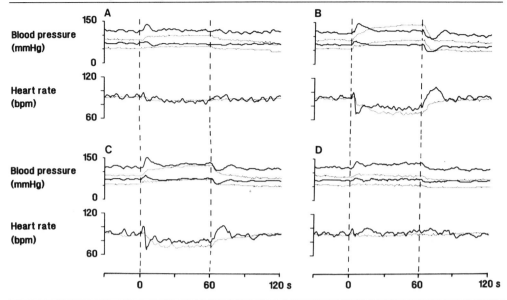

Figure 3. Circulatory effects on upright blood pressure of (A) leg-crossing, (B) squatting, (C) placing a foot on a chair, and (D) abdominal muscle contraction in healthy subjects ($N = 6$, continuous lines) and patients with orthostatic hypotension ($N = 7$, dotted lines). Subjects are standing quietly prior to the maneuvers. Vertical lines indicate duration of maneuvers. Note low upright pressure in the patients and the instantaneous increase in pressure induced by the maneuvers. Used with permission from Ten Harkel (unpublished).

heart and the brain and thereby enhances its perfusion. The two maneuvers together are measures taken also by normal humans when they experience orthostatic dizziness; treatment of fainting subjects traditionally consists of lowering the head between the knees. Also, immediately after a race, runners and speed skaters are often seen bending forward with their hands on their knees. If they remained in the upright position, they would sometimes experience a near-fainting response. Blunting of the vasoconstrictive responses in the exercised muscles by hyperthermia and local acidemia added to an instantaneous decrease in cardiac filling pressure due to the stopping of muscle pumping, causing the immediate drop in arterial pressure in the upright posture after heavy exercise.

Additional Useful Physical Measures

We encourage our patients to be as active as possible and to exercise leg and abdominal muscles. Prolonged recumbency during daytime should be avoided. Swimming is usually possible even in the most affected patients, but has the disadvantage, by the effects of prolonged whole body immersion, of inducing a marked polyuria after leaving the water with deterioration of orthostatic tolerance. With aerobic exercising in a swimming pool with the water at hip level (aquarobics) immersion effects can be expected to be less pronounced. Several of our patients have the experience that riding on a tandem bicycle is an enjoyable form of exercise. It enables them to pull up their legs and put them on the bicycle frame when they begin to feel uncomfortable. Finally, useful mechanical aids applied by severely affected patients are a small light-weight, portable **fishing chair** or a **derby chair,** which is a cane when folded but a seat when unfolded. This enables the patients to sit for brief periods when presyncopal symptoms develop.

Conclusion

Mechanical maneuvers such as leg-crossing, squatting, bending forward, and placing a foot on a chair are simple to perform and can increase the standing time of patients with orthostatic hypotension decisively. Their beneficial effect is an increase in mean arterial pressure, small in magnitude but sufficient to guarantee adequate cerebral blood flow. The underlying mechanism is an augmentation of thoracic blood volume. Instruction in these maneuvers should be part of a treatment program for patients with orthostatic hypotension.

References

1. Bannister R, Mathias JC. Management of postural hypotension. In: Bannister R, Mathias JC, eds. Autonomic failure. A textbook of clinical disorders of the autonomic nervous system. Oxford: Oxford University Press, 1992:622–45.
2. Fealy RD, Robertson D. Management of orthostatic hypotension. In: Low PA, ed. Autonomic disorders. Boston: Little Brown, 1993:731–46.
3. Ten Harkel ADJ, Van Lieshout JJ, Wieling W. Treatment of orthostatic hypotension with sleeping in the head-up position alone and in combination with fludrocortisone. J Int Med 1992;232:139–45.
4. Van Lieshout JJ, Ten Harkel ADJ, Wieling W. Combating orthostatic dizziness in autonomic failure by physical maneuvers. Lancet 1992;339:897–8.
5. Wieling W, Van Lieshout JJ, Van Leeuwen AM. Physical maneuvers that reduce postural hypotension in autonomic failure. Clin Auto Res 1993; 3:57–65.
6. Ten Harkel ADJ, Van Lieshout JJ, Wieling W. Effects of leg muscle pumping and tensing on orthostatic arterial pressure; a study in normal subjects and in patients with autonomic failure. Clin Sci 1994; 87:533–58.

66

Fludrocortisone

David Robertson
Vanderbilt University
Nashville, Tennessee

The addition of a fluorine atom to the cortisol molecular structure leads to a very potent mineralocorticoid with little glucocorticoid effect, **fludrocortisone.** The value of fludrocortisone for raising blood pressure in autonomic failure was first demonstrated by Liddle. Fludrocortisone has now been used for this purpose for 40 years.

There are several special features of fludrocortisone that complicate its successful use. First, most of its blood-pressure-raising effect is due to sodium retention, which develops over several days; therefore, the full pressor action of fludrocortisone is seen in 1–2 weeks, rather than on the day it is first administered. Doses should be altered at weekly or biweekly intervals, commencing with a dose of 0.1 mg po qd. Since patients usually expect a drug to work the first day, it is wise to discuss this delayed action so they are not disappointed by the lack of immediate salutary effect. They should also be aware that they will need to gain 5–8 pounds and experience mild ankle swelling in order for fludrocortisone to have its optimal favorable effect to raise their blood pressure.

It is important to be aware of **complications** of fludrocortisone therapy. Almost 50% of patients will develop **hypokalemia,** some within 1 week. About 5% will also develop **hypomagnesemia.** The former can be treated with potassium supplementation and the latter with small doses of magnesium sulfate. Usually correction of the hypokalemia will result in secondary correction of the hypomagnesemia.

Fluid retention is critical to fludrocortisone's beneficial effect. It should not be used in patients who are unable to tolerate an increased fluid load (e.g., congestive heart failure patients). In point of fact, congestive heart failure patients usually have increased (rather than reduced) orthostatic tolerance and we have seen patients with mild autonomic failure experience a lessening of their orthostatic hypotension when they develop congestive heart failure. We have never encountered a case of pulmonary edema in an autonomic failure patient undergoing treatment with fludrocortisone that did not respond immediately to assumption of the seated or upright posture. Weight gain of 15 pounds, however, should be avoided.

A common side effect of fludrocortisone is **headache.** This appears to be a greater problem in younger and healthier persons than in elderly or sick persons. Headache has limited the use of fludrocortisone in astronauts, who experience a very high incidence of **orthostatic intolerance** on return from space. Few patients with severe autonomic failure complain of **headache.** In patients who need fludrocortisone most of all, the headache is usually not noticed.

Very rarely, a patient who is receiving **warfarin** or a related drug for some well-established indication will, on development of autonomic failure, also need to be treated with fludrocortisone. A patient whose protime is well-controlled on warfarin may, when fludrocortisone is instituted, require a larger dose of warfarin to achieve the same effect. This does not occur in every patient, however.

Recently, there have been a number of improvements in our understanding of fludrocortisone actions. Whereas it was initially thought that mineralocorticoid receptors acted within the nucleus of the cell to alter gene transcription, it is becoming evident that some actions of mineralocorticoids are due to cell surface receptors that act through second messengers without requiring direct engagement of the DNA. Such mechanisms might be activated more rapidly than those requiring involvement of cellular transcription machinery. For this reason, a better understanding of the pharmacokinetic profile of fludrocortisone has been important. An assay for fludrocortisone has been developed recently, and has demonstrated that the drug is rapidly and nearly completely absorbed following oral administration and declines with a half-life of about 2 to 3 hr. Because of this relatively short half-life, it is probably more efficacious to give the drug in a twice-daily regimen rather than a once-daily regimen. However, many patients have clearly received benefit even with a once-daily regimen.

The dosage of fludrocortisone varies over a wide range in the published literature. It is unusual to have any benefit from a dosage smaller than 0.05 mg daily. In practice, 0.1 mg per day is usually the starting dose. That dose can be increased by 0.1-mg po increments at 1- to 2-week intervals. Few patients will require more than 0.4 mg po daily, but examples in the literature have included patients receiving 2.0 mg po qd. There appears to be little if any glucocorticoid effect at low (0.1–0.2 mg) daily doses of fludrocortisone, but ACTH suppression as manifested by reduced cortisol level can be seen following one oral dose of 2.0 mg fludrocortisone.

References

1. Chobanian AV, Volicer L, Tifft CP, Gavras H, Lian CS, Faxon D. Mineralocorticoid-induced hypertension in patients with orthostatic hypotension. N Engl J Med 1979;301:68–73.
2. Mitsky VP, Workman RJ, Nicholson E, Vernikos J, Robertson RM, Robertson D. A sensitive radioimmunoassay for fludrocortisone in human plasma. Steroids 1994;59:555–8.
3. Robertson D, Davis T. Recent advances in the treatment of orthostatic hypotension. Neurology 1995;45 (Suppl 4):S26–32.
4. Frick MH. 9-alpha-fluorohydrocortisone in the treatment of postural hypotension. Acta Med Scan 1966;179:293–9.
5. Seager LH. Pressor action of fluorohydrocortisone in orthostatic hypotension. Tufts Folia Med 1963;9:56–61.

67 *Midodrine and Other Pressor Drugs*

Roy Freeman
Harvard Medical School
Deaconess Hospital
Boston, Massachusetts

Treatment of Orthostatic Hypotension

Many patients respond to a combination of the nonpharmacological measures and fludrocortisone. For more severely afflicted patients further pharmacological intervention is required. Numerous agents from diverse pharmacological groups have been implemented in the treatment of orthostatic hypotension (see Table 1). Pharmacological measures include direct and indirect **sympathomimetic agents** and other pressors, **prostaglandin synthetase inhibitors, erythropoietin, dopamine blocking agents, vasopressin receptor agonists, antihistamines,** and **antiserotonergic agents.** Many of these agents, however, are of limited benefit and often have not been subjected to rigorous controlled trials.

An **ideal therapeutical agent** would have a consistent and sustained effect and would act preferentially on capacitance rather than resistance vessels, thus increasing venous return while limiting supine hypertension. Such an agent would take advantage of the presence of denervation supersensitivity and be responsive to alterations in posture. Unfortunately there is no agent that at present satisfies all these criteria. The therapeutic goal of all treatment endeavors

Table 1. Pharmacotherapy of
Orthostatic Hypotension

Mineralocorticoids
  9-α-Fludrocortisone
Sympathomimetic agents
  Ephedrine
  Pseudoephedrine
  Phenylpropanolamine
  Phenylephrine
  Methylphenidate
  Dextroamphetamine
  Tyramine (with monoamine oxidase inhibition)
  Midodrine
  Clonidine
  Yohimbine
  DL- and L-dihydroxyphenylserine (DL-DOPS)
Nonspecific pressor agents
  Ergot derivatives
  Caffeine
  Somatostatin analogs
β-Adrenergic blocking agents
  Propranolol
  Pindolol
  Xamoterol
  Prenalterol
Prostaglandin synthetase inhibitors
  Indomethacin
  Flurbiprofen
  Ibuprofen
  Naproxen
Dopamine blocking agents
  Metoclopramide
  Domperidone
V1 and V2 receptor agonists
  Desmopressin acetate (DDAVP)
  Lysine–vasopressin
Erythropoietin

is merely to ameliorate the symptoms of orthostatic hypotension while avoiding side effects. There is rarely the need to restore normotension.

Sympathomimetic Agents

These medications may be used alone or in combination with fludrocortisone. The immediate effectiveness of the sympathomimetic agents at low doses is most likely dependent on the increase in receptor number and affinity and the reduction in baroreceptor modulation that accompanies autonomic failure. The available α-1 adrenoreceptor agonists include agents with direct (e.g., midodrine, phenylephrine) and indirect (e.g., edphedrine, tyramine) effects.

Midodrine

The peripheral selective **α-agonist midodrine** shows promise in the treatment of orthostatic hypotension. The pressor effect of midodrine is due to both **arterial and venous constriction.** The efficacy of this agent has been demonstrated in both open-label and double-blind studies. Midodrine, the prodrug, is activated to de-glymidodrine the active α-receptor agonist. Absorption as the prodrug may theoretically minimize direct vasoconstriction of the gastrointestinal tract. The peak plasma concentration of midodrine occurs in 20–40 min and the half-life is 30 min. Patient sensitivity to this agent varies and the dose should be titrated from 2.5 to 10 mg three times a day. It is often wise to give most of the day's dose relatively early in the day, to avoid nocturnal hypertension. Potential side effects of this agent include pilomotor reactions, pruritus, supine hypertension, gastrointestinal complaints, and urinary retention. Central nervous system side effects occur infrequently. This agent is currently investigational.

In the past, ephedrine (25–50 mg three times a day), pseudoephedrine (30–60 mg three times a day), and phenylpropanolamine (12.5–25 mg three times a day) have been the most frequently prescribed agents. Because the effectiveness of the indirect agonists is at least in part due to the release of norepinephrine from the postganglionic neuron, these medications are in theory most likely to benefit patients with partial or incomplete lesions.

The use of all of the above medications is complicated by **tachyphylaxis,** although efficacy may be regained with a dose increase or after a short drug holiday. The sympathomimetic side effects such as anxiety, tremulousness, and tachycardia that accompany the use of some of these agents may be intolerable to patients. Severe **supine hypertension,** which occurs both as a consequence of baroreceptor denervation and as a side effect of treatment, often limits therapeutic intervention, although surprisingly, most patients tolerate sustained supine blood pressures without untoward effect. Raising the head of the bed 10 to 20° reduces supine hypertension and activates the renin–angiotensin–aldosterone system which decreases the nocturnal diuresis that is associated with autonomic failure. The cautious use of short acting antihypertensive agents at night (such as **topical nitrates, captopril,** or **nifedipine**) or ingestion of small amounts of alcohol before retiring may be of benefit. Orthostatic tolerance may be severely impaired by these endeavors should the patient need to leave the supine position.

There were initially optimistic reports on the use of the indirect acting agent **tyramine,** which releases norepinephrine from neuronal storage pools, in combination with a monoamine oxidase inhibitor to prevent breakdown of the released norepinephrine. The use of this combination of pharmacological agents is unfortunately limited by severe supine hypertension, an unpredictable response, and, in some cases, the failure to abolish orthostatic symptoms.

Prostaglandin Synthetase Inhibitors

The prostaglandin synthetase inhibitors such as indomethacin, flurbiprofen, and other nonsteroidal anti-inflammatory agents may also reduce orthostatic hypotension. These medications are rarely effective as monotherapy, but may be used to supplement treatment with 9-α-fluorohydrocortisone or a sympathomimetic agent. The probable mode of action of the prostaglandin synthesis inhibitors is to limit the vasodilating effects of circulating prostaglandins and arachidonic acid derivatives. These agents may also increase the central circulating blood volume and enhance vascular sensitivity to circulating pressor amines.

Caffeine

The methylxanthine caffeine has a well-established pressor effect that is in part due to blockade of vasodilating adenosine receptors. Caffeine improves orthostatic hypotension and attenuates postprandial hypotension in patients with autonomic failure. Typical caffeine doses are 100–250 mg three times a day, either as tablets or caffeinated beverages (one cup of coffee contains approximately 85 mg of caffeine and one cup of tea contains 50 mg of caffeine).

Somatostatin

Somatostatin analogs, such as the long-acting synthetic octapeptide **octreotide,** reduce the pancreatic and gastrointestinal hormone response to food ingestion and other stimuli. These agents attenuate the postprandial blood pressure fall and reduce orthostatic hypotension in patients with autonomic failure. Mechanisms of action for these medications include a local effect on splanchnic vasculature by inhibiting the release of vasoactive gastrointestinal peptides, enhanced cardiac output, and an increase in forearm and splanchnic vascular resistance. Subcutaneous doses of octreotide range from 25 to 200 μg. Side effects of nausea and abdominal cramps limit the use of these agents.

Dihydroxyphenylserine

DL- and L-**Dihydroxyphenylserine (DOPS)** are synthetic, nonphysiological, amino acid **norepinephrine precursors** that are decarboxylated by the ubiquitous L-amino acid decarboxylase to norepinephrine in both animals and man. The important role played by norepinephrine in the maintenance of upright blood pressure and the successful implementation of precursor therapy for

Parkinson's disease provide the rationale for the use of this agent to treat neurogenic orthostatic hypotension. Of the four stereoisomers D- and L-threo-DOPS and D- and L-erythro-DOPS, only L-**threo-DOPS** is pharmacologically and biologically active. Patients with dopamine β-hydroxylase deficiency are unable to synthesize norepinephrine and epinephrine in the central and peripheral nervous system. Because the conversion of DOPS to norepinephrine bypasses the β-hydroxylation step, DOPS is the ideal therapeutic agent for this inherited disorder. This agent may also be of benefit in patients with familial amyloid polyneuropathy, Parkinson's disease, multiple-system atrophy, and pure autonomic failure.

Dihydroergotamine

Dihydroergotamine, an ergot alkaloid that interacts with α-adrenergic receptors, has a selective **venoconstrictor** effect. This medication may increase venous return in patients with orthostatic hypotension without producing a significant increase in peripheral vascular resistance. Although dihydroergotamine is an effective pressor intravenously and intramuscularly, low oral bioavailability results in an inconsistent effect when taken orally.

β Blockers

Nonselective β blockers, particularly those with intrinsic sympathomimetic activity such as pindolol and xamoterolol, may have a limited place in the treatment of orthostatic hypotension despite the well-acknowledged negative chronotropy and ionotopy associated with these medications. The suggested mechanism of action of these medications is the blockade of vasodilating β$_2$ receptors, allowing unopposed α-adrenoreceptor-mediated vasoconstrictor effects to dominate. Congestive heart failure may be a serious side effect of this medication.

Vasopressin Analogs

The vasopressin analogs have a limited place in the treatment of orthostatic hypotension. The postural release of arginine–vasopressin is reduced in patients with autonomic failure, and patients with autonomic failure are supersensitive to exogenous vasopressin and vasopressin analogs. The synthetic vasopressin analog **desmopressin (DDAVP)** acts on the **V2 receptors** in the collecting ducts of the renal tubules and has no V1 receptor vasoconstricting potential. DDAVP, which can be taken via the nasal or intramuscular route, prevents nocturia and weight loss and reduces the morning postural fall in blood pressure in patients with autonomic failure. Fluid and electrolyte status should be carefully monitored during therapy to avoid hyponatremia. The vasopressor analogs of vasopressin (V1 receptor agonists), such as **lysine–vasopressin** nasal spray and intramuscular triglycl-lysine–vasopressin, may also increase blood pressure and peripheral vascular resistance and improve symptoms of orthostatic hypotension.

Clonidine

Clonidine is an **α-2 agonist** that usually produces a central sympatholytic effect and a consequent decrease in blood pressure. In patients with autonomic failure, who have little central sympathetic efferent activity, the effect of this agent on postsynaptic α-2 adrenoreceptors may predominate. These receptors may be more numerous on veins than arterioles. The use of clonidine (0.1–0.6 mg per day) could therefore result in an increase in venous return without a significant increase in peripheral vascular resistance. The use of this agent, at least theoretically, is limited to patients with severe central autonomic dysfunction in whom there is no ostensible effect of further sympatholysis and the peripheral effect may dominate. The hypertensive effect is inconsistent and in some patients residual sympathetic activity could be inhibited. The agent may cause profound hypotension in some patients with autonomic failure.

Yohimbine

Yohimbine is a centrally active, selective α-2 antagonist that increases sympathetic nervous system efferent output by antagonizing central or presynaptic α-2 receptors, or both. Yohimbine (8 mg three times a day) produces a modest pressor effect although theoretically patients should have some residual sympathetic nervous system output. Side effects of yohimbine include anxiety, tremor, palpitations, diarrhea, and supine hypertension.

Dopamine Antagonists

The dopamine antagonists **metoclopramide** and **domperidone** may also treat orthostatic hypotension. These agents most likely inhibit the vasodilating and natriuretic effect of dopamine or increase norepinephrine release due to blockade of prejunctional inhibitory dopaminergic receptors. The risk of tardive dyskinesia and other extrapyramidal side effects limits the long-term use of these agents.

Conclusion

Orthostatic hypotension is the most incapacitating symptom of autonomic failure. Most patients can be treated successfully with a combination of fludrocortisone and a sympathomimetic agent. Caffeine, prostaglandin synthetase inhibitors, erythropoietin, and, rarely, the other agents listed above may on occasion be used to supplement the treatment of patients who remain symptomatic. There is, however, a small group of patients who remain refractory to all therapeutic endeavors.

References

1. Bannister R, Mathias CJ. The management of postural hypotension. In: Bannister R, *et al.*, eds. Autonomic failure. Oxford: Oxford University Press, 1992:622–45.
2. Fealey RD, Robertson D. Management of orthostatic hypotension. In: Low PA, ed. Clinical autonomic disorders. Boston: Little Brown, 1993:731–43.

3. Freeman R, Miyawaki E. The treatment of autonomic dysfunction. J Clin Neurophysiol 1993;10:61–83.
4. McTavish D, Goa KL. Midodrine. A review of its pharmacological properties and therapeutic use in orthostatic hypotension and secondary hypotensive disorders. Drugs 1989;38:757–77.
5. Freeman R, Landsberg L. The treatment of orthostatic hypotension with dihydroxyphenylserine. Clin Neuropharmacol 1991;14:296–304.

68   *Erythropoietin in Autonomic Failure*

Italo Biaggioni
Vanderbilt University
Nashville, Tennessee

Animal studies suggest that the sympathetic nervous system modulates erythropoiesis. The reticulocyte response to acute blood-letting was greatly diminished in rats when their kidneys were functionally denervated. Intravenous administration of the **β-adrenergic agonist** salbutamol increased plasma concentrations of erythropoietin-like factor in rabbits. Conversely, β blockers blunted the erythropoietin response to hypoxia in rabbits and rats. Thus, **β2 adrenoreceptors** could positively modulate erythropoiesis by stimulating erythropoietin production.

Recent studies may potentially reveal the physiologic significance of these findings and their relevance to humans. Patients with severe autonomic failure have an unusually high incidence of anemia; if World Heath Organization criteria are followed (hemoglobin <120 g/liter for women and <130 g/liter for men), up to 38% of patients are anemic (1) without obvious cause. The **anemia of autonomic failure** is mild to moderate and is not accompanied by a compensatory increase in reticulocytes, suggesting an inadequate erythropoietic response. Furthermore, an inappropriately low serum erythropoietin is evident in those patients with lower hemoglobin levels.

Lack of sympathetic stimulation may thus result in decreased erythropoietin production and the development of anemia in patients with autonomic failure. In support of this hypothesis, it has been found that the magnitude of sympathetic impairment correlates with the severity of the anemia, and that plasma norepinephrine levels are lowest in patients with the most severe anemia. These results support the hypothesis that sympathetic innervation is required for an adequate erythropoietin response. However, acute renal denervation does not affect levels of mRNA encoding erythropoietin in animals. It is not certain, therefore, if the anemia of autonomic failure is solely due to the lack of sympathetic input to erythropoietin-producing cells in the kidney.

The fact that anemia can be associated with low erythropoietin levels in autonomic failure led to its treatment with **recombinant erythropoietin (epoetin alfa).** This therapy has successfully corrected anemia in all patients so far treated (1–3), even when used at lower doses (25–50 units/kg body wt, subcutaneously, three times a week) than those commonly employed for anemia of chronic disease. This response further confirms that inadequate erythropoietin production underlies anemia in these patients.

Recombinant erythropoietin also increases supine and upright blood pressure in autonomic failure patients (1–3), and may be effective in ameliorating orthostatic hypotension. This pressor response is not unexpected, since it is a well-documented side effect of erythropoietin treatment in chronic renal failure. The mechanisms by which erythropoietin increases blood pressure is not known. Erythropoietin increases the sensitivity to the pressor effects of **angiotensin II,** increases plasma **endothelin** levels, enhances **renal tubular sodium reabsorption,** and raises **cytosolic free calcium** in vascular smooth muscle. The relevance of these findings to its pressor effect in autonomic failure remains speculative. Additionally, there are other mechanisms that may be operative in these patients. Blood pressure is extremely sensitive to even small changes in intravascular volume in autonomic failure. It could be that the increase in red cell mass could directly mediate the increased blood pressure produced by erythropoietin (3).

Treatment of orthostatic hypotension remains a challenge in these patients. **Fludrocortisone** remains the first step in their treatment, but used alone it rarely resolves symptoms in severely affected patients. Vasoconstricting drugs are commonly used as second-line agents to improve upright blood pressure. While seemingly effective, it can be questioned whether peripheral vasoconstriction is the ideal approach to improve cerebral blood flow and provide symptomatic relief for orthostatic hypotension. An alternative approach would be to increase intravascular volume. Fludrocortisone increases plasma volume but only transiently and at the expense of expanding interstitial space. Treatment with erythropoietin, therefore, has the theoretic advantage of **selectively increasing intravascular volume.** Even though long-term, placebo-controlled studies are lacking, improvement of orthostatic hypotension by erythropoietin has been a consistent finding of published reports. Potential limitations of this therapy should be considered. Up to 50% of patients with severe autonomic failure also suffer from significant supine hypertension. Erythropoietin therapy has been reported to worsen supine hypertension in at least some patients (1–3). This side effect, however, is probably common to all therapies currently available. Other limitations include the inconvenience of injectable administration and the high cost of this medication. It is not known if erythropoietin will prove superior to currently available therapeutic alternatives.

In summary, patients with severe autonomic failure have a high incidence of anemia, which may contribute to their symptoms. Sympathetic failure can contribute to this anemia by blunting of the expected compensatory erythropoietin response. It is not clear if this phenomenon is the sole explanation for the anemia. Recombinant erythropoietin reverses anemia of autonomic failure and improves upright blood pressure. Preliminary evidence suggests that it also ameliorates symptoms of orthostatic hypotension. There are theoretical reasons why this approach may be of benefit in the treatment of autonomic failure. In the absence of controlled studies, a drug trial with erythropoietin in selected patients may be warranted.

References

1. Biaggioni I, Robertson D, Krantz DS, Jones M, Haile V. The anemia of primary autonomic failure and its reversal with recombinant erythropoietin. Ann Int Med 1994;121:181–6.
2. Hoeldtke RD. Streeten DHP. Treatment of orthostatic hypotension with erythropoietin. N Engl J Med 1993;329:611–5.
3. Perera R, Isola L. Kaufman H. Erythropoietin improves orthostatic hypotension in primary autonomic failure. Neurology 1994;44 (suppl. 2):A363.

Appendix
Consensus Statement on the Definition of Orthostatic Hypotension, Pure Autonomic Failure, and Multiple System Atrophy

American Autonomic Society and the American Academy of Neurology[1]

I. Definition

Orthostatic hypotension (OH) is a reduction of systolic blood pressure of at least 20 mm Hg or diastolic blood pressure of at least 10 mm Hg within 3 min of standing. It is a physical sign and not a disease. An acceptable alternative to standing is the demonstration of a similar drop in blood pressure within 3 min, using a tilt table in the head-up position at an angle of at least 60°.

[1] A consensus Conference was convened on November 16, 1995, at the Ritz–Carlton Hotel, Phoenix, AZ, with the specific aim of generating a consensus on the definition of three specific items: the definition of orthostatic hypotension, pure autonomic failure (Bradbury Eggleston syndrome, idiopathic orthostatic hypotension, progressive autonomic failure), and multiple system atrophy. The meeting was sponsored by the American Autonomic Society and cosponsored by the American Academy of Neurology.

Primer on the Autonomic Nervous System

Confounding variables to be considered when reaching a diagnosis should include food ingestion, time of day, state of hydration, ambient temperature, recent recumbency, postural deconditioning, hypertension, medications, gender, and age.

Orthostatic hypotension may be symptomatic or asymptomatic. Symptoms of OH are those that develop on assuming the erect posture or following head-up tilt and usually resolve on resuming the recumbent position. They may include lightheadedness, dizziness, blurred vision, weakness, fatigue, cognitive impairment, nausea, palpitations, tremulousness, headache, and neck ache. If the patient has symptoms suggestive of, but does not have documented orthostatic hypotension, repeated measurements of blood pressure should be performed. Occasional patients may not manifest significant falls in blood pressure until they stand for at least 10 min.

II. Pure Autonomic Failure (PAF)

Pure autonomic failure is an idiopathic sporadic disorder characterized by OH usually with evidence of more widespread autonomic failure. No other neurological features are present. Some patients with the manifestations of PAF may later prove to have other disorders such as multiple system atrophy. Reduced supine plasma norepinephrine levels are characteristic of PAF.

III. Parkinson's Disease with Autonomic Failure

A minority of patients with Parkinson's disease as defined by United Kingdom Parkinson's Disease Brain Bank criteria (1) may also develop autonomic failure, including OH. It is not known if these patients have a more serious prognosis than Parkinson's disease without autonomic failure.

IV. Multiple System Atrophy (MSA)

MSA is a sporadic, progressive, adult onset disorder characterized by autonomic dysfunction, Parkinsonism, and ataxia in any combination. The features of this disorder include:

A. Parkinsonism (bradykinesia with rigidity or tremor or both), usually with a poor or unsustained motor response to chronic levodopa therapy.

B. Cerebellar or corticospinal signs.

C. Orthostatic hypotension, impotence, urinary incontinence, or retention usually preceding or within 2 years after the onset of the motor symptoms.

Characteristically, these features cannot be explained by medications or other disorders.

Parkinsonian and cerebellar features commonly occur in combination. However, certain features may predominate. When Parkinsonian features predominate, the term striatonigral degeneration is often used. When cerebellar features predominate, the term sporadic olivopontocerebellar atrophy is often used. When autonomic failure predominates, the term Shy–Drager syndrome is often used. These manifestations may occur in various combinations and evolve with time.

Reference

1. Hughes, AJ, Daniel, DE, Kilford, L, and Lee, AJ. Accuracy of clinical diagnosis of idiopathic Parkinson's disease: A clinico-pathological study of 100 cases. J Neurol Neurosurg Psychiat 1992;55:181–4.

Participants

Sir Roger Bannister (Co-Chair), Pembroke College, Oxford, UK.

Irwin J. Schatz, M.D., (Co-Chair), Department of Medicine, University of Hawaii at Manoa, Honolulu, Hawaii, USA.

Roy L. Freeman, M.D., Division of Neurology, Deaconess Hospital, Boston, Massachusetts, USA.

Christopher G. Goetz, M.D., Department of Neurology, Rush Medical College, Chicago, Illinois, USA.

Joseph Jankovic, M.D., Department of Neurology, Baylor College of Medicine, Houston, Texas, USA.

Horacio C. Kaufmann, M.D., Department of Neurology, Mount Sinai School of Medicine, New York, New York, USA.

William C. Koller, M.D., Department of Neurology, University of Kansas, Kansas City, Kansas, USA.

Phillip A. Low, M.D., Department of Neurology, Mayo Clinic, Rochester, Minnesota, USA.

Christopher J. Mathias, M.D., St. Mary's Hospital, London, UK.

Ronald J. Polinsky, M.D., Sandoz Research Institute, East Hanover, New Jersey, USA.

Niall P. Quinn, M.D., University Department of Clinical Neurology, Institute of Neurology, The National Hospital London, UK.

David Robertson, M.D., Autonomic Dysfunction Center, Vanderbilt University, Nashville, Tennessee, USA.

David H. P. Streeten, M.D., Department of Medicine, Health Science Center, Syracuse, New York, USA.

Index